Hydroxyapatite and Related Materials

Editors

Paul W. Brown
Professor
Department of Materials Science and Engineering
The Pennsylvania State University
University Park, Pennsylvania

Brent Constantz
President and Chief Executive Officer
Chief Scientist
Norian Corporation
Mountain View, California

CRC Press
Boca Raton Ann Arbor London Tokyo

Library of Congress Cataloging-in-Publication Data

Hydroxyapatite and related materials / editors, Paul W. Brown, Brent Constantz.
p. cm.
Includes bibliographical references and index.
ISBN 0-8493-4750-5
1. Biomedical materials. 2. Hydroxyapatite--Physiological effect.
I. Brown, Paul W. (Paul Wenzil), 1943- . II. Constantz, Brent.
R857.M3H94 1994
612′.01524--dc20 93-47252
CIP

No claim to original U.S. Government works
International Standard Book Number 0-8493-4750-5
Library of Congress Card Number 93-47252
Printed in the United States of America 1 2 3 4 5 6 7 8 9 0
Printed on acid-free paper

ACKNOWLEDGEMENTS

The genesis of this volume was a symposium, *Hydroxyapatite and Related Compounds,* held April 13-15, 1993, at the Materials Research Society Meeting in San Francisco. The volume contains contributions from the symposium participants and from Walter Brown's colleagues at the ADA Fellowship. We are grateful to the Materials Research Society for providing the venue for the symposium. Funds supporting the symposium and the preparation of this volume were provided by:

Codman
Danek
DePuy
Howmedica
Norian
Osteonics
Smith and Nephew Richards.

We gratefully acknowledge their financial support. One of us (PWB) also wishes to acknowledge the support of NIDR Grant DE09421. Finally, we are deeply grateful to Wendy Bathgate, who was indispensible in assembling the volume.

Paul Brown
State College

Brent Constantz
Mountain View

THE EDITORS

Paul Brown, Ph.D., is a professor of Materials Science and Engineering at The Pennsylvania State University. He received a B.S. in Chemistry, an M.S. in Metallurgy, and a Ph.D. in Materials Science from the University of Wisconsin. Prior to joining the faculty at Penn State he was a materials engineer at the National Bureau of Standards (now NIST).

His professional interests include biomedical materials, chemical means to the formation of materials and composites, chemically bonded ceramics, multicomponent phase equilibria, and reaction kinetics. A particular interest is associated with the formation of hydroxyapatite and hydroxyapatite-based composites *in vivo*. He is the author of approximately 150 publications and holds one patent.

Professor Brown is the principal editor of *Cements Research Progress* and a member of the editorial board of *Advances in Cement Research*, and a contributing editor for *Phase Diagrams for Ceramists*. He is a member of the American Ceramic Society, the American Chemical Society, and the Biomaterials Society.

Professor Brown has been the recipient of various awards including the Deike Research Award and a Northwest University Consortium for Science (NORCUS) Fellowship. He was elected as a Fellow of the American Ceramic Society in 1992.

Brent R. Constantz, Ph.D., is the founder of Norian Corporation, an international leader in orthopaedic medical devices for skeletal repair.

Dr. Constantz received his B.A. from the University of California, Santa Barbara in Aquatic Biology and Geological Sciences in 1981. He received his M.S. and Ph.D. degrees in 1984 and 1986, respectively, from the Earth Sciences Department at the University of California, Santa Cruz. After doing post-doctoral work at the United States Geological Survey, Menlo Park, he was named a Fulbright Scholar assigned to the Weizmann Institute, Rehovot, Israel. Dr. Constantz incorporated Norian in 1987 and has been continuously employed there since that date.

Dr. Constantz is a member of the American Association for the Advancement of Science, The Orthopaedic Research Society, The Society of Biomechanics, The Biomaterials Society, The European Biomaterials Society, and The Materials Research Society.

He has been the recipient of a National Science Foundation Pre-doctoral Fellowship Award (1982 to 1985), a Fulbright Scholarship (1986 to 1987), and a National Science Foundation Small Business Innovative Research Award (1990). He has served as the Principal Investigator on several important corporate research contracts which Norian has completed with Pfizer Hospital Products Group.

Dr. Constantz is the inventor on 10 issued U.S. patents and has several more pending. He also has parallel patents which have issued or are pending internationally. He has presented numerous lectures at international meetings, national meetings, and guest lectures at universities, institutes, and corporations. He has published several important research papers. His current interests are biomineralization of bone, specifically calcium phosphate formation, and the body's cellular interactions with calcium phosphates and their biomechanical consequences.

DEDICATION

This volume is dedicated to the memory of Walter Brown. It is not possible to read the calcium phosphate literature without running across the tracks he has left. His knowledge of the chemistry of calcium phosphates was profound and his insight will be missed.

Paul W. Brown

Despite the central roles of calcium phosphates in biological mineralization, prior to 1960, calcium phosphates were an interest primarily to those concerned with soil sciences of geochemistry. In 1962, Dr. Walter E. Brown joined the American Dental Association (ADA) Health Foundation Paffenbarger Research Center (formerly Research Unit) at the National Institute of Standards and Technology (formerly National Bureau of Standards), thus becoming one of the early calcium phosphate scientists who were instrumental in bringing calcium phosphate research to the biological field. Prior to joining ADA, Dr. Brown had spent more than a decade at the Tennessee Valley Authority studying calcium phosphate chemistry. His knowledge in a broad range of basic properties of calcium phosphates, notably the crystal structure and property relationship, phase transformations of acidic calcium phosphates to hydroxyapatite in aqueous systems, and application of phase rules to thermodynamic solubility studies, enabled him to successfully develop a number of approaches for studying the physicochemical mechanisms of disease processes that involve calcium phosphates. His outstanding achievements in this area include a model that involves the formation of octacalcium phosphate as a precursor of biological apatite formation, a coupled diffusion-dissolution model for dental caries and other demineralization processes, and a new type of calcium phosphate biomaterial in the form of a self-hardening cement. Dr. Brown's passing on February 1993 marked an end of a period in which he has been an unfailing source of knowledge and inspiration to those who worked with him as well as to many other scientists in the field. In fact, Dr. Brown's work have impacted, in one way or another, the research of nearly all of the contributing authors of the Proceedings of the Symposium on Hydroxyapatite and Related Materials, and it is appropriate to dedicate the volume to him.

L. C. Chow

TABLE OF CONTENTS

Page

SECTION II. CONTRIBUTED PAPERS

Section I.

Invited Papers

BIOLOGICAL AND SYNTHETIC APATITES

Racquel Zapanta LeGeros
Department of Dental Materials
New York University of College of Dentistry

I. INTRODUCTION

The name 'apatite' describes a family of compounds having similar structure (hexagonal system, space group, $P6_3/m$) in spite of a wide range of composition.[1-3] The similarity of the x-ray diffraction (XRD) patterns of enamel, dentin and bone to those of mineral apatites (hydroxyapatite, HA, fluorapatite, FA)[3,4] together with chemical analyses showing calcium and phosphate as principal constituents led to the conclusion, as early as 1926,[3,4] that the inorganic phases of bone and teeth are basically calcium hydroxyapatite, HA, idealized as $Ca_{10}(PO_4)_6(OH)_2$. To date, the exact structure of biological apatites remain undefined. The submicroscopic dimensions of biological apatites precluded the use of single crystal analysis methods to determine their structure. Several observations which include the non-stoichiometry of these apatites and association of principal minor constituents, magnesium and carbonate, provided evidence that biological apatites are not pure HA and should be instead classified as carbonate apatites.[5-8]

In the area of basic research, the formation and physico-chemical properties of synthetic apatites (pure HA and calcium-deficient apatite) and biologically relevant or related calcium phosphates (e.g., amorphous calcium phosphate, $Ca_x(PO_4)_y$, ACP; brushite or dicalcium phosphate dihydrate, $CaHPO_4.2H_2O$, DCPD; monetite or dicalcium phosphate anhydrous, $CaHPO_4$, DCPA; octacalcium phosphate, $Ca_8H_2(PO_4)_6.5H_2O$, OCP, β-tricalcium phosphate, $Ca_3(PO_4)_2$, β-TCP), are investigated for a better understanding of the formation and properties of biological apatites.[6,7,9]

In the area of biomaterials, specifically, materials for bone repair, substitution or augmentation, the perceived similarity between bone apatite and HA provided the impetus for the development of commercial and non-commercial calcium phosphate materials including: ceramic HA[10-13] and non-ceramic HA;[14-19] coralline HA;[19] β-TCP;[20] biphasic calcium phosphates, BCP;[21-23] for dental and medical applications[10-12,20-26] and for coatings[18,27,28] on dental and orthopedic implants.

The purpose of this invited paper is to present some of the past and current studies on the formation and properties of synthetic apatites relevant to those of biological apatites.

0-8493-4750-5/94/$0.00 + $.50

II. BIOLOGICAL APATITES

A. OCCURRENCE

In biological systems, apatite or apatitic calcium phosphates occur as the principal inorganic constituent of vertebrate bone and tooth,[3-7,29] fish teeth,[30-32] some calcified fish scales,[30] and some species of shells.[33,34] They also occur as one of the major crystalline components in pathological calcification, e.g., dental and urinary calculi and stones,[5-7,35-38] some soft-tissue calcification;[6,7,39,40] and in marine phosphorites.[41,42] Ultrastructural studies of the interfaces between host bone and implanted calcium phosphate biomaterials showed the presence of apatite crystals[43,44] identified as carbonate apatite[7,22,45,46] similar to those of bone apatite.

B. COMPOSITION AND CRYSTALLOGRAPHIC PROPERTIES

1. Crystallographic Properties of Biological Apatites

The x-ray diffraction (XRD) pattern of enamel (Fig. 1A) shows sharp and well defined peaks compared to the broad ones in those of dentin (Fig. 1B) and bone (Fig. 1C) suggesting that the apatite crystals in enamel are much larger than those in either dentin or bone. Transmission electron microscopy (TEM) confirmed the size differences predicted from XRD analyses and demonstrated that the enamel apatite are long acicular crystals exhibiting a hexagonal cross-section[47] compared to the much smaller rod-shaped flatter bone apatite crystals. Human enamel apatite has significantly larger a-axis dimensions compared to pure HA (0.944 nm compared to 0.942 nm) while shark enamel apatite has a lower a-axis (0.9381nm) compared to pure HA and more similar to the dimensions of FA.[6,7,30,32]

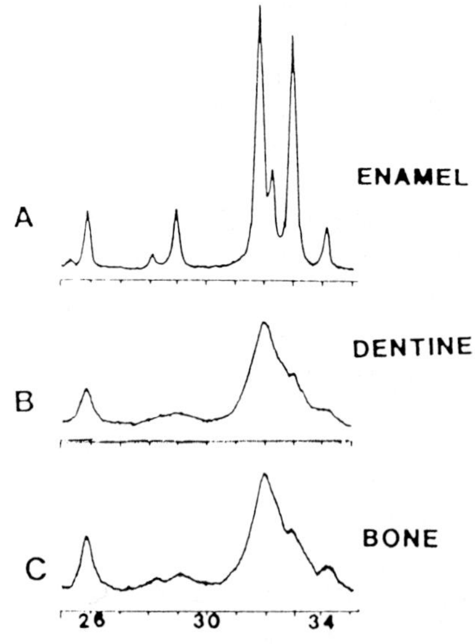

Figure 1. XRD patterns of powdered human enamel (A), dentin (B), and bone (C). The sharper diffraction peaks in (A) compared to (B) and (C) reflect the larger apatite crystals in enamel compared to those in dentin or bone.[5-7]

2. Non-stoichiometry or Calcium Deficiency of Biological Apatites

Biological apatites differ from the pure HA in composition, in crystal size and morphology (Fig. 2), and in stoichiometry.[6,7,48] The Ca/P molar ratio is 1.67 for pure HA, about 1.62 to 1.64 for human enamel and dentin apatite (Table

1). In bone apatite, the Ca/P increases with age.[7] Thus, in general, biological apatites are calcium-deficient or non-stoichiometric. The non-stoichiometry of these apatites is also reflected in the formation of β-TCP with HA after sintering[5,6,26,34] Other minor (e.g., magnesium, Mg; carbonate, CO_3; sodium, Na, chloride, Cl, acid phosphate, HPO_4, etc.) and trace (e.g., strontium, Sr; lead, Pb; etc.) elements are associated with these apatites.[5-8,29,48-54] From the XRD, Infrared (IR) and chemical analyses of biological apatites, they may be classified as either (a) *carbonate apatite* $(CO_3\text{-}AP)$ or (b) *fluor-carbonate apatite,* $(F,CO_3)\text{-}AP$, represented as: $(Ca,Na,Mg,K,X)_{10}(PO_4,CO_3,HPO_4)_6(OH,Cl,F)_2$, where X represents trace cations with concentrations less than 0.1 wt%. The minor elements, carbonate, magnesium and fluoride are believed to be responsible for the stability or instability of biological apatites.[5-7,32,51-59]

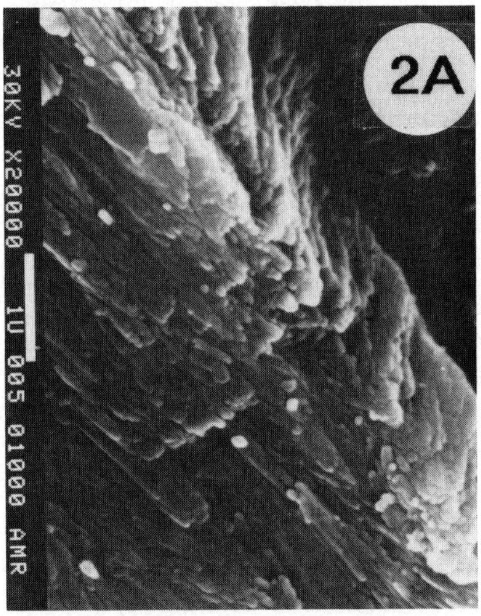

Figure 2. SEM of human enamel (A), precipitated calcium-deficient apatite (B), and ceramic HA (C).[6,7] The HA ceramic was prepared by precipitation and subsequent sintering at 1100°C. [SEM micrographs taken by Dr. Paul Shirra (B) and Professor T.V. Vijayaraghavan (C).]

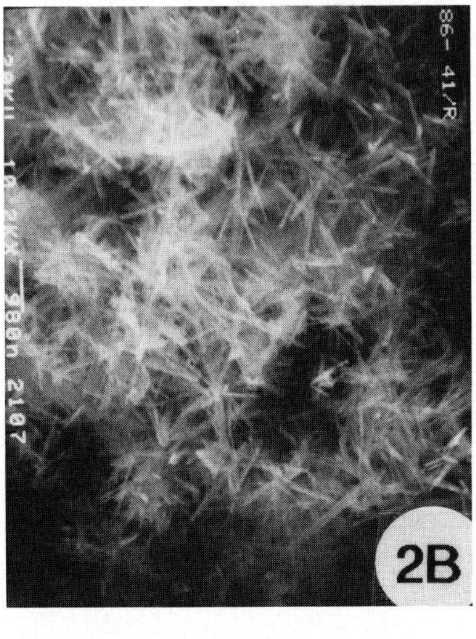

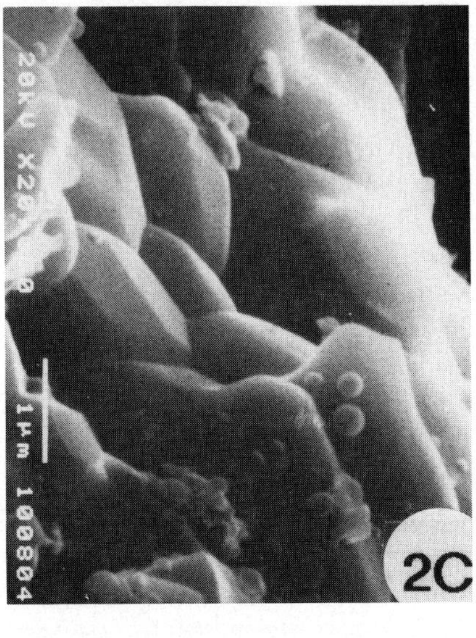

3. Carbonate in Biological Apatites

Carbonate, CO_3, is the principal minor constituent of biological apatites. The CO_3 concentration is least in human enamel apatites (about 3.5 wt%) and most in dentin and bone (Table 1). When present with fluoride, such as in enameloids of some species of fish, in some calcified fish scales and some species of shells, the CO_3 concentration in the apatite is much less. For example, the CO_3 content in shark enameloid which contains about 3.8 wt% F is about 1.5 wt% compared to that in human enamel, which contains about 0.1 wt% F.[30,32] The carbonate associated with biological apatites was first attributed to the presence of carbonate in non-apatitic phases, e.g., calcium carbonate, $CaCO_3$, or dolomite, $(Ca,Mg)(CO_3)_2$.[61] IR analyses of biological apatites (Fig. 3) demonstrated that the CO_3 vibration bands were different from those of simple

Table 1. Composition and Physical Properties of Apatites in Adult Human Enamel, Dentin and Bone.[6]

	Enamel	Dentin	Bone
Composition			
Calcium, Ca^{2+}	36.5	35.1	34.8
Phosphorous, as P	17.7	16.9	15.2
(Ca/P) molar	1.63	1.61	1.71
Sodium, Na^+	0.5	0.6	0.9
Magnesium, Mg^{2+}	0.44	1.23	0.72
Potassium, K^+	0.08	0.05	0.03
Carbonate, as CO_3^{2-}	3.5	5.6	7.4
Fluoride, F^-	0.01	0.06	0.03
Chloride, Cl^-	0.30	0.01	0.13
Pyrophosphate, $P_3O_7^{4-}$	0.022	0.10	0.07
Total inorganic (mineral)	97.0	70.0	65.0
Total organic	1.5	20.0	25.0
Absorbed H_2O	1.5	10.0	10.0
Trace elements: Sr^{2+}, Pb^{2+}, Zn^{2+}, Cu^{2+}, Fe^{3+}, etc.			
Crystallographic properties			
Lattice parameters (±0.0003 nm)			
a-axis	0.9441	0.9421	0.941
c-axis	0.6880	0.6887	0.689
'Crystallinity' index	70-75	33-37	33-37
Crystallite size (aver., nm)	0.13 x .03	0.0200 x .0040	0.025x .003
Ignition products (800°C)	β-TCMP* + HA	β-TCMP* + HA	HA + CaO

Weight analyses based on ashed samples except for CO_3 which was determined on unashed sample using an IR method. 'Crystallinity index' is determined from the ratio of coherent to incoherent scattering ratio in mineral OH-apatite (Holly Springs) taken as 100[5,7]. β-TCMP* -Mg-substituted b-tricalcium phosphate, or *whitlockite in biological systems, β-TCP is always Mg-substituted, $(Mg,Ca)_3(PO_4)_2$.]*

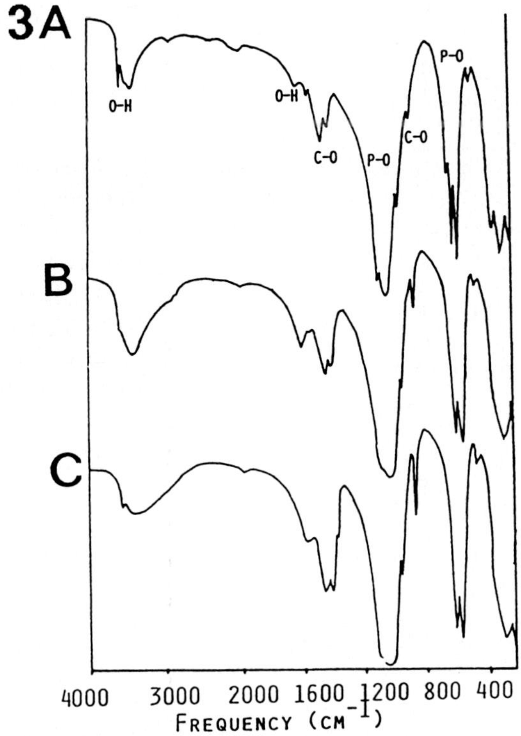

Figure 3. IR transmission spectra of powdered human enamel (A), dentin (B), and bone (C) showing the characteristic CO_3 vibration bands for biological apatites.[5-7]

carbonate compounds but similar to those of synthetic CO_3-apatites.[5-7,50,54,62] The CO_3 vibration bands in the IR spectra of biological apatites were found to be different from those of simple carbonates ($NaHCO_3$, Na_2CO_3, $CaCO_3$-calcite or aragonite form) but similar to those of synthetic CO_3-apatites with Type B (CO_3-for-PO_4) than with Type A (CO_3-for-OH) substitution[5-7,50,62] (Fig. 4). Types A and B CO_3-apatites are discussed further in Section IIB.

4. Magnesium in Biological Apatites

Like carbonate, magnesium is a principal minor constituent of calcified tissues.[3,4,50-53] It is still debated whether it is mostly associated with the organic[63] or a substituent in the inorganic phase[5-7,51] Like the carbonate, the magnesium concentration differs in different tissues, being least in enamel and most in dentin and bone[5-7,51] (Table 1).

5. Fluoride in Biological Apatites

Apatites in the enameloids of shark and of some species of fish species showed either very low (less than 0.3 wt%) or high (about 3.9 wt%) levels of F, apparently independent of the F concentration in the water of their origin[31] (Fig. 5). The apatite in some shells were also shown to contain F.[33] The F and CO_3 contents were inversely related: the higher the F, the lower the CO_3

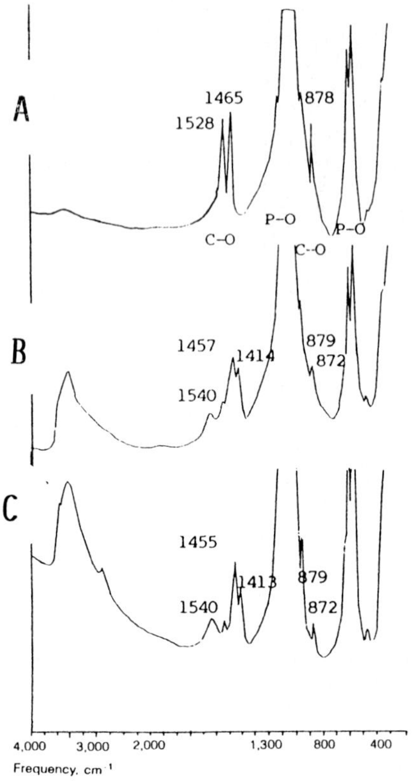

Figure 4. IR absorption spectrum of enamel (C) apatite compared with those of synthetic apaties showing two types of CO_3 substitutions: (A) Type A (CO_3-for-OH), and (B) Type B (CO_3-for PO_4 coupled with Na-for-Ca).[5-7,62]

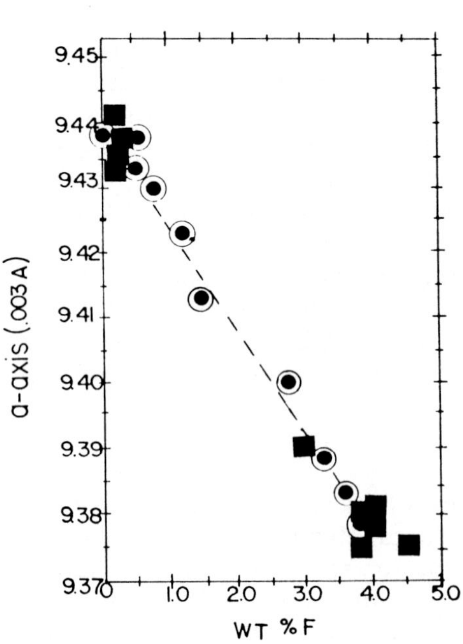

Figure 5. Effect of F substitution on the a-axis dimension for synthetic apatites (⊙) apatites from fish enameloid (□).[30]

content. The F content of bones was found to reflect the F intake and was related to its increase in crystallinity and decreased dissolution in acid buffer[60] and presumably also *in vivo*. Formation of (F,OH)- or F-apatite on tooth surfaces is believed to be one of the mechanisms for the cariostatic (caries-inhibiting) effect of F[55,57,58] applied systemically (from water supply) or topically (from dentrifices, gels, etc.), since these apatites are more resistant than the F-free apatites to dissolution by acids produced by the oral bacteria. The formation of a more stable F-apatite in bone is also one of the rationale for the use of F as one of the therapies for osteoporosis.

6. Precursor Phases: ACP, DCPD, OCP, β-TCP

The non-stoichiometry of biological apatites led to speculations that they could form from precursor phases such as ACP, DCPD, or OCP, which may initially form and then hydrolyze to apatite.[9,38,48,64-67] β-TCP as a precursor phase has also been suggested, however, pure β-TCP does not occur in biological systems and cannot be prepared from aqueous systems without the presence of Mg or other ions such as zinc.[5-7,68] All biologically occurring whitlockite or β-TCP are Mg-substituted and has been referred as b-TCMP.[5-7,35] The similarity in structure between OCP and HA was first shown by the late Dr. Walter Brown[64] and was the basis for his attractive OCP is the initial phase which hydrolyses to biological apatites.[48,64,65] However, these non-apatitic calcium phosphate phases (ACP, DCPD, OCP, β-TCMP) are usually found with or without the CO_3-apatite phase, in pathological calcification or diseased states[5-7,35-40,58,69] while principally CO_3-apatite is observed in the mineral or inorganic phases of normal calcification (enamel, dentin, bone). The transformation of one type of calcium phosphate phase to another is likely to occur in pathological calcification (e.g., dental calculi) or diseased states.

7. Dissolution/Precipitation Processes in Biological Systems

In synthetic systems, the transformation of one type of calcium phosphate to another and eventually to apatite, is believed to occur by a process of dissolution and precipitation.[7,9,16,69-73] In case of biological apatites, their extent of dissolution in acid buffers appear to be dependent on their composition. For example, the lower extent of dissolution for shark enameloid compared to that of human enamel may be attributed to its higher F and lower CO_3 contents[32]. During the caries process, the enamel or dentin apatite crystals are dissolved by the acid produced by the oral bacteria.[57] Several calcium phosphate phases may precipitate during this process: DCPD, OCP, (F,OH)-apatite, β-TCMP. All of these phases can form in acid conditions; the last two forming in the presence of F^- and Mg^{2+} ions respectively. The formation of β-TCMP with apatite in arrested dentin caries (Fig. 6) may have been due to the dissolution of the dentin apatite (which has a high Mg content) and precipitation of β-TCMP which can form under acid conditions when the Mg/Ca in solution exceeds a certain value,[7,51,69,74] or could have formed by hydrolysis of DCPD which formed initially and hydrolyzed to β-TCMP.[69] The formation of DCPD on enamel and dentin surfaces *in vitro* (Fig. 7) resulted from the dissolution of the enamel apatite in an acid solution containing phosphate and precipitation of DCPD, the stable calcium phosphate phase under this condition.[7,70]

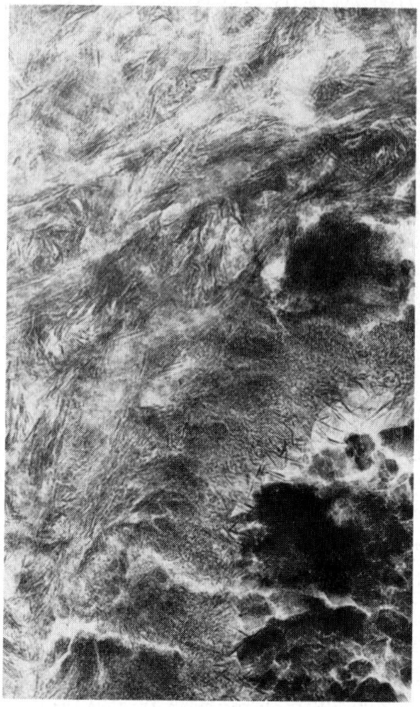

Figure 6. Transmission electron micrograph (TEM) of arrested dentin caries showing the presence of cubic crystals of β-TCMP (Mg-substituted β-TCP) and acicular (needle-like) crystals of apatite.[7,69]

II. SYNTHETIC APATITES

Synthetic apatites are prepared and investigated to understand the formation of biological apatites and some of their properties. Synthetic apatites for this purpose are prepared by precipitation in solutions containing different kinds and concentrations of elements, e.g., CO_3, F, Mg, Sr, Cl.[5-7,30,51,52,55,59,68,74-77] Dissolution properties of these apatites are of interest in relation to the coupled demineralization and remineralization processes associated with dental caries. However, for many years, the synthetic apatites used as prototype for enamel apatite were those precipitated and sintered at high temperatures or precipitated.[78] Only in recent years are synthetic CO_3-apatite being used as models for enamel apatite.[79,80]

Several types of synthetic apatites are now commercially available for use in bone repair, bone augmentation, bone substitution, and as coatings on dental and orthopedic implants. These apatites are prepared in different ways and available in different forms; used by themselves or as part of a composite; formed as a result of a reaction *in situ*, e.g., bone cements.

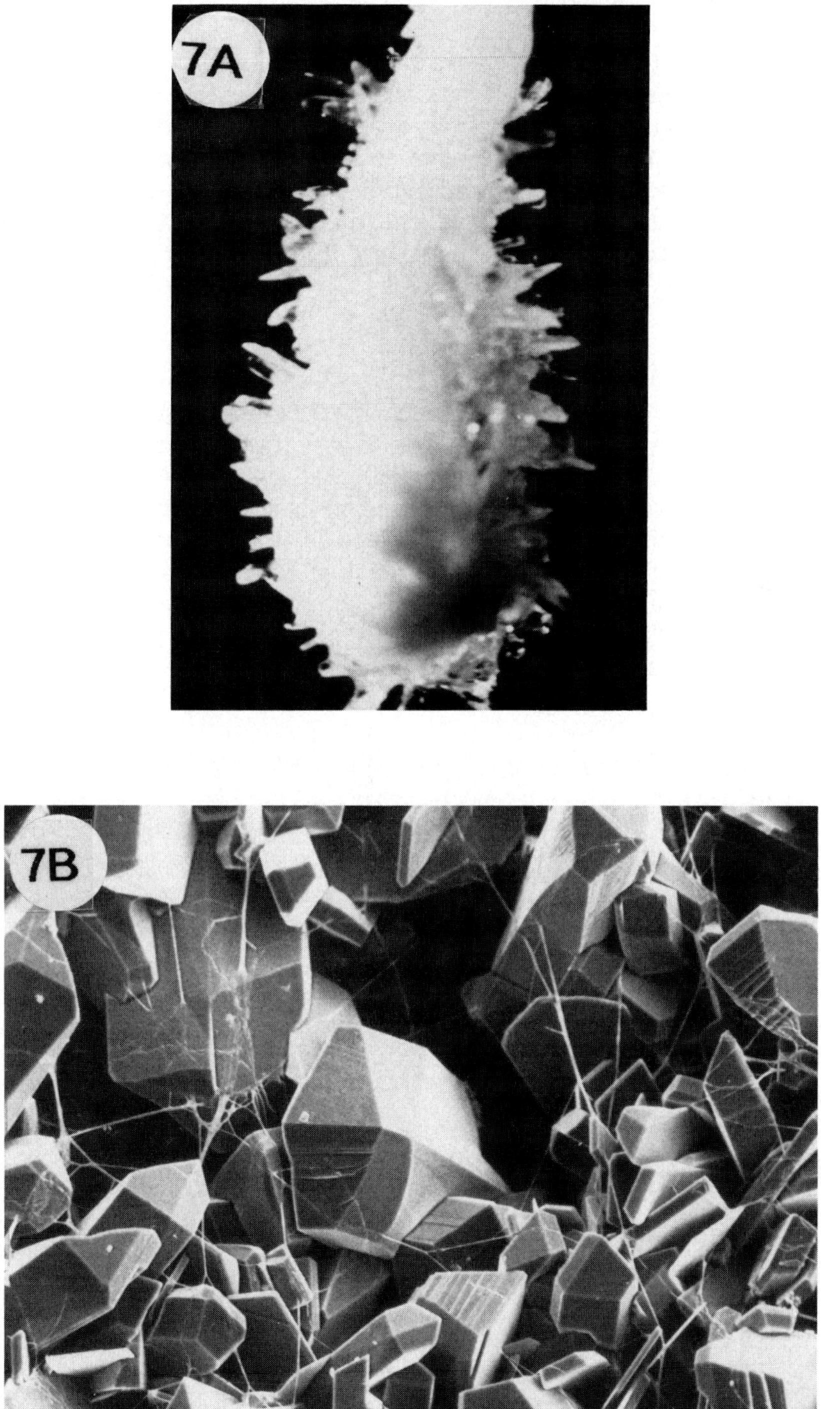

Figure 7. Photograph (A) and SEM (B) of DCPD crystals growing on tooth surfaces after immersion of tooth in phosphate-containing solution maintained at pH 3 (A) and at pH 6 (B).[7,70]

A. PREPARATION OF CALCIUM-DEFICIENT AND SUBSTITUTED APATITES

Synthetic apatite is prepared by different methods: precipitation under constant or changing composition conditions; hydrolysis; solution-mediated or heat-mediated reactions of solids; hydrothermal methods. The method of preparation, e.g., whether from non-aqueous (solid-state reaction) or aqueous systems determines the amount and type of substitution in the apatite. For example, the full incorporation of chloride, to form $Ca_{10}(PO_4)_2Cl$,[2] is facilitated in solid state reactions at high temperature, while only limited Cl incorporation, $(Ca,Na)_{10}(PO_4,HPO_4)_6(OH,Cl)_2$ is observed from reactions in aqueous systems.[5,7,52]

1. Precipitation Method

The crystallinity of precipitated apatites increase with increasing temperature of preparation (Fig. 8). It is observed that preparations made at temperatures lower than 80°C cannot really be described as apatite, but as 'apatitic.'[6] When precipitated at temperatures of 80° to 100°C, apatite is obtained from solution with initial pH of 4 to 11; the calcium deficiency of the apatite or 'apatitic' preparation decreasing with increasing pH. When prepared at lower temperatures, below 80°C, the pH/temperature dependence of the formation of different calcium phosphate phases (e.g., DCPD, DCPA, OCP) become is evident unless F is present which promotes the formation of (F,OH)-apatite.

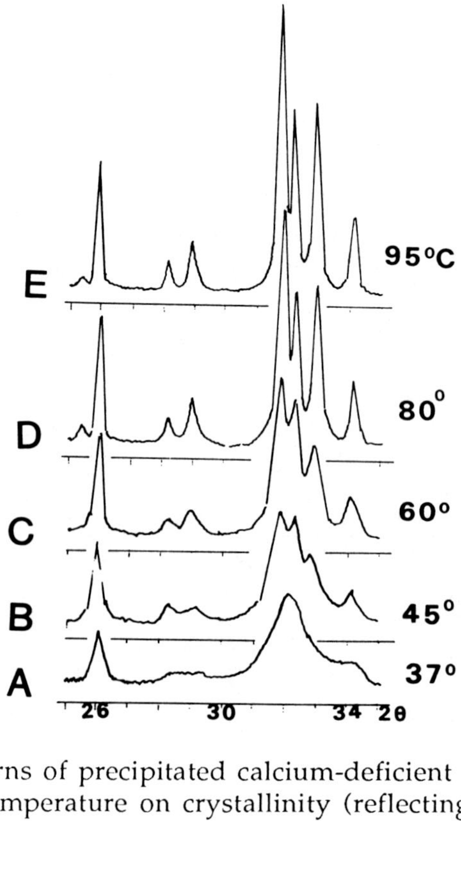

Figure 8. XRD patterns of precipitated calcium-deficient apatites showing the effect of temperature on crystallinity (reflecting crystal size and/or strain).[5-7]

2. Hydrolysis Method

Preparation of calcium-deficient or substituted apatites can also be accomplished by the hydrolysis of ACP, DCPD or DCPA, OCP, α- or β-TCP, or tetracalcium phosphate, $Ca_4(PO_4)_2O$, TTCP, in solution containing OH^- or HPO_4^{2-} ions at temperatures 37°C to 100°C. Hydrolysis of calcium phosphate phases (ACP, DCPD or DCPA, OCP, β-TCP) to apatite can proceed according to Fig. 9. The transformation of one calcium phosphate phase to apatite depends on the pH, temperature and presence of other ions besides calcium and phosphate. Thus, the hydrolysis of DCPD or OCP to AP is inhibited in the presence of Mg^{2+}, citrate or pyrophosphate ions but facilitated in the presence of F^- ions even in acid conditions, or in the presence of CO_3. In these cases, the ions become incorporated in the forming apatite (as shown in the reaction below). The hydrolysis reaction can also occur *in situ*. For example, hydrolysis of OCP to apatite resulted in formation of microcrystals of apatite following the outline of the original much larger OCP crystals[71] (Fig. 10).

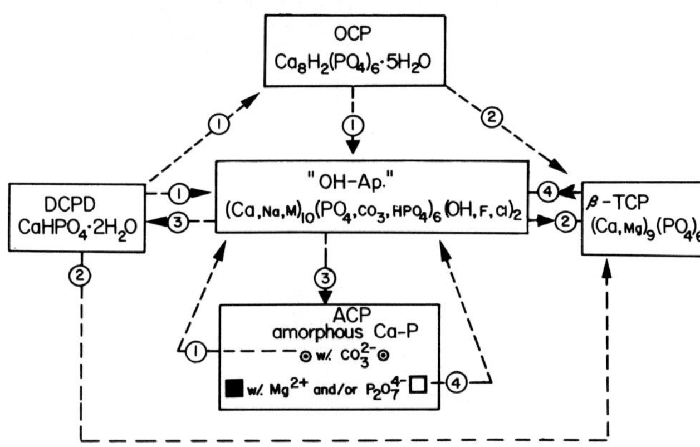

Figure 9. Schematic representation of the transformation from one type of calcium phosphate to another depending on pH, temperature and solution composition. However ACP containing critical amounts of Mg and/or P_2O_7 will not transform to apatite.

The hydrolysis method of preparing calcium-deficient or substituted apatites proceeds by the process of dissolution and precipitation according to the reaction below:

$Ca_x(PO_4)_y.nH_2O$ (ACP)
$CaHPO_4.2H_2O$ (DCPD) or $CaHPO_4$ (DCPA)
$Ca_8H_2(PO_4)_6.5H_2O$ (OCP) $\rightarrow$ $Ca^{2+} + HPO_4^{2-} + PO_4^{3-}$
$Ca_3(PO_4)_2$ (α- or β-TCP)
$Ca_4(PO_4)_2O$ (TTCP) $\swarrow$ (F, OH, or CO_3)

$(Ca,M)_{10}(PO_4,HPO_4,CO_3)_6(OH,F)_2$
Ca-def AP or F- or CO_3-AP

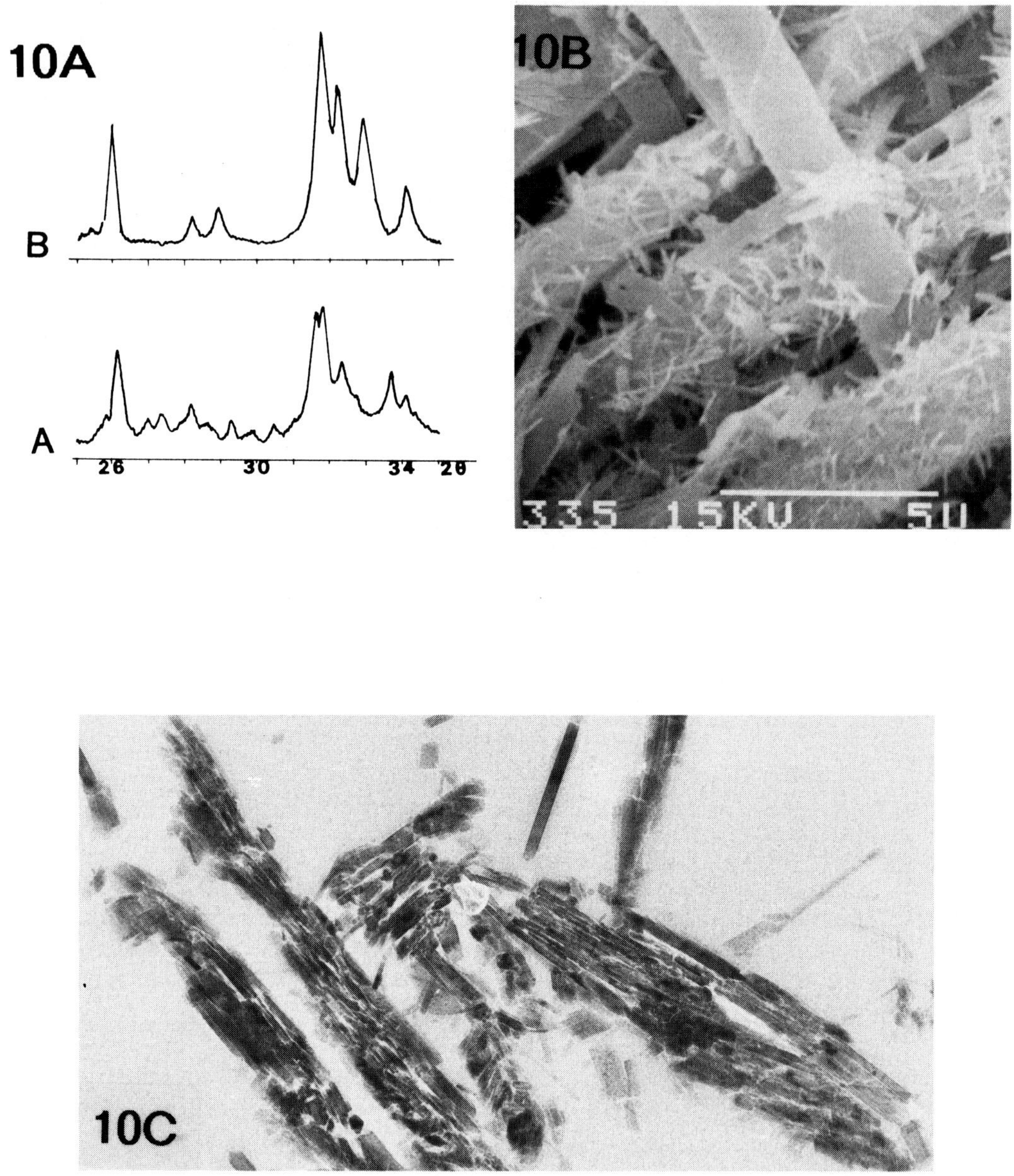

Figure 10. Hydrolysis of OCP to calcium-deficient apatite or $(F,OH)^-$ or CO_3-apatite in the presence of OH^-, F^- or CO_3^{2-} ions, respectively, as shown by XRD before (A) and after hydrolysis (B) in Fig. 10A; (Fig. 10B) SEM showing much smaller crystals of apatite growing on larger OCP crystals; (Fig. 10C) TEM showing micro-crystals of apatite growing end-to-end and side-to-side following the outline of the original OCP crystal.[7,71] (Magnification in 10C: 1,200,000X.)

Hydrolysis of non-phosphatic calcium compounds, e.g., $CaCO_3$ (calcite or aragonite form) or synthetic or biological (e.g., coral, shells) origin, or CaF_2 in solutions containing phosphate results in the formation to CO_3- or F- or (F,CO_3)-apatite.[41] The transformation of $CaCO_3$ (aragonite) to CO_3 or (F,CO_3)-apatite was speculated to be a possible reaction in the formation of marine phosphorites. The hydrolysis of CaF_2 to (F,OH)- or F- or CO_3-F-apatite is facilitated in the presence of phosphate and carbonate ions.[41] This is a possible reaction on the tooth surfaces after topical F application or high F concentrations in solutions promoting the formation of CaF_2.[7,81-83]

3. Solution-mediated reactions

Solution-mediated reactions of calcium compounds to form calcium-deficient apatites are especially investigated in the preparation of calcium phosphate cements,[15-18] in which case, the reactions take place at 25 or 37°C. The resulting apatite is usually calcium-deficient unless prepared in the presence of F when (F,OH)- or F-apatite is obtained (Table 2).

Table 2. Solution-mediated Reactions for Apatite Formation.

Reactions
$CaHPO_4$ + $CaCO_3$ (DCPA) (calcite)
$CaHPO_4.2H_2O + Ca_4(PO_4)_2O$ (DCPD) (TTCP)
$CaHPO_4$ + $Ca_4(PO_4)_2O$
$Ca(H_2PO_4)_2H_2O + Ca_4(PO_4)_2O + Ca(OH)_2$ (MMPCM) (TTCP)
$Ca_3(PO_4)_2$ + $Ca(OH)_2$ (α–TCP)
$Ca_3(PO_4)_2 + CaHPO_4.2H_2O + CaCO_3$ (β-TCP) (DCPD) (calcite)
Ca-def AP + $Ca(OH)_2$

B. EFFECTS OF SOME CATIONS AND ANIONS ON THE FORMATION AND PHYSICO-CHEMICAL PROPERTIES OF APATITE

When present in the solution, some cations or anions can inhibit the formation of apatite.[5-7,9,41,51,68,71,72] For example, hydrolysis of $CaHPO_4$ in solution containing citrate ions cause the formation of apatite of low crystallinity (Fig. 11B); and presence of pyrophosphate or molybdate ions or critical concentrations of magnesium, aluminum or stannous ions in the solution inhibits the hydrolysis to apatite (Fig. 11C), promoting instead the formation of ACP (Fig. 13C). Low concentrations of aluminum, magnesium, zinc, were shown to inhibit crystallization of apatite (Fig. 12) and promote the formation of substituted β-TCP.[68]

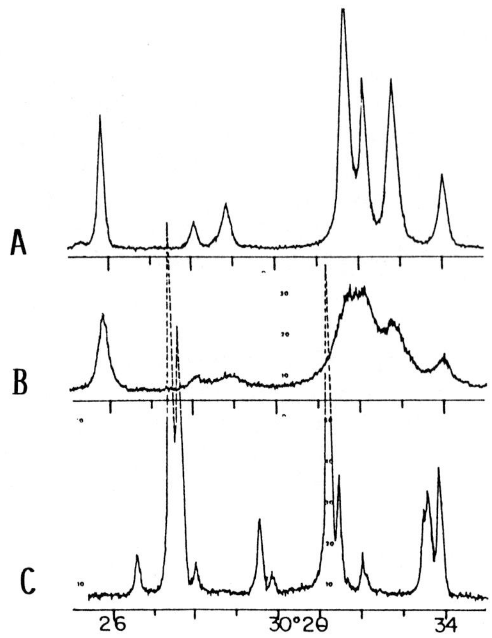

Figure 11. XRD patterns showing the effect of solution composition on the hydrolysis of $CaHPO_4$, monetite at 95°C. In basic solution (A); in solution containing citrate ions, apatite of poor crystallinity is obtained (B); and in solutions containing pyrophosphate or molybdate, no reaction took place (C).[6]

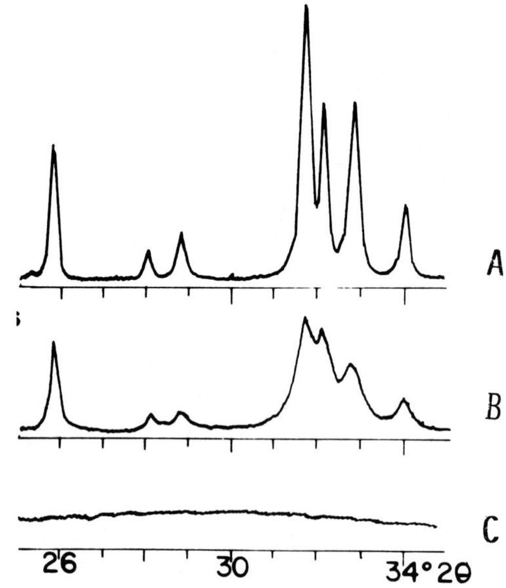

Figure 12. XRD patterns of calcium phosphate obtained with (B,C) and without (A) the presence of aluminum ions. The Al/Ca concentrations in solutions maintained at 95°C were: 0/100 (A), 5/95 (B), 15/85 (C). (C) gives an XRD of an amorphous calcium phosphate, ACP.[6,68]

13A

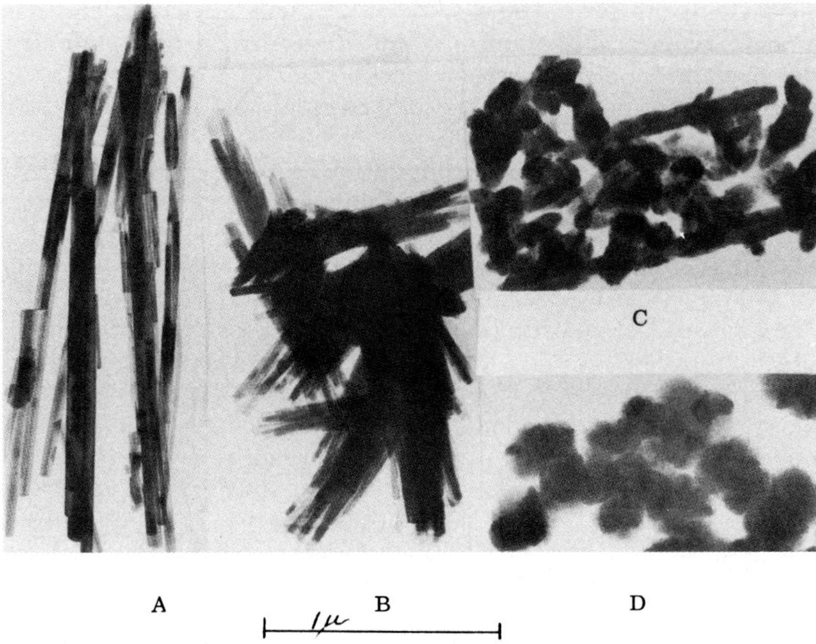

13B

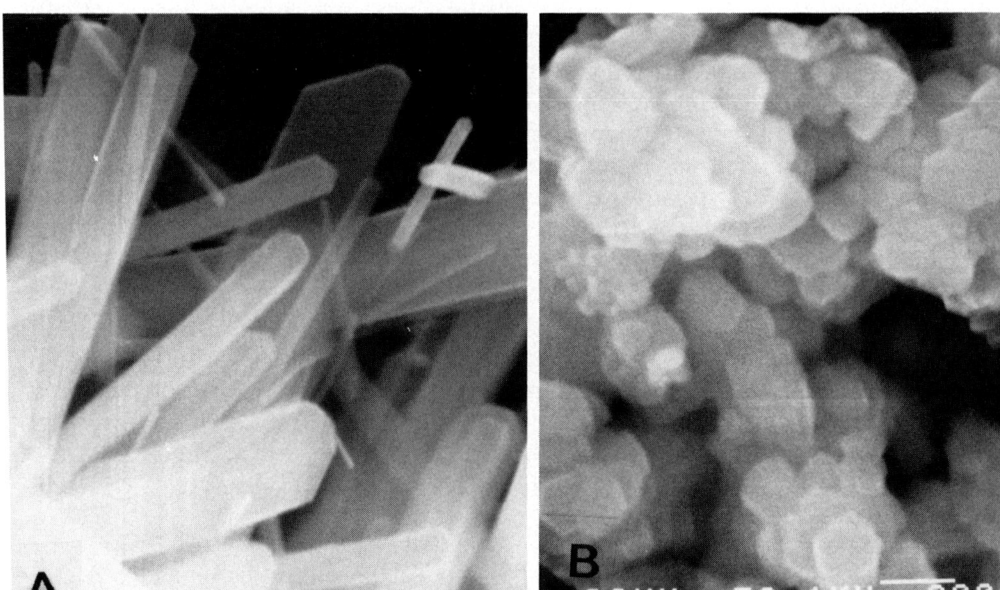

Figure 13. Effect of carbonate on reducing the crystal size and changing the morphology of CO_3-apatites[5-7,86-88] were shown by TEM (13A) and high resolution SEM (13B, 13C). Carbonate concentrations (wt %) in apatites shown in 13A: (A) 0.5; (B) 2.0; (C) 15.2 and (D) 17.2; in 13B, (A) 0.5, (B) 12.8. (TEM analyses in collaboration with Dr. Paul Shirra; high resolution SEM, with Ms. Jamie Schlottman.)

When the ions become substituents in the apatite, they cause changes in physico-chemical properties[5-7,54,55,84-88] which include changes in: lattice parameter (reflecting size and amount of substituent); crystallinity (reflecting crystal size and/or strain); crystal morphology; and dissolution properties. The substitutions of some of the biologically relevant ions are discussed below.

1. Carbonate

Synthetic CO_3-apatites showing two types of CO_3 substitution are prepared under two very different conditions. Type A (CO_3-for-OH) is obtained at high temperature and dry conditions.[54,85] Type B (CO_3-for-PO_4 coupled with Na-for-Ca) is obtained from aqueous systems at much lower temperatures (25 to 100°C), either by precipitation or hydrolysis methods.[5-7,48,62,65,71,72,86-88] The effect of CO_3 substitution on the lattice parameters depends on the type of substitution: Type A (CO_3-for-OH) causes expansion of the a- and contraction of the c-axis dimensions;[49,77,78] Type B (CO_3-for-PO_4 coupled with Na-for-Ca) causes contraction of the a- and expansion of the c-axis dimensions.[5-7,54,72] The characteristic vibration of the CO_3 groups occur at different absorption bands reflecting the difference in their structural environment. Type B CO_3-apatites most closely resemble biological apatites (Fig. 4). The CO_3 substitution was shown to cause reduction in crystallinity (decrease in crystal size) and change in shape from acicular to rod-shape to equi-axed flatter crystals[5-7,72,87-88] (Fig. 13). The CO_3 were shown to increase the extent of dissolution of synthetic apatites.[5-7,56]

2. Fluoride

Fluoride ions, when present in solution, readily gets incorporated in the forming apatite whether formed by precipitation or hydrolysis. F- or (F,OH)-apatite can form by the hydrolysis of DCPA or DCPD in solutions containing F.[5-7,60,70] F-containing apatites can also form by hydrolysis of CaF_2 in solutions containing phosphate ions[41] or by solution-mediated reaction of DCPD and CaF_2[89]. The F-for-OH substitution causes a contraction n the a-axis without significant effect on the c-axis (Fig. 5). Crystallinity is increased,[5-7,60] causing the formation of larger and thicker apatite crystals.[7] The incorporation of F in apatite imparts greater stability to the apatite, making it less soluble.[7,32,55,56,60] This is one of the mechanism for the observed cariostatic (caries-inhibiting) effect of F. In addition, F incorporation promotes higher Ca/P molar ratio, approaching stoichiometric value.[7,90,91] Synthetic apatites containing both fluoride and carbonate is prepared by precipitation or hydrolysis from solutions containing both F^- and CO_3^{2-} ions. Some biological apatites from fish enameloids or calcified fish scales or some species of shells contain both F and CO_3.

3. Magnesium and Other Substituents

Magnesium, chloride, and potassium ions were shown to substitute in apatite to a very limited extent.[7,51,52,92] Strontium can fully substitute for calcium,[5-7,76,77,93] the extent of substitution being pH dependent[6,7,76] Manganese can substitute as manganese or manganate ions.[68] Magnesium and strontium cause the apatite to be more soluble than the Mg- or Sr-free apatites.[7,51,76,77]

Table 3. Qualitative Effects on Lattice Parameters and Crystallinity of Apatites: Effect of Cations.

Cations	Ionic radius, A	a-axis	c-axis	Crystallinity
Barium	1.34	(+)	(+)	(-)
Potassium	1.33	(nc)	(nc)	(-)
Lead	1.20	(+)	(+)	(-)
Strontium	1.12	(+)	(+)	(nc)
Sodium	0.97	(nc)	(nc)	(nc)
Cadmium	0.97	(-)	(-)	(-)
Copper	0.97	(-)	(-)	(-)
Tin	0.93	am	am	am
Manganese	0.80	(-)	(-)	(-)
Zinc	0.74	(+)	(-)	(-)**
Iron	0.74	(+)	(+)	(-)**
Cobalt	0.70	(+)	(-)	(-)**
Nickel	0.69	(+)	(-)	(-)**
Lithium	0.68	(nc)	(nc)	(nc)
Magnesium	0.66	(+)	(-)	(-)**
Chromium	0.63	(+)	(-)	(-)

Precipitates obtained from solutions containing cation/Ca^{2+} =5/95 and 10/90; (+) = greater than; (-) less than that of unsubstituted calcium apatite; (nc) - no change. ** promotes formation of substituted β-TCP at the expense of *apatite; am –amorphous. For comparison, ionic radius of* Ca^{2+} *- 0.99.*

C. APATITES FOR BONE GRAFT MATERIALS AND COATINGS ON IMPLANTS

1. HA ceramic is usually prepared by precipitation under very basic conditions and sintering the precipitate at 950° to 1100°C. These ceramics can be prepared in dense or porous forms.[4-7,18,87] The crystals of ceramic HA are much larger than those of enamel or precipitated (non-ceramic) apatite (Fig. 2).

2. Coralline HA: Coralline HA is prepared by the hydrothermal conversion of coral (aragonite) in the presence of ammonium phosphate solution.[19] The conversion results in the formation of CO_3-apatite and small amount of β-TCMP (Mg-substituted β-TCP).[7,94-96]

3. 'Resorbable' HA: This preparation is an unsintered calcium-deficient apatite. The preparation of the commercial product is not known, However, as mentioned above, this type of apatite is a calcium-deficient apatite and can be prepared either by precipitation or hydrolysis methods.

4. Apatite from natural sources: Freeze-dried banked human bones and apatite from treated ones are also available.[7,95]

5. Calcium Phosphate Coatings on implants: Calcium phosphate coatings are applied either by electrodeposition,[28] ion-sputtering, or plasma-spraying[27] HA ceramic onto the metal implants. The composition of the coating depends on the method of coating: by electrodeposition or precipitation, apatite of poor crystallinity ('apatitic'); by ion-sputtering, ACP; and by plasma-spraying, HA and ACP as the major components mixed with other calcium phosphate phases, e.g., α- and β-TCP, TTCP, and sometimes with calcium oxide CaO.[7,27,28,98] A composition gradient was observed between the inner and outer layers of the coating: with the inner layer containing higher ACP/HA ratio.[7] Variations in composition of coatings can cause variations in their stability *in vivo* since the different calcium phosphate phases have different solubilities[7,9] decreasing in the order:

$$ACP > TTCP >> \alpha\text{-}TCP >> \beta\text{-}TCP >> HA \quad .$$

D. FORMATION OF CO_3-APATITE ON SURFACES OF CALCIUM PHOSPHATE BIOMATERIALS: A DISSOLUTION/PRECIPITATION PROCESS

Calcium phosphate biomaterials, like special glass ceramics, are described as bioactive and responsible for forming a uniquely high interfacial strength compared to other bioinert materials[98,99]. After implantation, these biomaterials were shown to form carbonate apatite on their surfaces,[22,43-46,99,100] (Fig. 14) intimately associated with an organic matrix[22,46,100] (Fig. 15). Such reactions *in vitro* and *in vivo* have been associated with bioreactivity.[99] The formation of carbonate apatite intimately associated with an organic matrix is believed to occur by the process of dissolution (from acids produced by cells on the material surface) and formation (either by direct precipitation or by hydrolysis of acidic calcium phosphate phases formed initially) of CO_3-apatite (the CO_3^{2-}, and, possibly, Mg^{2+} ions originating from the biological fluid) and become intimately associated with an organic matrix (Fig. 16).

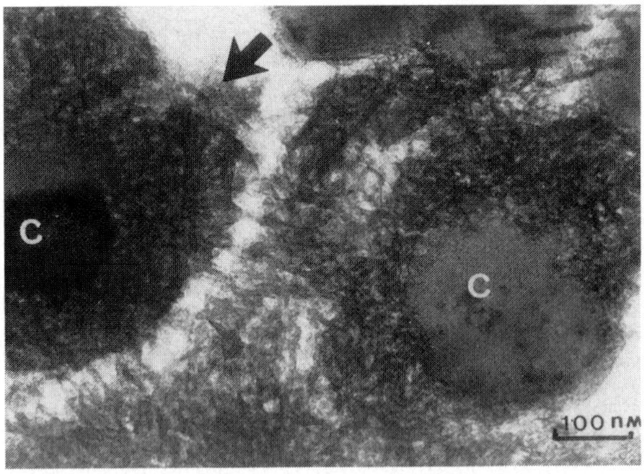

Figure 14. Formation of CO_3-apatite crystals on much larger HA ceramic crystals (c) after implantation.[7,22,45,46]

E. THE IDEAL CALCIUM PHOSPHATE BIOMATERIAL?

The focus on developing the ideal calcium phosphate biomaterial is very much on the forefront as evidenced by the number and variety of topics presented at this symposium. All the commercial phosphate materials are not similar to

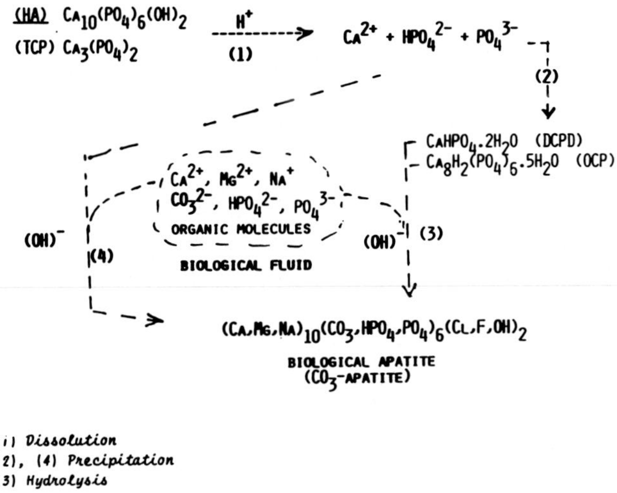

Figure 15. Transformation of HA ceramic to CO3-apatite associated with organic matrix is demonstrated in the IR spectra: (A) before implantation; material on core (B), and from the surface (C) of the retrieved HA ceramic implant; and material from bone furthest away from the implant site. C-O, P-O, O-H refers to the vibration bands of the CO3, PO4 and OH groups of the apatite. N-H refers to vibration bands of the organic matrix.[7,22,46]

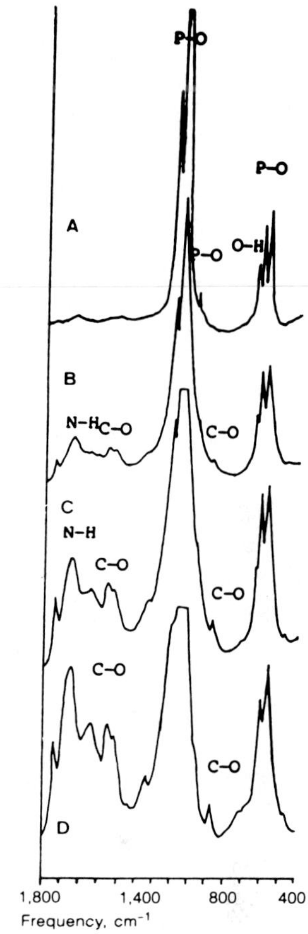

Figure 16. Schematic representation of the dissolution (1), precipitation (2,4) and (3) hydrolysis processes involved inthe formation of CO3-apatite crystals on surfaces of calcium phosphate (HA, β-TCP) biomaterials.

the bone mineral in composition, crystallographic and dissolution properties[7,26,94,103,104] as shown in Figs. 2, 14, 17 and 18. Many unanswered questions remain, these include: should the same or different types of material be used for different applications (bony defects vs. bone augmentation); should the material be more or less like the bone mineral in crystallinity, composition and resorbability; should the ideal coating on metal implants be principally

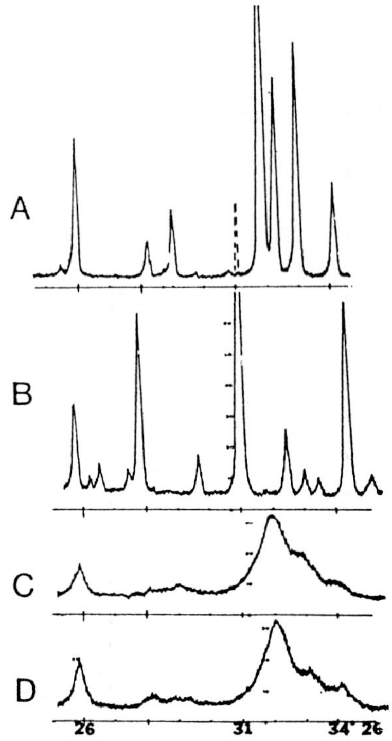

Figure 17. XRD patterns of commercial HA (A), and β-TCP ceramic (B) compared with the bone mineral (C) and experimental bone-mineral-like material (D).[14]

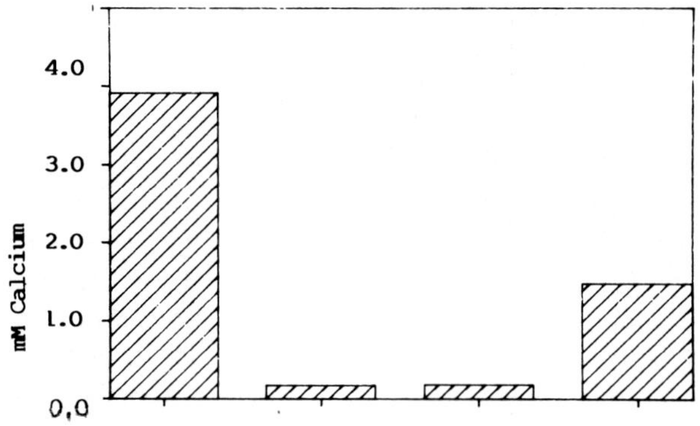

Figure 18. Comparative extent of dissolution of human bone (A); HA ceramic (B and C) and β-TCP (D) commercial ceramic materials. Dissolution in 0.1M KAc, pH 6, 37°C, 60 min. expressed as amount (mM/L) of Ca^{2+} ions released in the acid buffer.[14,26]

highly crystalline HA with limited dissolution rate or HA mixed with other calcium phosphate phases; should the ideal synthetic bone graft be a composite?[101,102]

Acknowledgements

The collaboration of several colleagues, especially Drs. G. Daculsi, I. Orly, J. P. LeGeros, R. Kijkowska, E. Nery, M. Heughebaert, S. Suga (deceased), W. P. Shirra, J. Schlottman, M. Tung; and the technical assistance of M. Retino, W. Torres, R. Zheng, D. Fan in some of the work cited in this paper is gratefully acknowledged. The assistance of Ms. Inna Shapiro and the support of NIH/NIDR Research Grant Nos. DE 04123 and DE 07223 and SO7RR07062 is acknowledged and appreciated.

The author specially acknowledges the encouragement received from the late Dr. Walter Brown, a great scientist and a great human being.

REFERENCES

1. Naray-Szabo, S., The structure of apatite $(CaF)Ca_4(PO_4)_3$. Z. Krist., 75,387-398.
2. Kay, M.I., Young, R.A., Posner A.S., Crystal structure of hydroxyapatite. Nature, 204, 1051-1052, 1964.
3. Mehmel, M., Uber die Struktur des Apatit, *Z. Krist.*, 75, 323-331, 1930.
4. De Jong, W.F., La substance minerale dans les os, *Res. Trav. Chim.*, 45, 445-448, 1926.
5. LeGeros, R.Z., Crystallographic studies of the carbonate substitution in the apatite structure. PhD Thesis, New York University, 1967.
6. LeGeros, R.Z., Apatites in Biological Systems, *Prog. Crystal Growth Charact.*, 4, 1-45, 1981.
7. LeGeros, R.Z., Calcium Phosphates in Oral Biology and Medicine. Monographs in Oral Science, Vol. 15, HM Myers (ed.) S. Karger, Basel, Switzerland., 1991
8. Featherstone, J.D.B., Mayer, I., Driessens, F.M.C., Verbeeck, R.M.H., Heijligers, H.J.M., Synthetic apatites containing Na, Mg and CO_3 and their comparison with tooth enamel mineral. Calcif. Tissue Int. 35, 169-171,1983.
9. Johnsson, M.S.-A., Nancollas, G.H., The role of brushite and octacalcium phosphate in apatite formation, *Critical Reviews in Oral Biology and Medicine*, 3(1/2), 61-82, 1992.
10. Jarcho, M., Calcium phosphate ceramics as hard tissue prosthetics, *Clin. Orthopaed.*, 157, 259-278, 1981.
11. De Groot, K., Ceramic of calcium phosphates: Preparation and properties. In: Bioceramics of Calcium Phosphate. ed. K. de Groot. Boca Raton, FL, 1983. 100-114.
12. Aoki, H., Kato, K., Ogiso, M. & Tabata, T., Studies on the application of apatite to dental materials, *J. Dent. Eng.*, 18, 86-89, 1977.
13. Bonel, G., Heughebaert, J-C., Heughebaert M., Lacout, J.L. & Lebugle A., Apatitic calcium orthophosphates and related compounds for biomaterials preparation. In: Bioceramics: Material Characteristic versus

In Vivo Behavior. eds. P. Ducheyne, and J.E. Lemons, *Ann. NY Acad. Sci.*, 523, 115-130, 1988.

14. LeGeros, R.Z., Properties of commercial bone grafts compared to human bone and new synthetic bone biomaterials, Ninth Annual meeting of the Society for Biomaterials, Birmingham, Alabama, Abstr. No. 86, April, 1983.
15. Brown, W.E., Chow, L.C., Dental restorative cement pastes, US patent No. 4, 518, 430, May, 21, 1985.
16. Fulmer, M.T., Martin, R.I., Brown, P.W., Formation of calcium deficient hydroxyapatite at near-physiological temperature, *J. Mater. Sci. Materials in Medicine*, 001-007,1992.
17. Mirtchi, A.A., Lemaitre, J., Munting, E., Calcium phosphate cements: study of the β-tricalcium phosphate—dicalcium phosphate—calcite cements, *Biomaterials*, 11, 83-88, 1990.
18. LeGeros, R.Z., Chohayeb, A., Shulman, A., Apatitic calcium phosphates: Possible restorative materials, *J Dent Res*, 61, 343, Abstr. 1482, 1982.
19. Roy, D.M. & Linnehan, S.A., Hydroxyapatite formed from coral skeleton carbonate by hydrothermic exchange, *Nature*, 247, 220-227, 1974.
20. Metsger, D.S., Driskell, T.D. & Paulsrud, J.R., Tricalcium phosphate ceramic--A resorbable bone implant: Review and current status, *J. Am. Dent. Assoc.*, 105, 1035-1038, 1982.
21. Hubbard, W., Physiological calcium phosphate as orthopedic implant material; PhD thesis, Marquette University, 1974.
22. LeGeros, R.Z., Daculsi, G., In Vivo transformation of biphasic calcium phosphate ceramics: ultrastructural and physico-chemical characterizations. In: Handbook of Bioactive Ceramics Vol.II. Calcium Phosphate Ceramics. Yamamuro N, Hench L, Wilson-Hench J (Eds.), CRC Press, 17-28, 1990.
23. Nery, E.B., LeGeros, R.Z., Lynch, K.L., Lee, K, Tissue response to biphasic calcium phosphate ceramic with different ratios of HA/βTCP in periodontal osseousdefects, *J. Periodontol.*, 63(9), 729-735, 1992.
24. Holmes, R.E., Bone regeneration within a coralline hydroxyapatite implant, *Plast. Reconstr. Surg*, 63, 626-636, 1979.
25. Wagner, J.R., A clinical and histological case study using resorbable hydroxyapatite for the repair of osseous defects prior to endosseous implant surgery. *J .Oral Implantol.* 15, 186-192, 1989.
26. LeGeros, R.Z., Calcium Phosphate Materials. In: NIH-NIDR State-of-the-Science Conference on Dental Materials, September 1986, Bethesda, *Adv .Dent. Res.*, 3, 164-180, 1988.
27. De Groot, K., Hydroxylapatite coatings for implants in surgery. In: High Tech Ceramics. ed. P. Vincenzini. Elsevier Science Publishers, B.V. Amsterdam, 381-386, 1987.
28. Ducheyne, P., Radin, S., Heughbaert M., Heughebaert, J.C., Calcium phosphate ceramic coatings on porous titanium: effect of structure and composition on electrophoretic deposition, vacuum sintering and in vitro dissolution, Biomaterials 11, 244-253, 1990.
29. McConnel, D., The applications of mineralogical theories to the "mineral" phase of teeth and bones, *Biochim. Biophys. Acta*, 17, 450-451, 1955.
30. LeGeros, R.Z., Suga, S., Crystallographic nature of fluoride in the enameloids of fish, *Calcif Tiss Int*, 32, 169-174, 1980.

31. Lee, D., LeGeros, R.Z., Microbeam electron diffraction and lattice fringe studies of defect structures in enamel apatites, *Calcif. Tiss. Int.*, 37, 651-658, 1985.
32. LeGeros, R.Z., Silverstone, L.M., Daculsi, G., Kerebel, L.M., In vitro caries-like lesion formation in F-containing tooth enamel, *J. Dent. Res.*, 62, 138-144, 1983.
33. LeGeros, R.Z., Pan, C.M., Suga, S., Watabe, N., Crystallo-chemical properties of apatites in atremate brachiopod shells, *Calcif. Tiss. Int.*, 37, 651-658, 1985.
34. Lowenstam, H. A., Weiner, S., Phosphatic shell plate of the barnacle Ibla (Cirripedia): A bone-like structure. *Proc. Natl. Acad. Sci. USA 89, 10593-10577, 1992.*
35. LeGeros, R.Z., Variations in the crystalline components of human dental calculus: 1. Crystallographic and spectroscopic methods of analyses, *J. Dent. Res.*, 53, 45-50, 1974.
36. LeGeros, R.Z., Morales, P., Renal store crystals grown in gel system, A preliminary report, *Invest. urol.*, 11, 12-20, 1973.
37. Pak, C.Y.C., Potential etiologic role of brushite in the formation of calcium (renal) stones, *J. Crystal Growth*, 53, 202-208, 1981.
38. Frondel, C. and Prien, E.L., Deposition of calcium phosphates accompanying senile degeneration and disease, *Science*, 103, 326-327, 1946.
39. LeGeros, R.Z., Contiguglia, S.R., Alfrey, A.C., Pathological calcification associated with uremia: two types of calcium phosphate deposits, *Calc. Tiss. Res.*, 13, 173-185, 1973.
40. McCarty, D.J., Lehr, J.R., Halverson, P.B.,Crystal populations in human synovial fluid, Arthritis and Rheumatism 26, 1220-1224, 1983.
41. LeGeros, R.Z., Go, P., Vandermaele, G.H., Quirlogico, G.B., LeGeros, D.J., Transformation of calcium carbonates and calcium phosphates to carbonate apatites: possible mechanism for phosphorate formation. In: Proc. 2nd International Congress on Phosphorous Compounds, Boston, 41-54, 1980.
42. Gulbrandsen R.A., Physical and chemical factors in the formation of marine apatite. *Econ. Geol.*, 64, 365. 1969.
43. Tracy, B.M., Doremus, R.H., Direct electron microscopy studies of bone-hydroxylapatite interface. *J. Biomed. Mat. Res.*, 18, 719-726, 1984.
44. Kay, J.F., Physiological Acceptance of a Ceramic Bone Implant Determined by Electron Optical Analysis, PhD. Thesis, Rensselaer Polytechnic Institute, 1977.
45. Daculsi, G., LeGeros, R.Z., Heughebaert, M., Barbieux, I., Formation of carbonate-apatite crystals after implantation of calcium phosphate ceramics. *Calcif. Tissue. Int.* 46, 20-27. 1990.
46. LeGeros, R.Z., Daculsi, G., Orly, I., Gregoire, M., Substrate surface dissolution and interfacial biological mineralization. In: The Bone Biomaterial Interface. JED Davies (Ed.), Univ. of Toronto Press, 76-88, 1991.
47. Nylen, M.U., Matrix-mineral relationships. A morphologist's viewpoint, *J. Dent. Res.*, 8(b), 922-926, 1979.
48. Brown, W.E., Chow, L.C., Chemical properties of bone mineral, *Ann. Res. Mater. Sci.*, 6, 213-226, 1976.
49. Arends, J., Davidson, C., The HPO_{4-2} content of sound and decalcified enamel, *Calcif. Tiss. Res.*, 18, 65-79, 1975.

50. Emerson, W.H. and Fisher, E.E., The infrared spectra of carbonate in calcified tissues, *Arch. Oral Biol.*, 7, 671-683, 1962.
51. LeGeros, R.Z., Incorporation of magnesium in synthetic and biological apatites: a preliminary report. In: Tooth Enamel IV, Rearnhead RW, Suga S (Eds.). Elsevier: Amsterdam: 32-36, 1984.
52. LeGeros, R.Z., The unit-cell dimensions of human enamel apatite: effect of chloride incorporation, *Arch. Oral Biol.*, 20, 63-71, 1974.
53. LeGeros, R.Z., Bonel, G., Types of 'H_2O' in human enamel and in precipitated apatites, *Calc. Tiss. Res.*, 26, 111-116, 1978.
54. Elliott, J.C., The Crystallographic Structure of Dental Enamel and Related Apatites. Thesis. University of London, 1964.
55. Moreno, E.G., Kresak, M. & Zahradnik, R.T., Physicochemical aspects of fluoride-apatite systems relevant to the study of dental caries, *Caries Res.*, 11 (suppl. l), 142-171, 1977.
56. LeGeros, R.Z., Tung, M.S., Chemical stability of carbonate and fluoride containing apatites, *Caries Res.*, 17, 419-429, 1983.
57. Nikiforuk, G., Understanding Dental Caries. 1. Etiology and Mechanisms. Basel, Karger, 1985.
58. LeGeros, R.Z., Chemical and crystallographic events in the caries process, *J. Dent. Res.*, 69, 567-574, 1990.
59. Sakae, T., LeGeros, R.Z.,Magnesium and carbonate concentrations in human enamel. J. Dent. Res. 69, 123, Abstr. no. 113, 1990.
60. LeGeros, R.Z., Singer, L., Ophaug, R., Quirolgico, G., The effect of fluoride on the stability of synthetic and biological (bone mineral) apatits: in: Menczel J., Robin GC (eds): Osteoporosis, New York, Wiley, pp. 327-341, 1982.
61. Posner, A.S., Duyckaerts, G., Infrared study of the carbonate in bone, teeth and francolite. *Experientia* 424-425, 1954.
62. LeGeros, R.Z., LeGeros, J.P., Trautz, O.R., Klein, E., Spectral properties of carbonate in carbonate-containing apatites, *Dev. Appl Spec*, 7B, 3-12, 1970.
63. Robinson, C., Weatherell, J.A. and Hallsworth, A.S., Distribution of magnesium in mature human enamel, *Caries Res.*, 15, 70-77, 1981.
64. Brown, W.E., Crystal structure of octacalcium phosphate, *Nature (Lond)*, 196, 1048, 1962.
65. Brown, W.E., Matthew, M., and Tung, M.S., Crystal chemistry of octacalcium phosphate, *Prog. Crystal Growth Charact.*, 4, 59-87, 1981.
66. Eanes, E.D., Posner, A.S., Kinetics and mechanism of conversion of non-crystalline calcium phosphate to crystalline hydroxyapatite, *Trans. N.Y. Acad. Sci. Ser. II*, 28, 233, 1965.
67. Francis, M.D., and Webb, N.C., Hydroxyapatite formation from a hydrated calcium monohydrogen phosphate precursor, *Calcif. Tissue. Res*, 6, 335-342, 1971.
68. LeGeros, R.Z., Taheri, M.H., Quirlogico, G.M., LeGeros, J.P., Formation and stability of apatites: effects of some cationic substituents. Proc. 2nd International Congress on Phosphorus Compounds, Boston: 89-103, 1980.
69. Daculsi, G., LeGeros, R.Z., Jean, A., Kerebel, B., Possible physico-chemical processes in human dentin caries. *J. Dent. Res.* 66, 1356-1359, 1987.

70. LeGeros, R.Z., Lee, D., Quirolgico, G., Shirra, W.P., Reich, L., In vitro formation of dicalcium phosphate dihydrate, $CaHPO_4$, *Scan. Electr Micros.*, 407-418, 1983.
71. LeGeros, R.Z., Daculsi, G., Orly, I., Solution-mediated transformation of OCP to apatite, *Scan. Electron Micros.*, 3, 129-138, 1989.
72. LeGeros, R.Z., LeGeros, J.P., Trautz, O.R., Shirra, W.P., Conversion of monetite, $CaHPO_4$, to apatites: effect of carbonate on the crystallinity and the morphology of apatite crystallites, *Adv. X-ray Ana.l*, 14, 57-66, 1971.
73. Ishikawa, K., Eanes, E.D., The hydrolysis of anhydrous dicalcium phosphate into hydroxyapatite, *J. Dent. Res.*, 72(2), 474-480, 1993.
74. Cheng, P., Grabher, J.J., LeGeros, R.Z., Effects of magnesium on calcium phosphate formation. *Magnesium J.*, 7, 123-132, 1988.
75. Boskey, A., Posner, A.S., Formation of hydroxyapatite at low supersaturation. *J. Phys. Chem.*, 80, 40-45, 1976.
76. LeGeros, R.Z., Kijkowska, R., Tung, M., LeGeros, J.P., Effect of strontium on some properties of apatites. In: Enamel Symposium V. RW Fearnhead, S Suga (Eds.), Elsevier Publishers, 393-401, 1989
77. Sillen, A., LeGeros, R.Z., Solubility profiles of synthetic apatites and of modern and fossil bones, *J. Archeol. Sci.*, 18, 385-397, 1991.
78. Higuchi, W.I., Gray, J.A., Hefferren, J.J., and Patel, P.R., Mechanisms of enamel dissolution in acid buffers, *J. Dent. Res.*, 44, 330-341, 1965.
79. Hsu, J., Fox, J.L., Higuchi, W.I., Powell, G.L., Otsuka, M., Quantitative relationship between carbonated apatite metastable equilibrium solubility and dissolution kinetics, *J. Colloid. Interface Sci.* (in press)
80. Budz, J.A., Lore, M., Nancollas, G.H., Hydroxyapatite and carbonated apatite as models for the dissolution behavior of human dental enamel, *Adv. Dent. Res.*, 1, 314-321, 1987.
81. LeGeros, R.Z., Zhang, R., Torres, W., LeGeros, J.P., Effect of phosphate on crystal growth of CaF_2, *Caries Res.*, 24, 407, Abstr. No. 41, 1990.
82. Ogard, B., Rolla, G., Helgeland, K., Uptake and retention of alkali-soluble and alkali-insoluble fluoride in sound enamel in vivo after mouthrinses with 0.05% or 0.2% NaF, *Caries Res.*, 17, 520-524, 1983.
83. Tung, M.S., Chow, L.C., and Brown, W.E., Hydrolysis of dicalcium phosphate dihydrate in the presence or absence of calcium fluoride, *J. Dent. Res.*, 64, 2-5, 1985.
84. Young, R.A., Elliott, J.C., Atomic scale bases for several properties of apatites, *Arch. Oral Biol.*, 11, 699-707, 1966.
85. Bonel, G., Contribution a l'etude de la carbonation des apatites, *Ann. Chim.*, 7, 65-88, 1972.
86. Zapanta-LeGeros, R., Effect of carbonate on the lattice parameters of apatite, *Nature*, 206, 403-404, 1965.
87. LeGeros, R.Z., Trautz, O.R., LeGeros, J.P., Shirra, W.P., Apatite crystallites: effect of carbonate on morphology, *Science*, 155, 1409-1411, 1967.
88. LeGeros, R.Z., LeGeros, J.P., Kijkowska, R., DeDeyn, B. and Schlottman, J., Effect of carbonate on the morphology of synthetic CO_3-apatites using high-resolution SEM, *J. Dent. Res.*, 68, 1003 Abstr. No. 1090, 1989.

89. Tung, M.S., Chow, L.C., Brown, W.E., Hydrolysis of dicalcium phosphate dihydrate in the presence or absence of calcium fluoride, *J. Dent. Res.*, 64, 2-5, 1985.
90. LeGeros, R.Z., Kijkowska, R., Jia, W.T., LeGeros, J.P., Fluoride-cation interaction in the formation and stability of apatites, *J. Fluor. Chem.*, 41, 53-64, 1988.
91. Ingram G.S., Nash, P.F., A mechanism for the anticaries action of fluoride. *Caries Res.*, 14, 298-303, 1980.
92. Rokbani, R., LeGeros, R.Z., Ayadi, M.T., Ariguib, N., Apatites in the System: $CaCl_2$-$Ca_3(PO_4)_2$-K_3PO_4-H_2O at 25°C, *J. Dent. Res.*, 72, 618, Abstr. 821, 1992.
93. Collins, R.L., Strontium-calcium hydroxylapatite solid-solutions preparation and lattice constants measurements. *J. Am. Ceram. Soc.*, 82, 5067-5077, 1960
94. LeGeros, R.Z., Materials for bone augmentation, repair and substitution. In: *Biomechanics in Orthopedics*. S Niwa, S. M. Perren and T. Hattori (Eds.). Springer Verlag, Tokyo, 147-174, 1992.
95. LeGeros, R.Z., Orly, I., Gregoire, M., Kazimiroff, J., Comparative Properties and in vitro reactions of HA Ceramic and coralline HS. In: *Proceedings First International Symposium on Apatite*, Mishima, Japan, July, 1991.
96. LeGeros, R.Z., Daculsi, G., unpublished results on bone apatite (BonAP), 1986.
97. LeGeros, J.P., LeGeros, R.Z., Edwards, B., Zitelli, J., Burgess, A., X-ray diffraction method for the quantative characterization of calcium phosphate coatings. *Characterization and Performance of Calcium Phosphate Coatings for Implants*, ASTM STP 1196, Emmanuel Horowitz and Jack E. Parr (Eds.), American Society for Testing and Materials, Philadelphia, 1993.
98. Osborn, F.J. & Newesely, H., The material science of calcium phosphate ceramic, *Biomaterials*, 1, 108-111, 1980.
99. Hench, L.L., Splinter, R.J., Allen, W.C., Greenlee, T.K., Bonding mechanisms at the interface of ceramic prosthetic materials. *J. Biomed. Mater. Res.* 2, 117-141 (1971).
100. Heughebaert, M., LeGeros, R.Z., Gineste, M., Physico-chemical characterization of deposits associated with HA-ceramics implanted in non-osseous sites, *J. Biomed. Mat. Res.*, 22, 257-268, 1988.
101. Doyle, C., Bioactive Composites in Orthopedics, In: Yamamuro T, Hench L, Wilson-Hench J (Eds.) *Handbook of Bioactive Ceramics*, Vol. II, CRC Press, Florida, 195-207, 1990.
102. LeGeros, R.Z., Penugonda, B., Potential use of calcium phosphate as fillers in composite restorative biomaterials. *Proc. Second World Congress on Biomaterials*, Washington DC., 1984.
103. Daculsi, G., LeGeros, R.Z., Mitre, D., Crystal dissolution of biological and ceramic apatites. *Calcif Tiss Int*, 45, 95-105, 1989.
104. Daculsi, G., LeGeros, R.Z., LeGeros, J.P., Mitre, D., Lattice defects in calcium phosphate ceramics. High resolution TEM ultrastructural study. *J. Appl. Biomat.* 2, 147-152, 1991.

CALCIUM PHOSPHATE APATITES IN NATURE

Deane K. Smith
Department of Geosciences and Materials Research Laboratory
The Pennsylvania State University
University Park, PA 16802

ABSTRACT

Apatite in the natural world comprises a major group of minerals which occurs in all geological environments. All the minerals of the group are hexagonal or monoclinic and based on a crystal structure which is hexagonal, a = 9.368Å, c = 6.844Å. Crystal chemical substitutions lead to a large variety of species in the group. Six species of calcium phosphate apatites are recognized.

Apatites occur in all geological environments usually as accessory minerals (<5%), but concentrations sufficient for economic interest other than gemstones are formed as sedimentary rocks and rarely as igneous segregations. Phosphate-rich deposits are exploited primarily for fertilizer. Museum quality specimens of fluorapatite are primarily from pegmatites, but unusually large crystals are found in skarn.

The closest apatite to bone apatite, carbonate- hydroxylapatite, is formed in very restricted environments usually by replacement of pre-existing organic matter or in guano deposits.

INTRODUCTION

Examining natural occurrences of minerals often suggests conditions which may be employed for their synthesis under laboratory conditions. This situation is certainly true for the apatite group minerals. Likewise, laboratory experimentation on mineral synthesis often improves our understanding of the natural environment.

Calcium phosphate apatites occur in all the principal rock-forming environments in the Earth's crust. Fluorapatite is found in igneous rocks from granite to peridotite, in the pegmatites and hydrothermal mineral deposits and in many sedimentary rocks both as primary particles and as a secondary phase forming the cement. Carbonate apatites are formed in sedimentary rocks primarily as a cementitious phase. Chlorapatite has the most restricted environment, being limited to gabbros and some pegmatites. Natural chemical substitutions in the calcium phosphate apatites are many. Some of these substitutions may be important in the formation of the specific apatite phase.

Apatite was first named as a mineral by Werner in 1786.[1] The name was derived from απαταειν, the Greek word to deceive, because it had been confused with several other minerals of similar appearance including: beryl, amethyst, olivine and fluorite. It had been suspected earlier by some workers to be a

0-8493-4750-5/94/$0.00 + $.50

distinct species, but its many color and habit variations limited its distinction from similar appearing minerals. Chemical analysis in 1788 by Proust and by Klaprota established apatite as a calcium phosphate and confirmed its similarity to calcined bone although the role of the OH, F and Cl was not recognized at this time.

An excellent review of apatites in nature, both geological and biological, has been prepared by McConnell.[2] Mineralogical information may be found in Ford;[3] Palache et al.,[4] and Deer et al.,[5] Fleischer and Mandarino,[6] and McClune.[7] Discussions of the crystal chemistry of the apatite group are found in McClelland[8] and Brown and Chow.[9] The extent of the literature on the apatite group is beyond the scope of this presentation, and no attempt will be made to cover it all.

Examples of apatites in several environments will be examined to indicate the conditions of formation. The modern nomenclature for the apatite group accepted by the International Mineralogical Association will also be reviewed.

CRYSTALLOGRAPHY AND CRYSTAL CHEMISTRY

The best characterized mineral in the apatite group is fluorapatite whose structure was first solved by Naray-Szabo[10] and Mehmel.[11] It forms spectacular crystals at several localities, and good samples are easy to acquire. The crystallographic parameters for this mineral are given in Table 1. Fluorapatite is hexagonal with the highest symmetry found among the apatite minerals. The crystal structure of fluorapatite is shown in Figure 1. The structure classifies as insular tetrahedral with two different cation sites and a unique anion site that forms a column along the c-axis. It is the behavior of the anion site with the substitution of Cl and OH for F which leads to atomic displacements that lower the crystal symmetry. Chlorine usually shifts off the mirror plane to lower the symmetry to $P6_3$ because it is larger than the F ion it replaces.

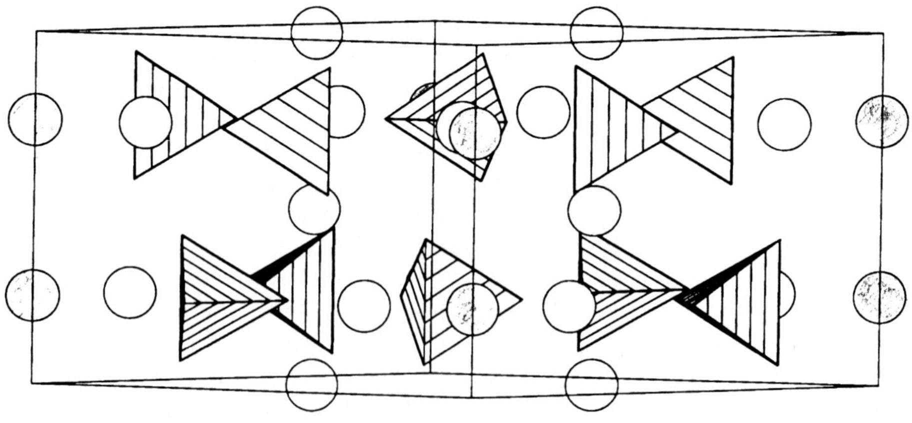

Figure 1. The crystal structure of fluorapatite. The fluorine atoms are shaded. The c-axis is vertical.

Table 1. Crystallographic Parameters for Fluorapatite.

Composition:	$Ca_5(PO_4)_3F$
Crystal System:	Hexagonal 6/m
Space Group:	$P6_3/m$
Cell Parameters:	a = 9.3684A, c = 6.8841A
Z and Density:	Z = 2, ρ = 3.20gm/cm^3
Optics: ε = 1.628, ω = 1.633, sign = (-)	

Swanson et al.;[12] Palache et al.;[4] McClune.[7]

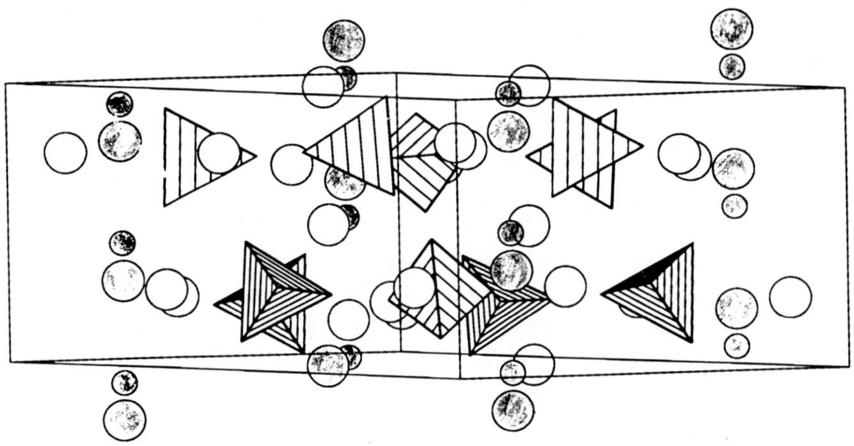

Figure 2. The crystal structure of hydroxylapatite. The OH ion is shown as the shaded pair of spheres with the H smaller. The c-axis is vertical.

The OH ion also is displaced off the mirror plane because of the electrostatic field of the H+ proton in the O^{2-} charge cloud. A combination of displacement and reversal of the $(OH)^-$ orientation causes most hydroxylapatites to be monoclinic $P2_1/m$. The structure of hydroxylapatite is shown in Figure 2. The main difference between the structures of fluorapatite and hydroxylapatite is the F^-, $(OH)^-$ substitution illustrated by the shaded circles.

The apatite minerals are all based on the fluorapatite structure which gives the structural formula

$$X_3Y_2(TO_4)Z$$

where:
X and Y are large sites with 7 and 9 coordination respectively,
T is a 4-coordinated tetrahedral site, and
Z is an anion site in a channel defined by the X sites where its coordination is 3 X cations.

Because of the accommodating nature of these structural sites, extensive ionic substitutions are allowed which lead to the wide variety of minerals which compose the apatite group in nature and to the many additional compounds which can be synthesized in the laboratory. The important substitutions in nature are given in Table 2.

Table 2. Crystal Chemical Substitutions in Natural Apatites.

X, Y = Ca, Sr, Ba, Re, Pb, U, Mn and rarely Na, K, Y, and Cu
T = P, As, V, Si, S, and C (as CO_3)
Z = F, Cl, OH, and O

Although the X and Y sites are of similar size, when there is more than one element occupying these sites, the larger ion tends to the larger Y site as long as it is divalent. Monovalent and trivalent ions tend to occupy the X site because the Z site as well as the T site can be involved in charge compensating substitutions.

It is the relative ease of ionic substitution which leads to the many species and varieties of the apatite group minerals. Many divalent cations with ionic radii in the range 1.0 to 1.6A can substitute in the X and Y sites. The trivalent lanthanides and quadrivalent actinides also commonly occur in these sites. The substitutions on the T and Z sites are more interesting to the bone and teeth scientists. The T site can be replaced by any element which forms a small tetrahedral oxyanion. The most common such ions in nature are AsO_4, VO_4, SO_4, and SiO_4. The most interesting substitution is CO_3 which is a planar, triangular oxyanion. It has been proposed by Borneman-Starinkevich and Belov[13] that CO_3 replaces PO_4 one-for-one with the triangular group positioning itself statistically in place of one face of the tetrahedron. The remaining O is replaced by either F^- or $(OH)^-$ to complete the spatial filling and to retain charge balance. This hypothesis has not been totally proven, but there are strong indications that at least some of the replacement is accomplished in this manner.

Substitutions on the Z site play a very important role in the crystallography of the specific species. The Z site lies in the channel formed by the X sites. In fluorapatite, the F is just the right size to fit between three X atoms, and it lies on the (001) mirror planes to yield the space group $P6_3/m$. When Cl substitutes for the F, the Cl is too large to fit on the mirror plane, so it is displaced along the c-axis and the space group becomes $P6_3$. (OH) substitution is even more complex. The (OH) ion is not spherically symmetric because of the H proton imbedded in the charge cloud of the O. The H causes a displacement of the O off the mirror plane, the H-O orientation tends to align in a given channel, but adjacent channels may have different displacements and orientations. The result is that well-crystallized hydroxylapatites usually are monoclinic with space group $P2_1/m$ or $P2_1$.

NOMENCLATURE OF THE APATITE GROUP

The nomenclature of the apatite minerals is very confusing because many of the names were initially applied to ill-defined varieties which did not deserve species status. Table 3a lists the calcium phosphate species which are currently recognized by the International Mineralogical Association, IMA, Commission on New Minerals and Mineral Names, CNMMN (Fleischer and Mandarino[6]). Table 3b lists the other apatite minerals that are recognized. The term "apatite" is now reserved as the group name, and should not be used to indicate any specific mineral.

There are many historical names that still appear in the literature, both old and new, which are no longer accepted by the IMA/CNMMN. Many of these names are listed in Table 4 along with their modern equivalent. The role of the IMA/CNMMN is to promote consistent usage of a reasonably logical set of species names especially for the mineralogical community and hopefully for any one else using mineral names. Recent years have seen many new restrictions on what defines a species with a concomitant simplification of the related nomenclature. For example, in a solid- solution series, only two unique mineral names are used for the end-member compositions with less than 10% substitution of the other ion. Between 10% and 50% substitution, the end-member name is used along with an adjectival modifier indicating the substitution. This rule has resulted in many old, well-established names being dropped from modern usage. A specific example is the feldspar plagioclase series where albite and anorthite are the end members; oligoclase and andesine are replaced by calcian albite, and labradorite and bytownite by sodian anorthite.

The IMA nomenclature is very specific with respect to the calcium phosphate apatites. The names have been simplified using the chemical characteristics of the principal substitutions that define the five (six?) recognized species. Chlorapatite, fluorapatite, and hydroxylapatite do not present much of a problem, as the names have been used for some time. They are often abbreviated Cl-AP, FAP and HAP, respectively. The IMA recommends that the commonly used "francolite" and "dahllite" be dropped and replaced by "carbonate-fluorapatite" and "carbonate-hydroxylapatite" respectively. There is considerable doubt concerning the existence of "oxyapatite" (voelckerite), but the name has been retained until the true situation is resolved. Although the recommendations may upset some old-timers in apatite research, the new nomenclature certainly assists new readers to keep the specific species intended straight in spite of the longer names. They are usually abbreviated CFAP, CHAP, and OAP, respectively. The world community, both mineralogists and non- mineralogists, should adopt these recommendations.

"Hydroxylapatite" is a different problem. It is not a question of species designation, but rather one of proper spelling. A survey of the literature shows that the non-mineralogists tend to use "hydroxyapatite" rather than "hydroxylapatite" in spite of the fact that it is the (OH)-, hydroxyl, ion that substitutes in this species. All researchers should adopt the IMA spelling to be consistent. The IMA does represent the international community when it comes to proper use of mineral nomenclature, and their decisions are not made without considerable debate among the members of the CNMMN.

Throughout the rest of this paper, the abbreviations will be used where appropriate. The term "apatite" will be used to indicate the series of mineral species or where the specific species has not been identified.

Table 3. Accepted Apatite Group Minerals (IMA/CNMMN).

A. Ca-Phosphate Apatites

Carbonate-fluorapatite	$Ca_5(PO_4,CO_3F)_3F$	CFAP
Carbonate-hydroxylapatite	$Ca_5(PO_4,CO_3OH)_3OH$	CHAP
Chlorapatite	$Ca_5(PO_4)_3Cl$	Cl-AP
Fluorapatite	$Ca_5(PO_4)_3F$	FAP
Hydroxylapatite (not hydroxyapatite)	$Ca_5(PO_4)_3OH$	HAP
Questionable		
Oxyapatite	$Ca_{10}(PO_4)_6O$	OAP

B. Non-Ca-phosphate apatites

Alsforsite	$Ba_5(PO_4)_3Cl$
Belovite	$(Sr,Ce..)5(PO_4)_3OH$
Britholite-Ce	$(Ce,Ca..)_5(PO4)3(OH,F)$
Britholite-Y = Abukumalite	$(Y,Ca..)_5(PO_4)_3(OH,F)$
Caracolite	$Na_3Pb_2(SO_4)_3Cl$
Cesanite	$Na_3Ca_2(SO_4)_3OH$
Chlorellestadite	$Ca_5[SiO_4,PO_4,SO_4]_3(Cl,F)$
Clinomimetite	$Pb_5(AsO_4)_3Cl$
Fermorite	$(Ca,Sr)_5[AsO_4,PO_4]OH$
Finnemanite	$Pb_5(AsO_4)_3Cl$
Fluorellestadite	$Ca_5[SiO_4,PO_4,SO_4]_3(F,OH,Cl)$
Hedyphane	$Pb_3Ca_2(AsO_4)Cl$
Hydroxylellestadite	$Ca_5[SiO_4,PO_4,SO_4]_3(OH,F,Cl)$
Johnbaumite	$Ca_5(AsO_4)OH$
Mimetite	$Pb5(AsO_4)_3Cl$
Morelandite	$(Ba,Ca,Pb)_5[AsO_4,PO_4]_3Cl$
Pyromorphite	$Pb_5(PO_4)_3Cl$
Strontium-apatite	$Sr_5(PO_4)_3(OH,F)$
Svabaite	$Ca_5(AsO_4)F$
Turneaurite	$Ca_5[AsO_4,PO_4]_3Cl$
Vanadinite	$Pb_5(VO_4)Cl$

Table 4. Archaic Apatite Mineral Names.

Not recognized by IMA/CNMMN	
Apatite	= now a group name
Dahllite	= carbonate-hydroxylapatite
Francolite	= carbonate-fluorapatite
Staffelite	= carbonate-fluorapatite
Voelckerite	= oxyapatite
Kurskite	= carbonate-fluorapatite
Quercyite	= carbonate-hydroxylapatite
Wilkeite	= sicicatian strontian apatite
Manganapatite	= manganoan fluorapatite
Moraxite	= greenish-blue from Norway
Lasurapatite	= blue (with lapis) from Siberia
Asparagus-stone	= yellow-green from Spain
Naurite	= colloidal from Nauru Is., Pacific
Eupychroite	= fibrous carbonate-fluorapatite
Podolite	= carbonate-fluorapatite
Dehrnite	= sodian hydroxylapatite
Lewistonite	= potassian hydroxylapatite
Saamite	= strontian apatite
Varietal name	
Collophane	= massive cryptocrystalline apatite

GEOCHEMISTRY OF PHOSPHORUS IN THE EARTH

Phosphorus is the eleventh most abundant element in the Earth's crust,[14] usually considered to compose 0.10 weight percent. The apatite minerals are the most abundant phosphorus-containing minerals and form the tenth most abundant mineral group in the Earth's crust. Thus, it should not be surprising that the apatite minerals are commonly encountered in all geological environments. FAP is a common accessory mineral (<5%) in all types of igneous rocks from granites to ultra basics. It is especially common in pegmatites where it may form large crystals (>10cm.) crystals. In fact the largest fluorapatite crystal ever recorded is 2.13 m. long by 1.22 m. in diameter weighing 6458 kg. from the Aetna pegmatite mine, Quebec, Canada, as cited in Rickwood.[15] In high-temperature hydrothermal ore deposits, FAP, HAP, and Cl-AP may occur as gangue along with metallic sulfides and oxides. FAP is a minor accessory mineral in most metamorphic rocks, but in skarn (metasomatic contact metamorphic deposits), FAP is associated with calcite and Ca-silicates. FAP occurs in massive deposits associated with magnetite which were formerly considered skarn but are now known to be an igneous segregation. FAP and Cl-AP are also found in car bonatites. In sedimentary rocks, carbonate apatites are associated with marine shales, limestones and chert (opal). Some lime stones may contain considerable P, and rocks with apatite concentrations over 50% are termed "phosphorites."

Geological processes at the surface of the Earth move vast amounts of phosphorus around from the land to the rivers and oceans. In ocean waters, the phosphorus content is highly variable depending on the temperature and acidity of the water, but the average value is usually quoted as 70ppb.[16] Average river water contains about 20ppb which increases significantly in estuaries to 20-120ppb. Animals with chitinous skeletons account for much of the phosphorus in the organic component of the Earth. The residence time of phosphorus at the surface of the ocean is short, 2 to 6 years; but at depth, the residence time is long, $\approx 10^6$ years. Although the river water concentration is low, the rivers still supply 1.7×10^{12} g/year to the oceans. In addition to the rivers, the atmosphere carries phosphorus and supplies 1.4×10^{12} g/year of which more than 10% is soluble and is deposited in solution rather as particulate matter. The details of the phosphorus cycle are still not well understood.

OCCURRENCES OF APATITE MINERALS

It is not the purpose of this paper to review all the occurrences of apatite minerals in nature because that would be too massive an undertaking. What will be presented will be short discussions of the manner in which the apatite forms in each major geologic environment along with a few examples.

IGNEOUS ROCKS

Igneous rocks are formed by the solidification of silicate melts from high temperatures. Because the crystallization follows the liquidus-solidus phase relations, minerals in low abundance normally will be the last to crystallize, but diorite and granodiorite melts may have enough P present for the FAP phase field to intersect the liquidus and allow early FAP to form. An example of euhedral early crystallized apatite is shown in Figure 3. Late-crystallizing phases should form in the interstices between the early-crystallizing phases which will result in the crystals being anhedral (without crystal facets). Some alkali- rich igneous rock may form an immiscible phosphate-rich liquid phase which leads to large late-stage segregations of FAP some of which are associated with magnetite.

Where the P content is very low, the P may remain in the fluid phase, and the apatite will then form at the time that the rock re-reacts with this fluid. This reaction is termed pneumatolitic, and the crystals that form will be small, are often euhedral (with crystal facets), and may be included inside pre-existing mineral grains. This situation is often encountered in granites and other related siliceous igneous rocks. An example is illustrated in Figure 4. Concentrations of the apatite minerals in igneous rocks is rarely sufficient to yield a source for mining the deposit for the phosphorus content. An exception is the Khibiny deposits of Russia which are magmatic segregations where the presence of significant P in the melt lowers the melting temperatures to below 800°C and allows a late stage melt phase to concentrate FAP along with magnetite.

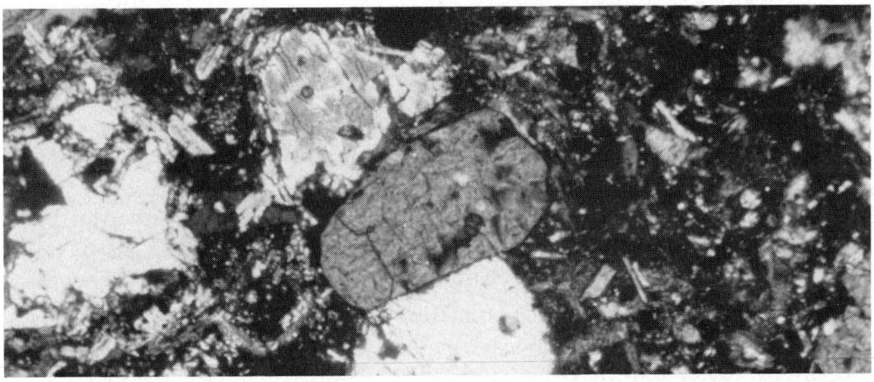

Figure 3. Apatite phenocrysts in an augite biotite phonolite from Crazy Mountains, Montana. The apatite is the euhedral crystal in the center of the field. It represents primary crystallization.

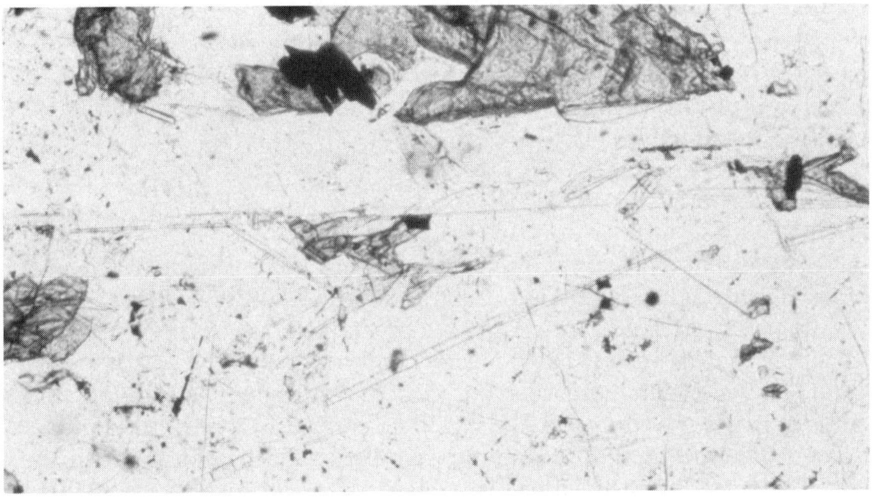

Figure 4. Thin needles of apatite in an olivine dolerite from Sonora, Mexico. These crystals represent late-stage reaction and crystallization.

Carbonatites are an unusual rock type, which often have significant concentrations of apatite. They are also classified as igneous. These rocks may represent carbonate-rich melts that have segregated in the crust or mantle, and they usually have rare-earths, niobium, tantalum and other rare elements in the associated minerals. The apatite which occurs with this rock is FAP rather than CFAP because the CO_3 will not substitute in the fluorapatite structure at the high temperatures of formation.

PEGMATITES

Pegmatites are rocks which form from the late-stage fluids that separate from the igneous or metamorphic source and become injected into fracture systems in the cooler surrounding rocks. In the pegmatitic stage, there are two liquids: a silica-rich melt and a water-rich fluid. The water-rich fluid significantly lowers the viscosity of the mixture, and the melt-fluid complex can move quickly into the fractures. Because the fractures are of relatively small dimensions, the pegmatite will cool rapidly and crystallize, but because the viscosity is relatively low, ionic migration is rapid and crystals can grow to very large dimensions.

Apatites that form in pegmatites can develop very large crystals. The concentration of the P as well as F and OH is much higher than in the source rocks because of the earlier crystallization of non P-containing minerals. FAP and hydroxylian FAP are common in this environment, and Cl-AP will form if Cl is available. Because of the higher elemental concentrations, the apatite phase will form in the middle of the crystallization sequence. Sometimes it forms euhedral crystals, and sometimes it forms anhedral crystals depending on the abundance and proximity of adjacent mineral grains in the pegmatite.

Because of the high concentration of water in these late stage rocks, all the silicate-rich liquid may solidify before the water-rich fluid is incorporated into crystallizing minerals. Large pockets will form into which unusually well-developed crystals may grow undisturbed by surrounding crystals. It is in these pockets that some of the spectacular museum-quality crystals are found. The apatite in these rocks is usually associated with many silicate minerals. Pegmatites rarely have enough apatite to allow mining unless they contain significant quantities of substituted lanthanide or actinide elements. Some specimens are used for gem purposes.

HYDROTHERMAL ORE DEPOSITS

Hydrothermal deposits are those rocks that have formed from water-rich fluids moving through pre-existing rocks and open fracture systems. These fluids could be the residual fluids from igneous crystallization, or they could be other ground water that is heated by some thermal source in the Earth's crust. This hot water may contain considerable concentrations of dissolved elements. Quantities of P along with F and OH could be carried in these fluids into a cooler environment where the apatite minerals would crystallize along with the other minerals that form. Usually, there is a high metal content to these fluids, and the associated minerals are metal sulfides, oxides, fluorides and some silicates. The apatite is not of economic interest in these deposits, unless it is of gem grade, and it is considered part of the gangue.

METAMORPHIC ROCKS

Metamorphic rocks are those rocks which have formed by altering a pre-existing rock through reactions induced by heat, pressure, and/or the introduction of new elements. The pre-existing rock will have to contain significant P for an apatite to form unless the P is added during the metamorphism. Some marine shales and limestones do contain abundant P, and apatite will develop or recrystallize from its original dispersed micro crystals into larger easily recognized grains. Many marbles have millimeter-sized apatite crystals along with graphite and phlogopite. An example is shown in Figure 5. Pelitic P-rich marine shales may metamorphose to schists with significant apatite as illustrated in Figure 6.

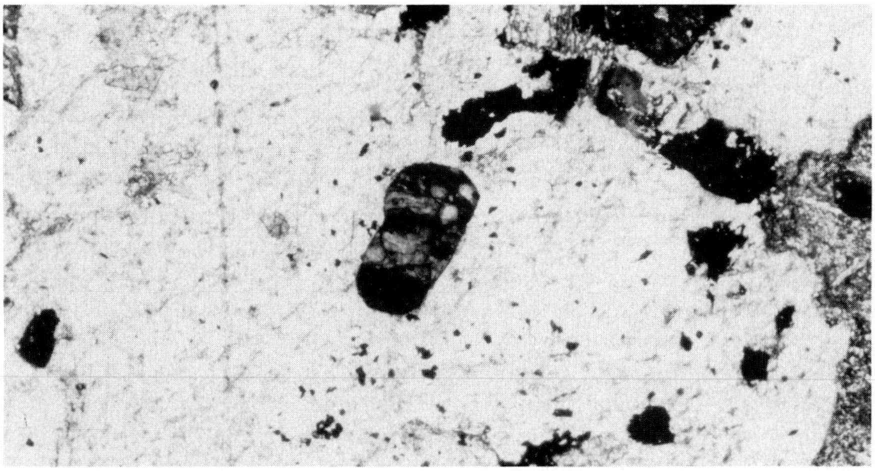

Figure 5. Apatite crystals in a calcitic marble associated with phlogopite and graphite from the Adirondack Mountains, New York.

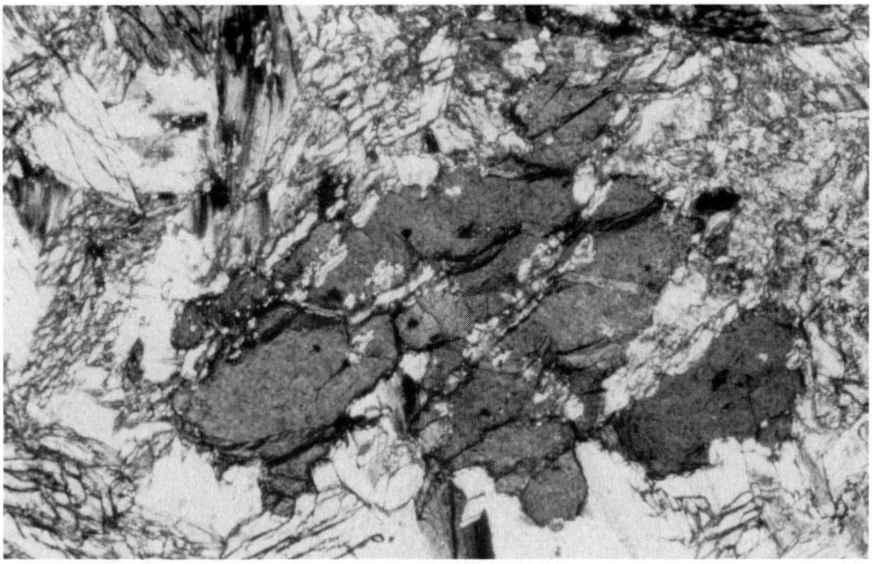

Figure 6. Cluster of apatite grains in a chlorite, glauconite schist from Healdsburg, California. The rock is a metamorphosed shale.

Metasomatic (elements added) metamorphism may develop unusual concentrations of apatite. Such deposits are termed skarn, and form when igneous melts are injected into cooler rocks and the melt has a high content of water and volatile elements. Where these fluids encounter limestones in particular, extensive reactions may occur, and the limestone is replaced by newly formed minerals. Apatite minerals will form in these rocks along with many unusual silicate minerals. CFAP and CHAP form in limestone skarn. Cl-AP is known in some Cl-rich rocks that also contain scapolite.

SEDIMENTARY ROCKS

Sedimentary rocks are those rocks which have formed at the surface of the Earth as a result of atmospheric effects and water. The highest concentrations of phosphorus are in the oceans or in guano accumulations from animals. Thus, other than fossilized guano, marine shales and carbonates are the rocks which contain the most P averaging 400 to 700 ppm, respectively. Phosphate-rich rocks may contain up to 37% P_2O_5 usually as CFAP or CHAP. Such rocks are termed "phosphorites," and they are widely distributed in the world. The most common form of apatite encountered in these deposits appears to be CFAP. The details of apatite formation in phosphorites is still in doubt, but it is recognized that there are both inorganic and organic processes that lead to the apatite.

Phosphorites are usually formed in shallow marine environments such as the Mediterranean Sea, but they commonly associate with deep-sea sediments like cherts and opal. The suggestion that is most accepted is that deep ocean water with higher concentrations of P rise into the shallow environments and deposition results. The evidence suggests that apatite does not precipitate directly from the sea water, but follows a complex path which may involve trace elements, organic intermediates, changes in Eh and pH, temperature and pressure. The complex nature of sea water has precluded experimentation and modeling to establish the important reactions which lead to apatite formation.

Some phosphorites are the result of replacement of carbonate shell or are the concentration of organic materials such as guano, bones, teeth and fish scales. These deposits are usually small but can be locally important economically. The most common mineral in these deposits seems to be CHAP. Another type of phosphorite is where fragments of phosphatic materials are concentrated as detrital particles along with limestone and silicates. An example is shown in Figure 7.

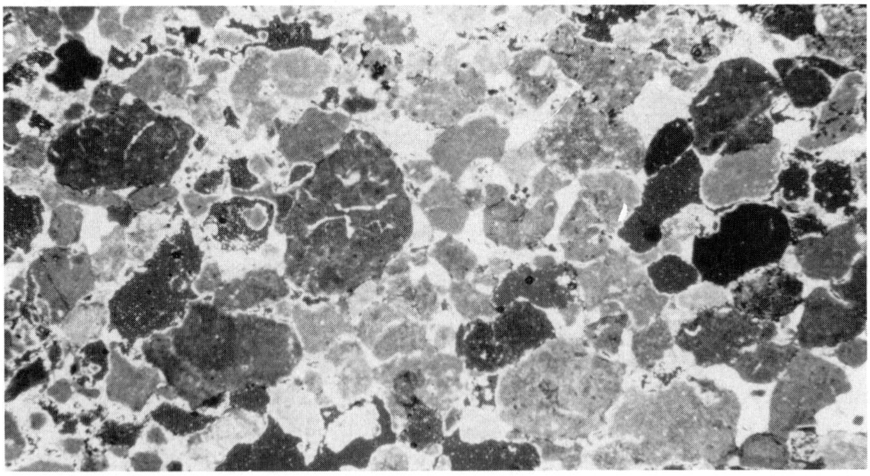

Figure 7. A pellet limestone with numerous phosphorite grains from Council Grove, Kansas. All the grains were derived from a pre-existing limestone and phosphorite.

Because the most closely related natural apatites to bone mineral are found in phosphorites, a few additional comments are valuable here. As indicated above, CHAP appears to be more common from deposits derived from organic phosphate sources, and CFAP appears to be more common in marine phosphorites. The reasons for this distribution are not clear. Bentor[17] has reviewed this phosphorite problem along with many others. Some of the points brought up by Bentor as "Unsolved Problems" include: 1. What is the true mineral in a phosphorite, and is it always the same? 2. What is the significance of the association of phosphorite with chert (opal) and organic matter? 3. How is the rate of deposition of apatite related to and controlled by Eh, pH and water depth? 4. What is the role of Mg and trace elements such as the rare-earths and uranium in the formation of apatite? 5. Where does the P actually originate? 6. What is the relation of the mixing of shallow and deep ocean water to deposition and to the distribution of phosphorite deposits around the world? Obviously, there is much work to be done yet to understand phosphorites in nature.

Terrestrial sediments may also have apatite either as single-crystal or phosphorite grains. One example is given in Figure 8. Most commonly the apatite acts as the cement in a clastic rock. The source of the apatite is unknown, but the P is at least partially mobilized from the associated rocks by the moving ground water in the pore spaces. Apatite crystals are also found in opal as radiating clusters suggesting that it formed while the opal was still in the gel state.

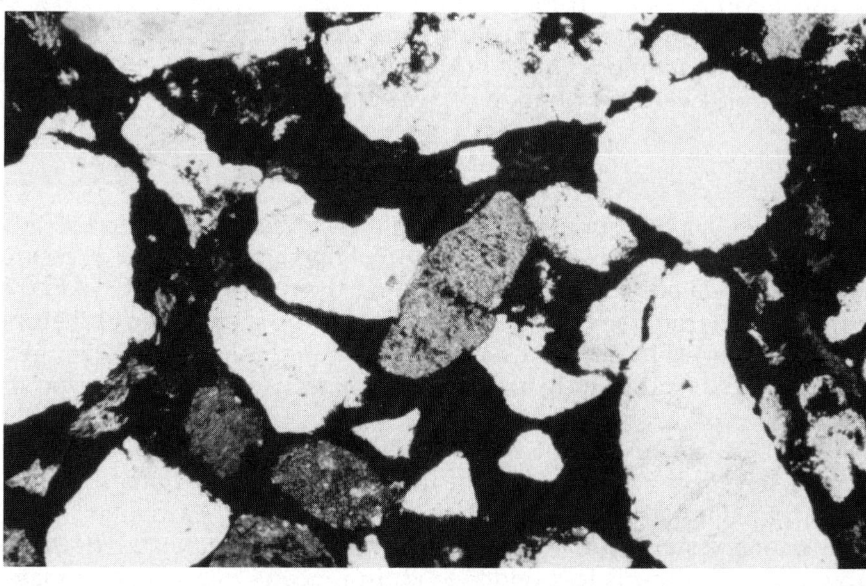

Figure 8. An apatite grain in a hematitic quartzite from Winfield, Pennsylvania. The apatite is a fragment from a pre-existing phosphorite which was deposited along with the other detritus.

Most of the commercial deposits of phosphate are from sedimentary deposits. Although the earliest work on phosphorites dates from 1847, it was around 1930 when extensive exploration for deposits began. Since then, considerable exploration and research on phosphorites has been done. Current important phosphorite localities are listed in Table 5, Notholt.[16]

Table 5. Important Localities for Economic Phosphate Deposits.

Locality	Type
United States	
Florida	Phosphorite
Tennessee	Phosphorite
Western states	Phosphorite
Russia	
Khibiny Tundra	Segregation
Kazahkstan	
Karatau	Phosphorite
Mediterranean	
Morocco	Phosphorite

NOTABLE OCCURRENCES

The most famous localities for apatite minerals are due to museum quality specimens that the localities have produced. Most of the well-developed crystals are FAP. FAP occurs in many colors because of the chemical substitutions. Manganese usually results in a blue color for FAP but may cause a yellow in Cl-AP. A violet color is also common, but the color is not stable suggesting that it is in part due to color centers. Other colors are caused by rare-earth elements and actinides. Some of the famous localities are listed in Table 6 showing the worldwide distribution of apatite.

SUMMARY

This paper has been prepared to bring this conference back to Earth where apatite was first prepared by Mother Nature. Although most of the research on apatite today is related to bone replication and the formation of CHAP, there is still much to learn from the occurrences in nature. The wide range of distribution of apatite occurrences in different rock types and in markedly different geologic environments needs more study to relate the occurrences and the specific species that form.

The general principles of the crystallography and crystal chemistry of the mineral species is well known, but there are still many details on the less-well crystallized apatites that need to be studied. In particular, the exact mechanism for the substitution of CO_3 for PO_4 needs more work. The chemistry of apatite crystallization is less understood. In igneous rocks, apatite may form as a primary crystallization product or as the result of late stage rock-fluid reactions. In sedimentary rocks, there is evidence that the apatite is not a direct precipitation product but the result of several intermediate steps.

The closest mineral matter to bone apatite is in the phosphorite deposits. Because of the economic value of phosphorus in modern agriculture, there is a renewed effort to study the formation and distribution of phosphorites. This effort coupled with the many studies on the synthesis of bone apatite should ultimately lead to new discoveries and a better understanding of the formation of CHAP.

Table 6. Famous Localities for Fluorapatite.

Locality	Occurrence
Russia	
Khibiny Tundra, Kola Peninsula	Segregation
Taka River, Ural Mountains	Metamorphic
Misak, Ilmen Mountains	Igneous
Czechoslovakia	
Pisek, Bohemia	Pegmatite
Schlaggenwald, Bohemia	Pegmatite
Germany	
Epprechstein, Waldstein, Bavaria	Pegmatite
Laacher See, Rhein	Igneous
Ehrenfriedersdorf, Saxony	Veins
Austria	
Knoppenwand, Salzburg	Veins
Zidertal, Tyrol	Veins
Italy	
Biella, Piedmont	Syenite
Elba	Pegmatite
Spain	
Jumilla, Murdia	Andesite
Caceres, Estremadura	Veins
Switzerland	
Gletsch	Igneous
St. Gotthard, Aar	Veins
France	
Villeder	Veins
England	
Cornwall	Veins
Wheal Franco, Tawstock, Devonshire	CHAP
Sweden	
Gellivara	Veins
Nordmark	Skarn
Mexico	
Durango	Skarn
United States	
Mt. Apatite, Auburn, Maine	Pegmatite
Adirondack Mountains, New York	Skarn
Franklin, New Jersey	Metamorphic
Magnet Cove, Arkansas	Skarn
Canada	
Ottawa Co., Quebec (>500 pound crystals)	Skarn
Lanark Co., Renfrew Co. Fronterac Co., Ont.	Pegmatite

ACKNOWLEDGEMENTS

The author would like the thank Paul Brown for the invitation to participate in this conference. Charles P. Thornton was considerable help in providing the thin sections for the photographs and in critically reading the manuscript.

REFERENCES

1. Werner, Gerhard's Grundr., 281, 1786.
2. McConnell, D., Apatite, Its Crystal Chemistry, Mineralogy, Utilization, and Geologic and Biologic Occurrences, Springer-Verlag, New York, pp. 111, 1973.
3. Ford, W. E., Dana's Textbook of Mineralogy, 4th. Ed., J. Wiley and Sons, 703-706, 1946.
4. Palache, C., Berman, H., and Frondel, C., Dana's System of Mineralogy, J. Wiley and Sons., 877-889, 1951.
5. Deer, W. A., Howie, R. A., and Zussmann, J., Rock-Forming Minerals, Volume Five: Non Silicates, Longmans, London, 323-338, 1962.
6. Fleischer, M. and Mandarino, J. A., Glossary of Mineral Species, The Mineralogical Record, 1991.
7. McClune, W. F. The Powder Diffraction File Sets 1 - 44, International Centre for Diffraction Data, Newtown Square, PA. 1994.
8. McClelland, G. H. and Lehr, J. R., Crystal Chemical Investigation of Natural Apatites, Amer. Mineral., 54, 1374-1391, 1969.
9. Brown, W. E. and Chow, L. C., Chemical Properties of Bone Mineral, in Annual Review of Materials Science, R. A. Huggins, Ed., Annual Reviews, Inc. Palo Alto, CA. 213-236, 1976.
10. Naray-Szabo, S., The Structure of Apatite, Zeit. Krist., 75, 387, 1930.
11. Mehmel, M., Uber die Struktur des Apatits, Zeit. Krist., 75, 323, 1930.
12. Swanson, H. E., Morris, M. C., Evans, E. H. and Ulmer, L., Standard X-ray Diffraction Powder Patterns, National Bureau of Standards Monograph 25 [3], 22-23, 1964.
13. Borneman-Atarinkevich, I. D. and Belov, N. V., Carbonate-apatites, Dokl. Akad. Nauk SSSR, 90, 89-92, 1953.
14. Mason, B., and Moore, C. B., Principles of Geochemistry, J. Wiley and Sons, 1982.
15. P. C. Rickwood, The Largest Crystals, *Am. Min.* 66:85-97 (1981).
16. Notholt, A. J. G., Phosphorite Resources in the Mediterranean (Tethyan) Phosphogenic Province: A Progress Report, Sci. Geol. Mem., 77, 9-21, 1985.
17. Bentor, Y. K., Phosphorite—The Unsolved Problems, in SEPM Special Publication No. 29, 3-18, 1980.

HYDROTHERMAL PROCESSING OF HYDROXYAPATITE: PAST, PRESENT, AND FUTURE

Masahiro Yoshimura and Hiroyuki Suda
Research Laboratory of Engineering Materials
Tokyo Institute of Technology
4259 Nagatsuta Midori-ku
Yokohama, 227 JAPAN

1. INTRODUCTION

Apatite is a common mineral in igneous, sedimentary and metamorphic rocks,[1] which has the general chemical formula of $A_{10}(BO_4)_6X_2$, where A is Ca, Sr, Ba, Pb, Cd, and many rare earth elements, BO_4 is PO_4^{3-}, VO_4^{3-}, SiO_4^{4-}, AsO_4^{3-}, CO_3^{2-}, X is OH^-, Cl^-, F^-, CO_3^{2-}. Water also has been reported to exist in the apatite structure in several forms.[2-4] The presence of the elemental phosphorus which is a major component of apatite was first detected in 17th century and the phosphorus in mineral pyromorphite (lead apatite) was discovered in 1779.[5,6] Since the first synthesis of apatite was done in the middle of the 19th century,[7] a large number of studies in the geochemical, crystallochemical, biological, and other fields have been conducted. Some physico-chemical properties of apatites determined by these studies are summarized in Table 1, with reference to books,[1,5,6,8] review articles,[2,9-11] and basic research papers.[12-18] Most of the geochemical and crystallochemical studies were performed using natural apatites, whereas biological or recent studies were mainly done using synthesized apatites. The generally used "gem-grade" natural apatite single crystal (Durango, Mexico) shown in Figure 1 has prismatic shape, greenish color, and is considered to be formed under a hydrothermal condition. Apatite is also well known as the main inorganic constituent of hard tissues of human and animals. Because it is recognized to be one of the best biocompatible materials, there have been many reports on the biological aspects (e.g. Refs. 19-21). Various preparation methods for HAp including the hydrothermal method have been used for such studies. The hydrothermal method has priority over the other methods in the synthesis of ideal ceramic powders, due to the effects of hydrothermal fluid on solid materials. In the present paper, hydrothermal processing, which has been recognized to be an excellent method for the preparation of ideal ceramic powders,[22,23] is described and its application to HAp is reviewed.

The processing of hydroxyapatite is reviewed from the perspective of past crystallochemical, geochemical and phase stability studies and ongoing investigations of the processing of ideal fine crystals for ceramics with tailored

0-8493-4750-5/94/$0.00+$.50

microstructures. Recent developments, such as the synthesis of hydroxyapatite whiskers, coatings, and solvothermal method, are also described.

Table 1. Physico-chemical properties of synthetic hydroxyapatite or natural fluorapatite.

Properties	Values	Comments	References
Theoretical Formula	$Ca_{10}(PO_4)_6(OH)_2$	composition varies with sample preparation	1, 5, 6, 8-11
Space Group	P6$_3$/m (hexagonal) P2$_1$/b (monoclinic)	mono. ↔ hexa. transition may occur at ca. 200°C	1, 8-11, 34-43
Lattice Parameters	a=9.41-9.44 Å c=6.84-6.94 Å	large discrepancies in L.P. of " Wet Chemically" HAp	1-4, 8-11, 18-20, 34-43
Theoretical Density	3.16 g/cm^3	varies with composition	1, 8-11
Moh's Hardness	3 (CO_3-Ap) 5 (HAp)	water &CO_3 in apatite lattice lower hardness	1, 8
Heat Capacity	184.07 cal/K·mol at 298.16K 180.16 cal/K·mol at 298.15K	"wet " HAp following calcined at 950 °C "wet" HAp following calcined at 1100°C	12 13
Thermal Expansion Coefficient	11-14 x 10^{-6} K^{-1}	"wet" HAp expands non-linearly	3, 4, 18
Melting Point	1614 °C	"synthetic" HAp, hot-stage microscope method	16
Surface Energy	S(001)=95±25MPa S(100)=480±30MPa	Natural FAp, slow cleavage method	14
Stiffness Coefficient at R.T. (Mbars)	C11=1.434, C33=1.805 C44=0.415, C12=0.445 C13=0.575, C66=0.495	Natural FAp, ultrasonic pulse superposition	15
Dielectric Constant	7.40-10.47	varies with composition	8
Refractive Indices	n_w=1.649-1.651, n_e=1.642-1.644	relationship between indices & composition is shown in ref.1	54
Optical Frequency	2.71 (//c) 2.69(⊥c)	varies with composition	1, 8

2. PREPARATION METHODS FOR HYDROXYAPATITE

The first synthesis of apatite was that of Daubrée in 1851[7] who obtained HAp by passing phosphorus trichloride vapor over red hot lime. Since then, a number of preparation of HAp have been reported, and the results prior to 1951 were reviewed by Jaffe.[24] Preparative methods for HAp are largely divided into three classes, Table 2. First is the conventional **solid state reaction method** at high temperature, the second is the **wet chemical method** at relatively low temperature, and the third ,which is a very important method today, is the **hydrothermal method** using high temperature-high pressure aqueous solutions.

The **solid state reaction method** has generally been used for the processing of ceramic powders and for studying phase stabilities. The powders prepared by this method, however, usually have irregular forms with a large grain size, and often exhibit heterogeneity in composition due to incomplete reaction resulting from small diffusion coefficients of ions within solids.

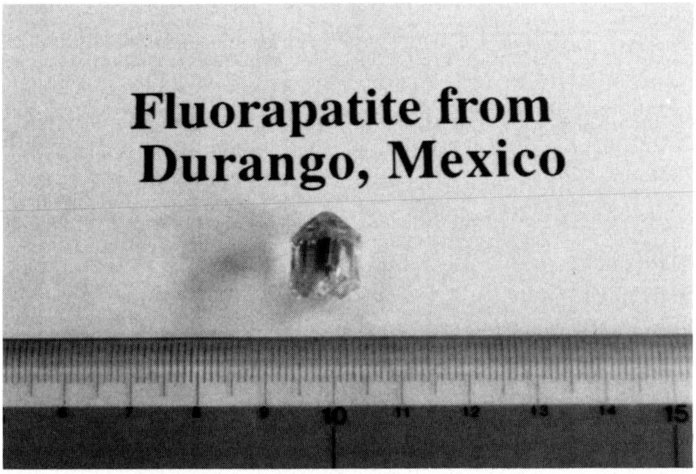

Figure 1. Photograph of natural fluorapatite single crystal mined at Durango, Mexico.

Since the **wet chemical method** is relatively easy to conduct, HAp has frequently been synthesized by this method. In particular, since reactions in any living thing occur in aqueous solutions at low temperatures, many experiments on the preparation of HAp by this method have been reported in order to investigate the formation mechanism of calcium phosphates *in vitro* and *in vivo*. The powders prepared by this method, however, seem not to be appropriate as the starting materials for ceramics, because they are usually poorly crystallized, inhomogeneous in composition and irregularly formed.

On the other hand, the **hydrothermal method** enables us to prepare well crystallized, compositionally homogeneous, uniform and easily sinterable powders due to the effects of the high temperature-high pressure aqueous solutions, which will be discussed in a later section in detail.

Other methods in order mainly to grow large single crystals have also been reported. The **gel growth method** was used for the growth of calcium phosphates.[25] The **melt growth method**[26] was used for the preparation of single crystals of apatite from a stoichiometric melt. Those crystals grown from the melt at high temperatures, however, are usually severely strained due to the large temperature gradients existed during growth. The **flux growth method**[27] is excellent from this point of view, since the fluxes, such as CaF_2, $CaCl_2$, and $Ca(OH)_2$ mixed with the starting apatite powders reduce the liquidus temperature far below needed for the melt growth method, resulting in the production of less strained apatite crystals. Similarly, hydrothermal growth also gives less strained crystals. The sol-gel method,[28] the polymerized method[29] have also been utilized for the processing of apatites.

Table 2. Preparation techniques for hydroxyapatite.

Techniques	Starting Materials	Synthetic Conditions	Comments	References
Solid State Reaction	$Ca_3(PO_4)_2$+ $CaCO_3$ $Ca_2P_2O_7$ + $CaCO_3$	900-1300°C, usually with water vapor flowing	Ca/P=1.67, large grain size, irregular forms, inhomogeneous	many works
Wet Chemical Method	$Ca(NO_3)_2$ + $(NH_4)_2HPO_4$ $Ca(OH)_2$ + H_3PO_4	R.T.- 100°C pH: 7-12	Ca/P < 1.67 fine irregular crystals with low crystallinity inhomogeneous	many works
Hydro-thermal Method	wet chemically prepared HAp, other calcium phosphates, seeding	100-200°C (1-2 MPa), 300-600°C (1-2 Kbar)	Ca/P=1.67 homogeneous, fine single crystals or large crystals	51-62, 67 81, 85-87
Gel Growth Method	Gel + Ca^{2+} + PO_4^{3-}	R.T. - 60 °C pH: 7-10	large Monetite, Brushite, OCP, but small HAp	25
Melt Growth Method	$Ca_3(PO_4)_2$ - CaF_2, $CaCl_2$	1650 °C	large crystals with lattice strain	26
Flux Growth Method	CaF_2, $CaCl_2$ as flux $Ca(OH)_2$ as flux	1325°C (FAp, ClAp) HAp	large crystals with little lattice strain	27 59

Sol-gel, alkoxide, and the other chemical methods have also been used. CVD, plasma spray method and the other (electro) chemical methods have been mainly used to form HAp layers on substrate.

3. HYDROTHERMAL PROCESSING

Reactions which occur under the conditions of high temperature-high pressure (>100°C, >1 atm) aqueous solutions in a closed system are generally called **hydrothermal reaction.** The use of hydrothermal methods for the crystal growth of quartz (SiO_2) began in 1905 by Spegia.[30] The earliest systematic hydrothermal research on phase equilibrium studies was that of Morey in 1913.[31] The first international symposium on hydrothermal reactions was held in 1982 at Tokyo Institute of Technology, where physicists, chemists, and mineralogists from all over the world discussed the subject.[32]

Aqueous solutions under hydrothermal conditions play an important roles in the occurrence and formation of many minerals in nature. Aqueous solutions and vapor are continuous under high temperature-high pressure conditions and are supercritical fluids above the critical point (T_c = 374.2°C, P_c = 22.1 MPa, and ρ_c = 0.32g/cm^3 for pure water, Fig. 2[33]). High temperature–high pressure solution, vapor and supercritical fluids might be called **hydrothermal fluids**. Actions of hydrothermal fluids on solids are categorized in the following four classes corresponding to the degree of interactions, that is, physical to chemical (Table 3 and Fig. 3).

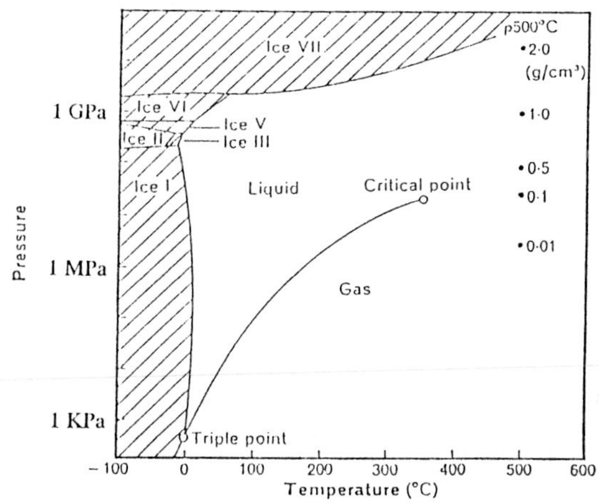

Figure 2. Pressure-temperature phase diagram for pure water. The density of water for several pressures at 500°C is shown, and the pressure is plotted on a logarithmic scale. The vapor pressure curve begins at the triple point and ends at the critical point (T_C=374.2°C, P_C=22.1 MPa, ρ_C=0.32g/cm^3).[33]

Table 3. Actions of hydrothermal fluid on solid materials.

Classification	Actions	Application
(*a*) ***Transfer Medium***	transfer of heat, pressure, and kinetic energy	erosion, machining abrasion, HIP, forming, etc.
(*b*) ***Adsorbent***	adsorbed, desorbed at the surface	surface diffusion, catalyst, dispersion, crystallization, sintering, ionic exchange, etc.
(*c*) ***Solvent***	dissolution and precipitation	synthesis, extraction, growth, modification, degradation, etching, corrosion, etc.
(*d*) ***Reactant***	formation of materials, quality changing	formation and decomposition of hydrates, hydroxides, and oxides, corrosion hydration of cements

(a) **Transfer medium.** The hydrothermal fluid physically transfers heat, pressure and mechanical energy to the solid material. This action can be applied to erosion, machining, abrasion from limited directions or to forming or HIPing when it is applied isostatically.

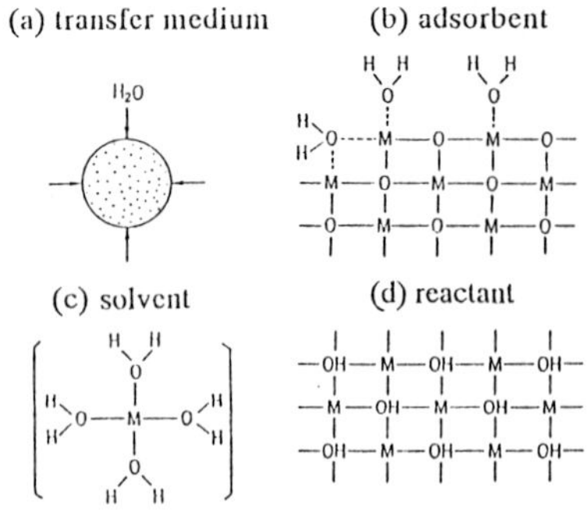

Figure 3. Schematic illustration of four actions of hydrothermal fluid on solid state materials: (a) transfer medium, (b) adsorbent, (c) solvent and (d) reactant.

(b) **Adsorbent**. The hydrothermal fluid or its one components is adsorbed and/or desorbed on the surfaces of solids. These processes accelerate surface diffusion and surface reaction, therefore they are important in catalysis, dispersion, crystallization, sintering, ion exchange, etc.

(c) **Solvent**. Hydrothermal fluid can dissolve one or more components of the solid materials to form molecular clusters, and/or ionic species including complexes, which can transport the components long distances. Dissolved components can be precipitated in the reverse reactions. Thus, the action promotes the rearrangement of ionic species through dissolution and precipitation. The solvent action of hydrothermal fluids can be applied in the synthesis, extraction, growth, modification, etching, and bring about degradation and corrosion of solid materials.

(d) **Reactant**. Hydrothermal fluids can react with solids to form other solid products such as hydrates, hydroxides, oxides, hydrides etc. This action is closely related to the hydration of cements, the synthesis of those materials, and to the corrosion of them.

Considering above four actions, we can conclude that the hydrothermal processing is an extension of solution processing to high-temperature and high-pressure. Thus, hydrothermal processing can be used in place of almost any solution processing technique. It should be noted that the hydrothermal processing involves (1) high energy, (2) accelerated processing, and (3) improved accessibility to equilibrium. Therefore it results in more highly crystallized products and in acceleration in corrosion and degradation.

These features facilitate the fabrication of fine crystals which are homogeneous in size, shape and composition. In particular, multi-component crystals are not always easy to fabricate by conventional solution methods, because the processes of solvent-removal or solvent-separation frequently causes inhomogeneities even if the starting solution is homogeneous. On the other hand, hydrothermal processing can produce homogeneous fine crystals. Therefore, we can conclude here that the hydrothermal processing is one of the most suitable processes to prepare fine powders with controlled size, shape, crystallinity and composition. The crystals formed typically have high densities with no porosity and are homogeneous in composition. This is important because most powders prepared from solutions are generally mixtures even though they are homogeneous. Furthermore, crystals with controlled shape and size are almost non-aggregated, because their surfaces have the lowest surface energies. These characteristics are very important for ceramic powders. They should be the ideal powders for ceramics made through sintering. The above mentioned advantages of the hydrothermal method of powder processing were compared by Dawson[22] as shown in Table 4. Thus the *hydrothermal synthesis allows superior compositional and morphological control, powder reactivity, and eliminates the calcination and milling steps.*

Table 4. Advanced oxide powder process comparison.[22]

	Conventional	Sol-gel	Coprecipitation	Hydrothermal
Cost	Low–moderate	High	Moderate	Moderate
State of development	Commercial	R&D	Commercial/ demonstration	Demonstration
Compositional control	Poor	Excellent	Good	Good–excellent
Morphology control	Poor	Moderate	Moderate	Good
Powder reactivity	Poor	Good	Good	Good
Purity (%)	<99.5	>99.9	>99.5	>99.5
Calcination step	Yes	Yes	Yes	No
Milling step	Yes	Yes	Yes	No

4. HYDROTHERMAL PROCESSING OF HYDROXYAPATITE

4.1 CRYSTALLOCHEMICAL, GEOCHEMICAL AND PHASE STABILITY RELATED STUDIES, BY THE USE OF NATURAL OR SYNTHETIC LARGE SINGLE CRYSTALS

Many researchers in the past mainly concerned with crystallochemical, geochemical and phase stability related aspects of apatite, by the use of natural or hydrothermally synthesized large single crystals.

The **crystal structure** of fluorapatite (FAp) was first determined by Náray-Szabo [34] and by Mehmel,[35] independently in 1930. Later, the structure was re-examined in detail by Hendricks et al.,[36] Beevers et al.,[37] Posner et al.,[38] Kay et al.,[39] Sudarsanan et al.,[40] Elliott et al.,[41] Hughes et al.,[42] and Sänger et al.[43] In most of those studies, natural apatite (mainly fluorapatite, mined at Durango, Mexico, as shown in Figure 1) were used. The general agreement on the crystallographic aspects is as follows:

1. apatite shows ionic bonding character, and it is made up by close packing of large oxygen ions, resulting in the hexagonal crystal system.[10]
2. the space group of fluorapatite (FAp) is $P6_3/m$.[34-39]
3. although the space group of hydroxyapatite (HAp) is believed to be $P6_3/m$, HAp prepared at high temperature is $P2_1/b$ (monoclinic) at room temperature,[41] nearly identical with chlorapatite (ClAp).
4. a phase transition in hydroxyapatite is suggested to occur at ca. 200°C, probably due to the order-disorder orientation of OH^- ions along c-axis.[17,41]

Just recently, it was concluded that $P6_3/m$ describes only a time/space average for HAp.[43]

The physico-chemical properties summarized in Table 1 have been reported using mostly natural apatite single crystals.[14,15] Crystallographic dependence of these properties can be determined only by the use of natural or synthesized large single crystals.

Natural apatites have also been used for the most **geochemical scientific research.** For example, the kinetics of oxygen and strontium diffusion in natural fluorapatite (Durango, Mexico) have been determined under hydrothermal conditions to study the potential application of those data to the determination of its thermal history.[44] Shemesh et al.[45] measured oxygen isotope ratios ($\sigma^{18}Op$) in natural francolite (F,CO_3-Ap) samples ranging in age from early Proterozoic to Recent in order to investigate the geochemical functions of oxygen and carbon on the formation of apatites.

The determined by the **phase diagram** is very important for the understanding of the reaction mechanism occurred in vivo at low temperatures and in magmas under high-temperature and high-pressure region. The phase equilibria in the system CaO-P_2O_5-H_2O have been extensively studied by solid state reactions method under atmospheric pressure of water vapor by van Wazer,[46] and in aqueous systems at lower temperature than 100℃ by Brown et al.[47] The latter studies related to the phase stability at low temperature aqueous solutions are of great importance because of their relevance to biological tissue growth process, however, it is a problem whether the true equilibrium is attained or not, particularly at low temperatures. The phase stability studies conducted up to several hundred degrees have the same problem. Therefore, it is necessary to accelerate the reaction under hydrothermal conditions. Skinner[48] and Feng et al. used the hydrothermal method for the study of phase diagram in the system CaO-P_2O_5-H_2O under 1700kPa (1.7 MPa) at 200℃ and under 2000 bars (200 MPa) over the range 300-600℃, respectively, mainly to accelerate reactions to achieve equilibrium (Fig. 4). These phase diagrams show that the region where only HAp forms becomes narrower with increasing temperature. Appearance of β-$Ca_2P_2O_7$ at 600℃ instead of $CaHPO_4$ at 200℃ is also shown. Young et al.[50] also used the hydrothermal method to promote the homogeneous distribution of ionic species in HAp powders prepared by solid state reaction.

There are a large number of papers[51-62] on the preparation of **large HAp single crystals** (Table 5). The attempt to grow HAp crystals made by Morey and Ingerson in 1937[51] may be the earliest work. Since then, many studies have been reported. Rathje[52] and Hayek et al.[53] obtained large HAp crystals in 1941 and 1955, respectively. In 1956, Perloff et al.[54] prepared well-crystallized HAp crystals with 0.3 mm in length by the hydrolysis of synthetic $CaHPO_4$ in a platinum-lined, Morey-Ingerson type hydrothermal bomb at 300℃, 1250 lb/in^2 (8.6 MPa) for 10 days. In 1966, Jullmann et al.[55] prepared HAp crystals 2.35 mm in length and 0.2 mm in diameter by crystallization of wet chemically prepared HAp at 500℃, 354 bars (35.4 MPa) for 10 days. Kirn et al.[56] briefly reviewed the efforts to grow large single crystals of HAp. In 1971, Roy[57] grew prismatic single crystals of HAp up to 4 mm length hydrothermally from melts in the system $3CaO{\cdot}P_2O_5$-$Ca(OH)_2$ and $3CaO{\cdot}P_2O_5$-$Ca(OH)_2$-H_2O. In 1973, Mengeot et al.[58] succeeded preparing HAp single crystals of up to 7x3x3 mm in size by controlling the temperature gradient. They stated for the first time that HAp exhibited **retrograde solubility** in hydrothermal fluids between 300℃ and 670℃ under pressures of 45000 to 60000 psi (310-414 MPa). After the appearance of this report, most of the researchers set nutrients at colder region (dissolution occurs) and HAp seed crystals at hotter region (crystallization occurs), respectively in order to grow larger HAp single crystals. In 1973, Eysel et al.[59]

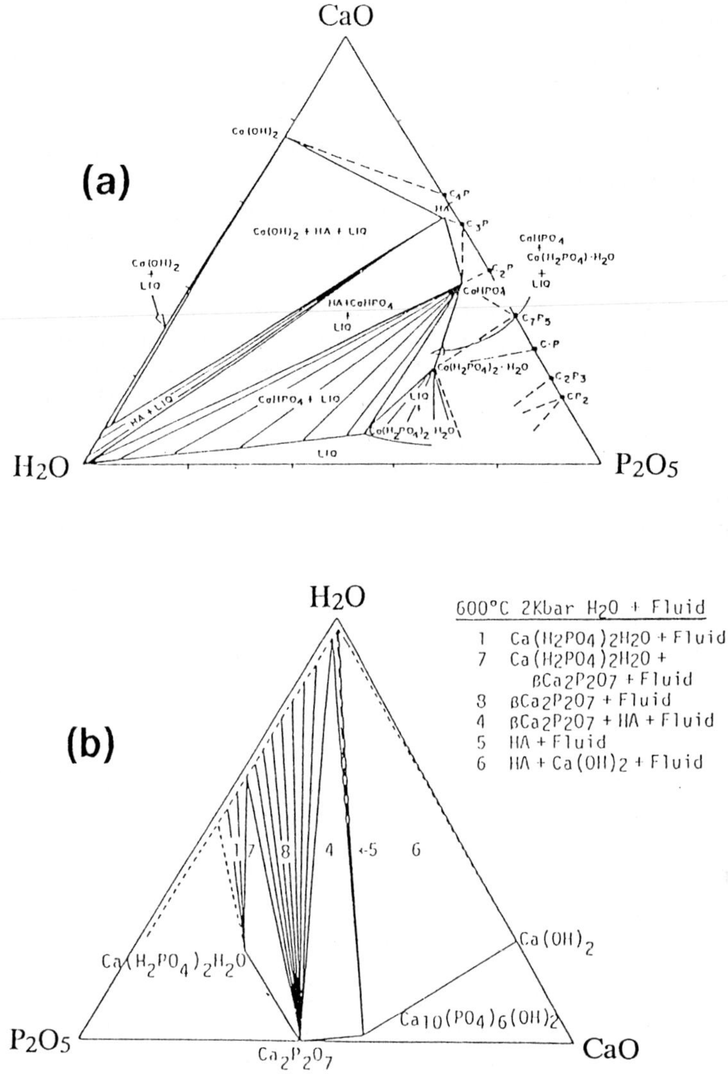

Figure 4. Phase diagram in CaO-P_2O_5-H_2O system under hydrothermal conditions of: (a) 200°C, 1.7 kPa,[49] and (b) 600°C, 2 kbar.[48]

grew large single crystals of HAp up to 8 x 0.5 mm by a hydrothermal method using $Ca(OH)_2$ as a flux and employing the oscillating temperature technique. In 1973, Aoki et al.[60] prepared crystals up to 0.1 mm in length by the hydrolysis of $CaHPO_4{\cdot}2H_2O$ under hydrothermal conditions, and found that HAp grew larger in weak acidic conditions. In 1979, Arends et al.[61] confirmed the **retrograde solubility** of HAp and prepared HAp single crystals up to 3.5 mm in length using procedure with three different stages: wet chemical preparation, a Soxhlet extraction at 100°C, then a hydrothermal recrystallization at 2 kbar (200 MPa) in the temperature range 430-500°C. They also found effects of CO_3^{2-} on the morphology of the crystals. Needle-like crystals were dominant if the carbonate content was higher than 0.1 %, whereas the equiaxial crystals in the case of below 0.1 % carbonate content. Hata et al.[62] synthesized Cd hydroxyapatite single crystals partly substituted with the first series transition elements for Cd ion to investigate the substitution effects on the crystal growth and the structural changes. Those crystals grow into hexagonal prisms or thin plates with the sizes up to 0.5 mm. They form a superstructure which belongs to $P6_3$ and have more distorted PO_4 tetrahedra than the structure of pure Cd hydroxyapatite. Although the experimental evidence for the **retrograde solubility** of HAp under hydrothermal conditions has been reported,[58,61] neither systematic experiment nor theoretical study have been conducted as far as we know. In this regard, Vereecke et al.[63] reported the calculation of the solubility diagrams and the effects of some parameters such as temperature (< 100℃), pH, partial CO_2 pressure and ionic strength. According to this report, the solubility of HAp becomes lowered with temperature, indicating the **retrograde solubility** of HAp below 100℃. Experimental or theoretical studies on the **retrograde solubility** under hydrothermal conditions are necessary, for the purposes of crystal growth and fundamental research.

Table 5. Hydrothermal synthesis of hydroxyapatite large single crystals.

Starting Materials	**Synthetic Conditions**	**Comments**	**References**
Morey et al. (ref.51, 1937) and Rathje (ref.52, 1941) may be the earliest workers.			
$CaHPO_4$	300°C, 1250 lb/in^2, for 10 days	0.3 mm in length	54
wet chemically prepared HAp	500°C, 354 bars, for 10 days	2.35 mm in length, 0.2mm in diameter	55
$CaHPO_4$	350°C, 100 MPa	2 mm	56
$Ca_3(PO_4)_2{\cdot}Ca(OH)_2$ or $Ca_3(PO_4)_2{\cdot}Ca(OH)_2$-$H_2O$ system	15000 psi, held at 850-900 °C, then cooled 20 °C/h. to ~750°C, quenched	4 mm in length	57
synthesized HAp as nutrient & HAp seed	300-670°C, 45000-60000 psi	7 x 7 x 3 mm, identify the retro grade solubility of HAp	58
$Ca_3(PO_4)_2{\cdot}Ca(OH)_2$-$CaCO_3$-$H_2O$ system, $Ca(OH)_2$ as flux	oscillating temperature technique, 750- 880 °C,14500-17500 psi	8 x 0.5 mm	59
$CaHPO_4 \cdot 2H_2O$	100-300 °C, 20hs.	0.1 mm	60
wet chemically, followed by Soxhlet extracted HAp	430-500°C, 2 kbar	3.5 mm, check the retrograde solubility of HAp	61

4.2 HAP FINE CRYSTALS AND THEIR APPLICATIONS TO CERAMICS WITH TAILORED MICROSTRUCTURES

Much effort has been devoted to improve the mechanical properties of hydroxyapatite ceramics as is shown in Table 6. Most of them were made from calcined powders previously precipitated by solution methods. In 1972, Aoki et al.[20,64] succeeded in the fabrication of hydroxyapatite ceramics by a hot-press technique. In 1976, Jarcho et al.[65] fabricated highly translucent HAp ceramics by calcining the filter cake-like HAp prepared by a solution method. The HAp ceramics had close to theoretical density and were free of fine pores and second phase, resulting in the high compressive and tensile strength. De With et al.[66] and many other researchers also obtained nearly fully dense HAp ceramics from commercial powders or wet chemically prepared HAp. Those calcined powders, however, were aggregated and had some heterogeneity in their compositions. Furthermore, those ceramics required firing temperatures of 1100°C to 1200°C in order to attain the theoretical density, resulting in the enlargement of grain size.

Table 6. Fabrication of HAp ceramics and composites.

Starting Materials	Properties of Products	References
In 1972, Aoki et al. [64] succeeded in sintering HAp by hot-press technique.		
filter cake-like precipitated HAp, calcined at 1100°C	translucent HAp, 99.6% R.D., good mechanical properties	65
hydrothermally prepared fine crystals, HIPed at 1000°C, 200MPa of Ar	translucent HAp 99.9% R.D., grain size: 0.6 μm E= 133 GPa	68
"**hydrothermal**" HAp & commercial HAp with different sizes HIPed at 1000°C, 200MPa of Ar	gradient ceramics with *dense / porous* layers	69
"**hydrothermal**" HAp homogeneously dispersed with ZrO_2, HIPed at 1050°C	fracture toughness: 2.5 times as high as that of pure HAp ceramics	70, 71
"**hydrothermal**" HAp homogeneously dispersed with Si_3N_4 whisker, HIPed at 1000°C	fracture toughness: 3 times as high as that of pure HAp ceramics	72
dense HAp ceramics by **hydrothermal hot pressing** at 300°C, followed by calcination at 1050°C	relative density of 95 %, grain size : 0.5 μm	73
dense non-stoichiometric HAp (Ca/P=1.55) by **hydrothermal hot pressing** at 350°C, 50MPa	relative density of 80 %, decomposition of HAp into TCP does not occur	74
transparent dense HAp ceramics (Ca/P:1.55-1.67) by HIP at 100°-800°C, 320-850MPa	lowest temperature of densification (at 600 MPa) : 300°C (Ca/P=1.55), 400°C (1.60), 800°C (1.67)	75
"**hydrothermal** " HAp homogeneously dispersed with *SiC platelet*,	HAp dispersed with SiC platelet, hardness: 1.3 times higher	76
TZP-dispersed HAp composite through filter-cake forming, and HIPed at 800-1150°C, 100MPa, 2h	strength and toughness: 20% and 100% higher than that of "pure" HAp ceramics	77

As pointed out in the former section, well crystallized HAp crystals which need no calcination process can be obtained by the use of **hydrothermal technique**. In 1988, Ioku et al.[67] successfully synthesized such HAp crystals under relatively mild hydrothermal conditions at 200°C under 2 MPa, which was sufficient for complete crystallization of HAp but not for the further crystal growth. The apparatus used and the resulting powders are shown in Figures 5 and 6, respectively. Well crystallized HAp fine crystals as indicated by x-ray diffraction patterns (Fig. 7) are uniform, non-aggregated, and have the size of 25 x 25 x 90 nm. A Williamson-Hall plot (Fig. 8) for as-received commercial HAp powder and hydrothermally treated HAp crystals indicates that the former has the lattice strain and/or compositional fluctuation, while the latter does not. Furthermore, hydrothermally prepared HAp does not contain any other crystalline/amorphous phases than HAp, whereas wet chemically prepared HAp would have such phases revealed by the exothermic peak at ca. 300°C on the DTA curve,[67] which may indicate the crystallization of amorphous phase. HAp prepared wet chemically at low temperatures would be under unstable state, because "...materials formed at temperatures so low that atom and ion mobility within the precipitated solid would be too low for the minimum free-energy configuration to be reached" as stated by Holcomb et al.[3] On the other hand, the re-arrangement of ionic constituents into a stable state with minimum free-energy is promoted under hydrothermal conditions. This is one of the attractive features of the hydrothermal processing mentioned in the former section.

Since the HAp fine crystals prepared hydrothermally are homogeneous in composition and have high crystallinities, desired sizes with narrow size distribution, desired shape and good sinterability, they are the optimum HAp

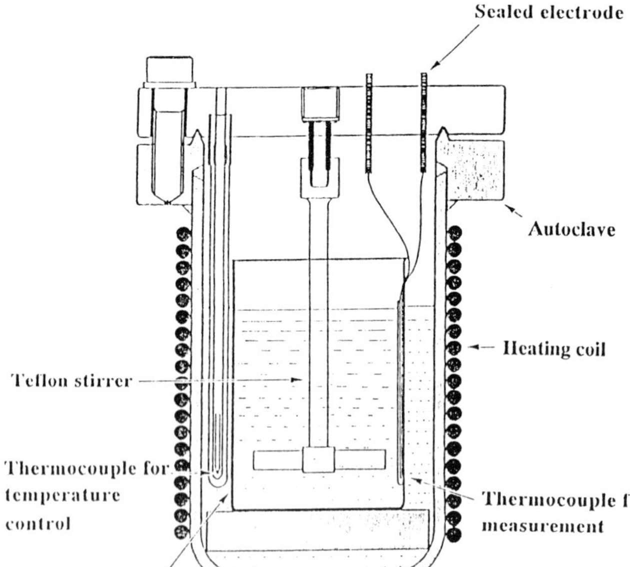

Figure 5. Schematic illustration of reaction apparatus used for the synthesis of hydroxyapatite fine crystals.[67]

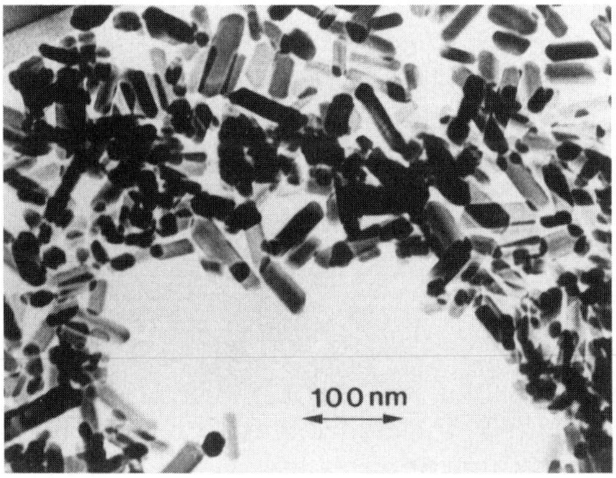

Figure 6. TEM photograph of the hydroxyapatite fine crystals synthesized hydrothermally at 200°C, under 2MPa for 10h.[67]

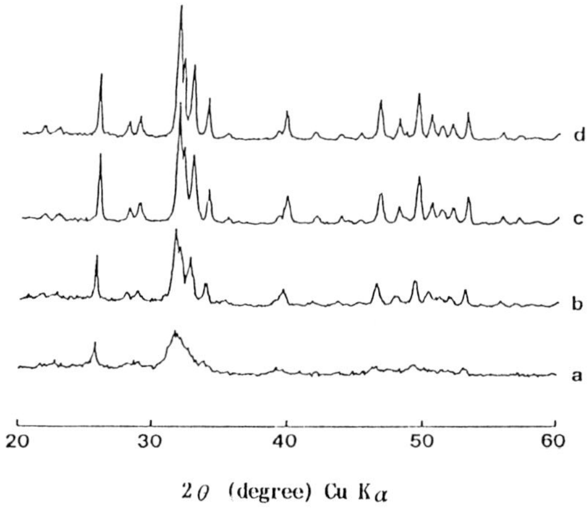

Figure 7. X-ray diffraction of hydroxyapatite powders: (a) prepared wet chemically at room temperature for 10h, and synthesized hydrothermally for 10h; (b) at 100°C under 0.1 MPa, (c) at 150°C under 0.5 MPa, and (d) at 200°C under 2 MPa.[67]

powder for ceramics and for structural-chemical studies. Not only biocompatibility but microstructure, e.g. grain size, pore size and porosity, must be tailored for the utilization of HAp ceramics as an implant material. In 1988, transparent HAp ceramics with fracture toughness of 1.1 $MPa{\cdot}m^{1/2}$ (Fig. 9) were prepared by HIP (Hot Isostatic Pressing) treatment of the hydrothermally prepared HAp fine crystals at 1000°C.[68] HIP treatment of two types of HAp powders with different sizes and sinterabilities (Fig. 10) enabled them to fabricate dense/porous layered HAp ceramics as shown in Figure 11.[69]

Although pure HAp ceramics have excellent biocompatibility, their mechanical strength are insufficient. One of the most effective methods to

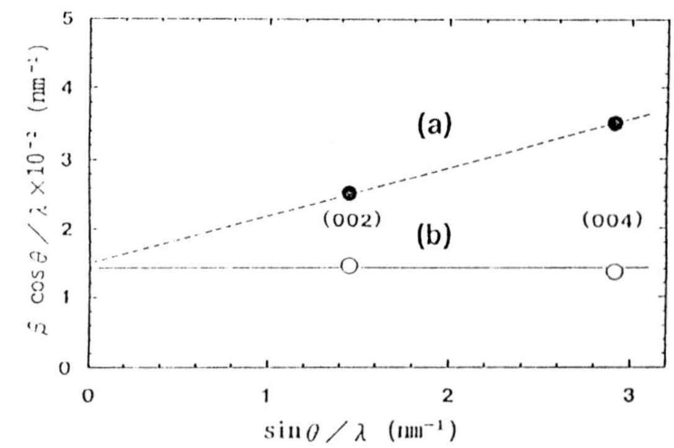

Figure 8. Williamson-Hall Plot for: (a) commercial hydroxyapatite powders (as-received) and (b) hydroxyapatite crystals prepared by the hydrothermal treatment of "sample (a)" at 200°C under 2 MPa for 10h.

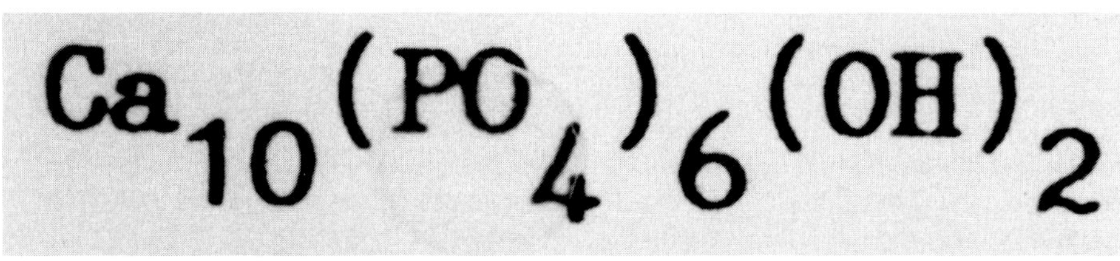

Figure 9. Post-sintered apatite ceramics obtained by HIP at 1000°C under 200 MPa of Ar gas for 1h, after which sintering in air at 1050°C for 3h.[68]

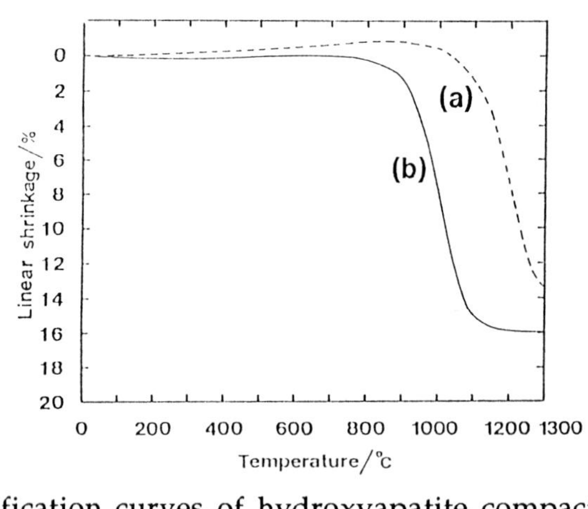

Figure 10. Densification curves of hydroxyapatite compacts CIPed under 200 MPa (heating rate: 10°C/min): (a) commercial HAp powder with size of 0.2 × 2μm, and (b) hydrothermally synthesized HAp fine crystals with size of 0.025 × 0.09μm.

improve the mechanical properties is to fabricate the **composites**. This requires the preparation of homogeneously dispersed powder mixtures, followed by sintering. HAp powders homogeneously dispersed with tetragonal zirconia (t-ZrO_2) have been synthesized hydrothermally.[70,71] After HIPing at 1050°C, the product has an almost pore free microstructure, resulting in the fracture toughness of 2.8 MPa·m$^{1/2}$, which value is 2.5 times higher than that of transparent pure HAp ceramics.[70,71] This improvement in fracture toughness was caused by the crack deflection toughening mechanism and probably by a transformation toughening mechanism. The important point is that the homogeneous mixing of powders could be attained by the hydrothermal technique. In contrast, aggregated t-ZrO_2 powders were observed in case of the conventional mechanical mixing with HAp powders.[70,71] Similarly, HAp powders homogeneously dispersed with Si_3N_4 whiskers (Fig. 12) were also synthesized hydrothermally.[72] After HIPing at 1000°C, the products possessed almost pore free microstructures consisting of HAp and TCP matrices and Si_3N_4 whiskers. The value of fracture toughness was 3.1 MPa·m$^{1/2}$, which was 3 times as high as that of the transparent HAp ceramics.[72] Fabrication of a "pure" HAp composite, that is, HAp fine crystals reinforced by HAp whiskers, is also under investigation in our laboratory.

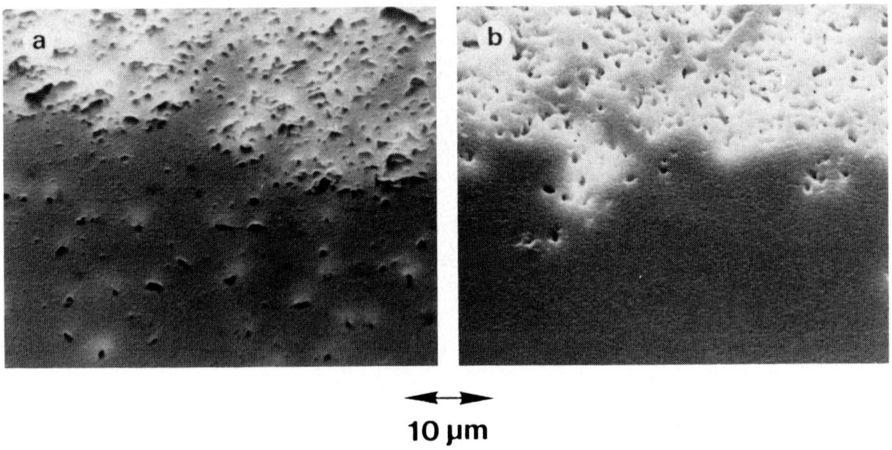

Figure 11. SEM photographs of the polished and thermally etched cross section of the dense/porous layered HAp ceramics: (a) before HIPing, normal sintering at 1050°C for 3h, and (b) after HIPing at 1000°C under 200 MPa or Ar gas for 1h.[69]

Hydrothermal sintering method, which has been developed to obtain the dense sintered ceramics at lower temperatures than for normal sintering, is appropriate for materials that undergo a phase transition, decomposition, evaporation,and grain growth at high temperature, because the hydrothermal sintering can be done under milder conditions than normal sintering. This hydrothermal sintering method was modified into a **Hydrothermal Hot Pressing Method** by Yamasaki's group,[73,74] where uniaxially compressing of powders under a hydrothermal condition is performed, resulting in the densification of powders at relatively low temperatures. It has been applied to the densification of stoichiometric HAp fine crystals.[73] This modified technique also allows the synthesis of dense non-stoichiometric Ca-deficient HAp ceramics,[74] by the treatment at a temperature as low as 350°C (thereby preventing HAp decomposition into β-$Ca_3(PO_4)_2$). Such a non-stoichiometric HAp ceramic (Ca/P=1.55) prepared at 350°C, 50MPa, 2 hours has the relative density of about 80%. Densification of Ca-deficient HAp powders by Hot Isostatic Pressing method has also been reported,[75] where much higher pressures as 320-850 MPa were applied. The lowest temperature for the densification decreased with a decrease of Ca/P ratio and with increase in crystal water content.

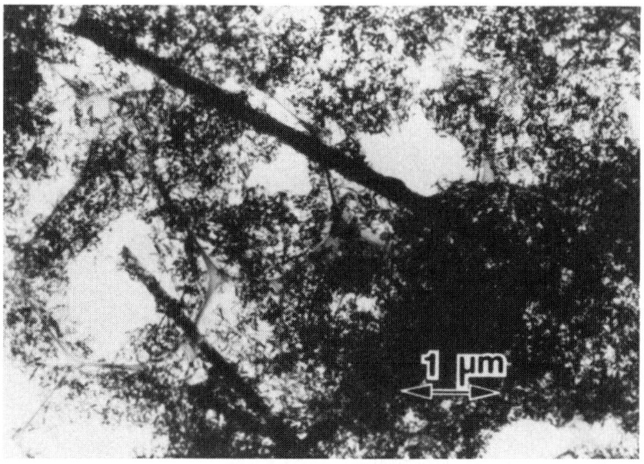

Figure 12. TEM observation of the homogeneously dispersed mixtures of hydroxyapatite fine crystals and Si_3N_4 whiskers prepared at 200°C under 2 MPa for 10h.[72]

4.3 MORPHOLOGICALLY CONTROLLED HAP CRYSTALS AND WHISKERS

Morphological control of HAp crystals is a stringent requirement in many applications. For example, HAp has been used as the filler for column-chromatography and in the other fields as well as the substitute material for hard tissues. One of the reasons why HAp has been proposed as the potential material for a filler is that it adsorbs proteins with high efficiency. In particular, c-plane (perpendicular to c-axis) and ab-plane (parallel to c-axis) of HAp crystals were reported to preferentially adsorb acidic and alkaline proteins, respectively.[78] Thus, morphological control of hydroxyapatite crystals, especially with elongated along a- or c-axes is expected to raise efficiency. There are some reports[60,79-87] on the synthesis of HAp needle-like crystals or fibers (Table 7). Recently, Nagata et al.[88] reported hydrothermal synthesis of plate-like apatite crystals. Extensively elongated HAp crystals[81,83,85-87] can be expected to have great potential as new "biocompatible whiskers" which will substitute for the "biohazardous fiber," such as asbestos and for other whiskers or fibers. Fibers as SiC, Si_3N_4, etc., are considered to be bioinert but not biocompatible. Biocompatible HAp whiskers, therefore, have great potential for use in composites containing organic and inorganic materials, and ceramics and metals dispersed with whiskers. HAp whiskers are a promising material for the applications to reinforcing filler, insulating agent, packing media for column chromatography, and the other biomedical fields. Although various methods for preparation of HAp such as wet chemical methods at low temperature, solid state reaction, hydrothermal methods, and the other methods are well known, it is relatively difficult to obtain morphologically controlled HAp by the other methods than the hydrothermal method. It is now possible to obtain morphologically controlled needle-like HAp fine crystals by the hydrothermal treatment of wet chemically prepared HAp by using various additives as shown in Figures 13 and 14.[85] **HAp whiskers** were successfully prepared by the hydrothermal treatment of β-$Ca_3(PO_4)_2$ with or without additives.[86,87] In particular, chelating agents such as EDTA, citric acid and lactic acid effect the elongation of HAp crystals. Since HAp is thermodynamically stable at ambient temperature, we can obtain HAp powders by the transformation of other calcium phosphates ($CaHPO_4$, $CaHPO_4{\cdot}2H_2O$, $Ca_8(PO_4)_6{\cdot}4H_2O$, α-$Ca_3(PO_4)_2$, and β-$Ca_3(PO_4)_2$) in aqueous solution systems. Similarly, those calcium phosphates can be used as raw materials for the synthesis of HAp whiskers.[86,87] As shown in figure 15, the HAp whiskers are about 30-50 µm in length and 0.1-1 µm in width, and are single crystals elongated along c-axis as revealed by the selected electron

Table 7. Preparation of HAp whiskers and fibers.

Starting Materials	Synthetic Conditions	Shape and Size	References
$CaHPO_4$ + NaOH	100~300°C, 20hs., pH 5 **(Hydrothermal)**	***Needle*** 10~20 µm	60
α-$Ca_3(PO_4)_2$ + $Ca(OH)_2$, HNO_3	80 °C, 2~3 hs., pH 4 ~10	Plate-like, ***Needle***, 3~5 µm	79, 80
$CaHPO_4$ + Urea	90°C, 71 hs., pH: 4-7	***Needle*** 0.3 x 10 µm	82
$Ca(NO_3)_2$ + $(NH_4)_2HPO_4$ + Urea	80~100 °C, 0.5 ~170 hs., pH: 2-6	Fiber or ***Whisker*** (?) 3 x 50 µm	83 (a)
$Ca(NO_3)_2$ + $(NH_4)_2HPO_4$ in agar system	R.T. pH: 4 ~ 9	***Fibrous*** HAp composed of hollow ovals	84
$CaCl_2$ +EDTA + $(NH_4)_2HPO_4$ + NH_4OH	200 °C, 30 hs., pH : 5.8 - 7.5 **(Hydrothermal)**	agglomerated ***Whiskers*** with lattice strain	81
$Ca(NO_3)_2$ + $(NH_4)_2HPO_4$ + Urea	120 ~ 150 °C, 0 ~ 6 hs. **(Hydrothermal)**	Fiber or ***Whiskers* (?)** 0.2 x 50 µm	83 (b)
wet chemically prepared HAp + additives	200°C, 2 MPa, 5 hs. **(Hydrothermal)**	***Needle*** fine crystals 0.03 x 0.33 µm	85
ß-$Ca_3(PO_4)_2$ + Citric Acid, EDTA Lactic Acid	200°C, 1 ~10 hs., pH : 3 ~4 **(Hydrothermal)**	***Whiskers*** (single crystals), 0.1-1 x 20-30 µm	86, 87

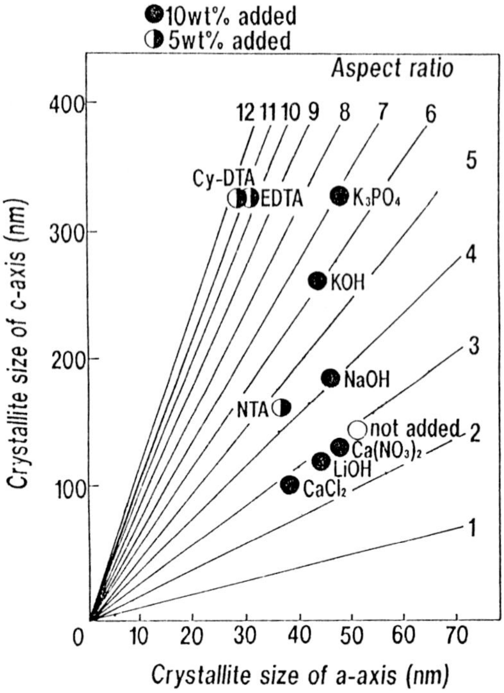

Figure 13. Changes of crystallite size and aspect ratio (c/a) of hydroxyapatite crystals synthesized hydrothermally at 200°C under 2 MPa for 5h with 5 or 10 wt% of various additives.[85]

diffraction pattern. Hydrothermal decomposition of Ca-chelates followed by the reaction of free Ca ions with phosphate ions in solution produces them. Recently, we investigated the factors affecting the formation of HAp whiskers in the $Ca(OH)_2$-H_3PO_4-citric acid or lactic acid systems.[89]

4.4 HAp COATINGS

The insufficient strength of hydroxyapatite prevents its direct use for implantation in load-bearing applications. One of the most effective methods to overcome its disadvantage is to **coat** ceramics or metal substrates with a hydroxyapatite layer (Table 8).

Many studies have been reported on the fabrication of such coatings by physical or chemical vapor deposition (PVD, CVD) techniques.[90-92] They include D.C. plasma spraying, R.F. plasma spraying, sputtering, and flame spraying techniques. The main problems associated with these techniques are the appearance of unidentified crystalline or amorphous phases and off-stoichiometry of HAp. Extreme high temperatures up to 20000 K within plasma arc should change the state of HAp crystalline powders into partially molten or plastic materials,[90] and may cause dehydration. Even if the temperature of the surface to be coated is kept below 100° to 150°C,[90] a portion of the layer remains in the molten state. Therefore, the coated layer needs to be heat treated at 800°C in order to increase its crystallinity.[90] High temperature plasma torch also causes the decomposition of HAp into tetracalcium phosphate and α−tricalcium phosphate.[91]

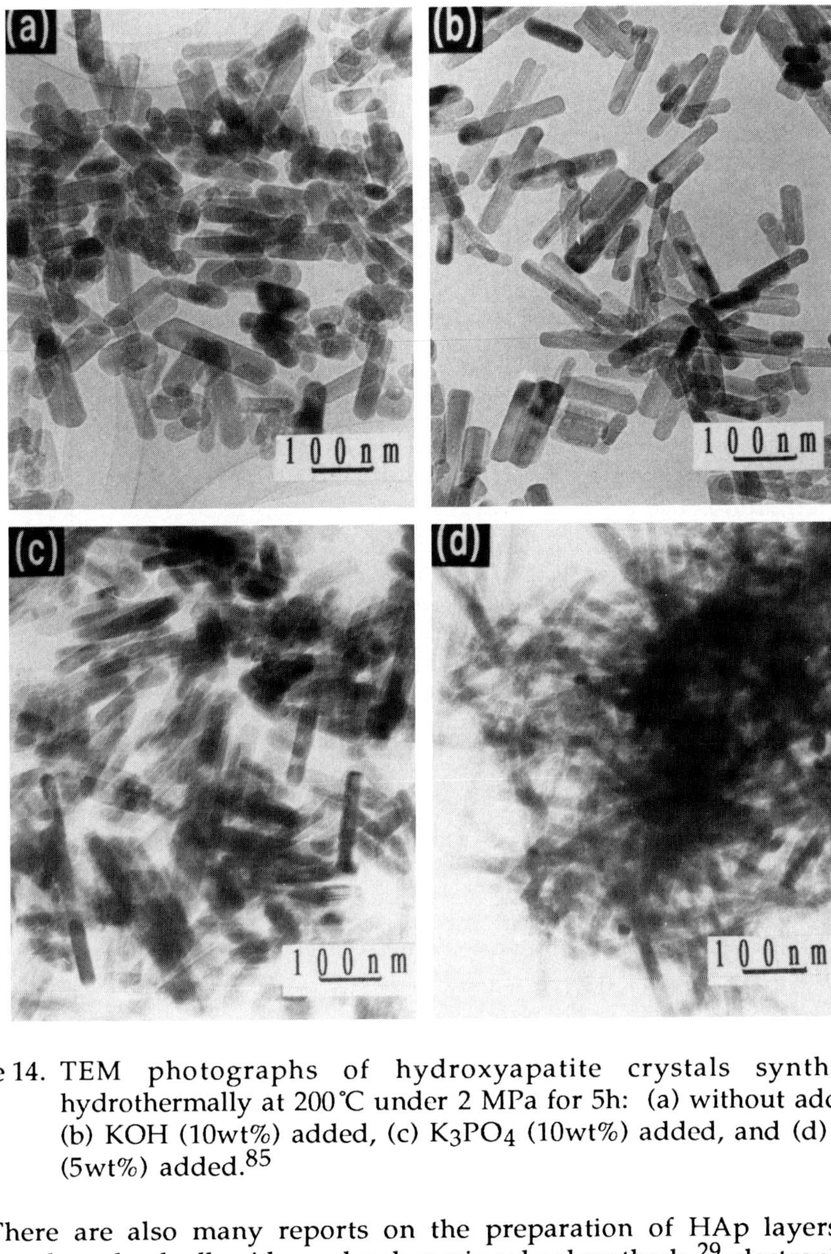

Figure 14. TEM photographs of hydroxyapatite crystals synthesized hydrothermally at 200℃ under 2 MPa for 5h: (a) without additives, (b) KOH (10wt%) added, (c) K_3PO_4 (10wt%) added, and (d) EDTA (5wt%) added.[85]

There are also many reports on the preparation of HAp layers from solutions by sol-gel, alkoxide, and polymeric sol-gel methods,[29] electrophoretic deposition,[95] electrochemical deposition[99] spark discharge,[93] electrochemical,[98] and hydrothermal methods.[92,94,97] Alkoxide and polymerized sol-gel methods, however, enable us only to form poorly crystallized HAp on substrates. Calcination processes at high temperatures which are necessary to improve the crystallinity lower mechanical properties due to the occurrence of the breaking and/or cracking of the layers and solid state reaction of layers with substrate. For example, Brendel[29] reported that HAp layers prepared by the polymeric route and dip coating method, followed

Table 8. Recent works on HAp coating.

Techniques	Comments	References
Plasma Spray Coating	HAp layer of 50 μm on rods, heating it at 800°C increases its crystallinity	90
Radio-Frequency Thermal Plasma Process	HAp layers on ZrO_2 ceramics	91
Hydrothermal transformation of plasma sprayed α-TCP	coated layer with needle HAp crystals onto Ti	92
Deposition of HAp by **spark discharge** in electrolyte	10-50 μm HAp porous layer onto Ti	93
Hydrothermal decomposition of Ca-EDTA in [P] aq.	needle HAp crystals deposited onto Ti	94
Electrophoresis deposition of HAp	HAp layers on ZrO_2, Al_2O_3 ceramics	95
HAp layer prepared in a simulated body fluid	chemical bonded HAp layers induced by silica or titania gel	96
Polymeric route using [Ca]+$C_6H_5PCl_2$ + acetone	dip coated thick and highly porous layers on Al_2O_3 and Ti	29
Hydrothermal treatment of anodic TiO_2 with ß-TCP	coated layer with needle-like HAp crystals onto anodic TiO_2	97
Electrochemical synthesis of HAp in a simulated body fluid	coated layer with fine HAp powder onto Ti	98
Electrochemical deposition of Ca-deficient Ap	coated layer with HAp (Ca/P~1.50, 45 x 8 μm) onto SUS, Ti	99

by calcination were revealed not to be "pure" hydroxyapatite based on anomalous lattice constants, XRD profiles, and IR spectra. Therefore, it is necessary to prepare the HAp layers through *"in-situ" or chemical process without calcination at high temperatures.* HAp layers formed in this way are expected to bond chemically with substrate, resulting in the better adhesion properties. In this regard, Kokubo et al.[97a-c] have developed an excellent coating process, resulting in the formation of the chemical bonding between HAp and substrate and pointed out that silica or even titania gels could initiate the nucleation of "bone-like" apatite in a simulated body fluid at 37°C. In 1993, Monma[99] reported the deposition of Ca-deficient HAp crystals with interesting morphologies on metal substrates at 20°-90°C by an electrochemical deposition technique. Preciptation is facilitated by the electrolysis of water to give an alkaline solution. Thus, the coverage and adhesion of HAp to the substrate might not be sufficiently strong. Similar disadvantages can be expected in HAp coatings prepared by the electrophoresis deposition method.[95] On the other hand, "the **hydrothermal electrochemical process**," which is the in-situ synthesis of HAp layers on a substrate by electrochemical reaction, should have a great advantage, as indicated previously in the coating of dielectrics.[100] Study of the HAp coatings on metal substrate by this hydrothermal electrochemical method is now under investigation in our laboratory.

4.5 SOLVOTHERMAL METHOD

Both hydrothermal and solvothermal, using high temperature non-aqueous solvents, method will be applied to the synthesis of apatites. Basic properties of non-aqueous solvents such as alcohol, NH_3, N_2O_4, SO_2, HCN, etc., and their application to material syntheses have been extensively studied.[101-106] These non-aqueous solvents are expected to be used also in the synthesis of apatites. For example, **alcohothermal method** might be effective for the synthesis of apatites, because the solubility of apatite may be changed in alcohol-water system. The change in property of water such as the weakening of the ions hydration sphere and bonding can be expected to result in the enhancement of dehydration of Ca and P ions. Such modifications may have promoted effects on the crystallization kinetics of HAp, as pointed out by Lerner et al.,[105] who reported the effects of ethanol (C_2H_5OH) on the crystallization of HAp crystals. As another example, Inoue et al.[106] reported the synthesis of HAp by a **glycothermal method**, where Ca acetate and phosphoric acid (or triethyl phosphate) dispersed in 1,4-butandiol (or ethylenglycol) was treated at 300°C for 2 hours in an autoclave. The resulting HAp had high crystallinity with crystallite size of 56 nm by the use of other starting materials than ethylene glycol. The ease in breaking the C-O chemical bond in $PO(O\text{-}(CH_2)_nOH)_3$ was considered to be an important factor in the crystallization of HAp. This type of research has just been started, so we shall wait to see what the future holds.

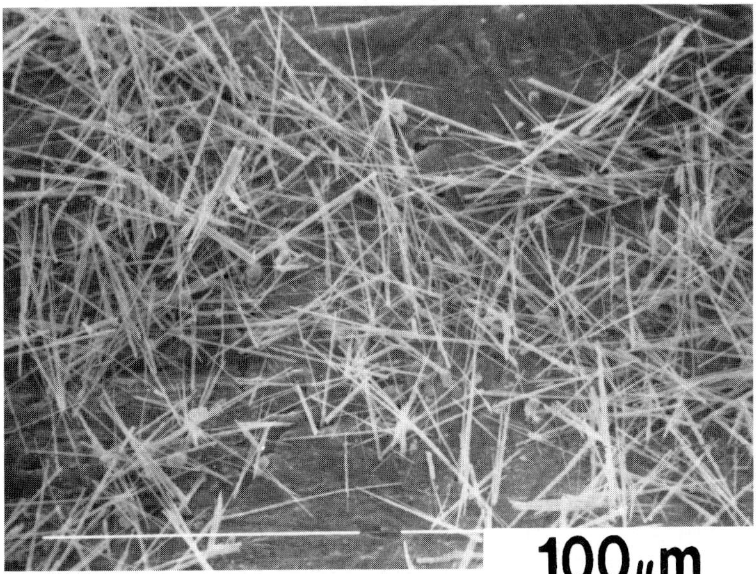

Figure 15. SEM photograph of hydroxyapatite whiskers synthesized by the hydrothermal treatment of β-tricalcium phosphate (TCP) with citric acid at 200°C under 2 MPa for 5h.

SUMMARY

The hydrothermal method can be used to prepare both large and small well crystallized hydroxyapatite crystals. Such crystals have been and will be used for crystallochemical, geochemical and phase stability studies, as ideal powders for ceramics and composites with biocompatibility and bioactivities. Furthermore, hydrothermal processing can be applied to the synthesis of whiskers, coatings and extended to non-aqueous solvothermal methods.

We believe the hydrothermal method can be applied in a wide variety of fields.

ACKNOWLEDGEMENT

Natural single crystal (Durango, Mexico) was kindly given by Professor R. C. Bradt, Mackay School of Mines, University of Nevada-Reno.

REFERENCES

1. W.A. Deer, R.A. Howie and J. Zussman, eds., Rock-Forming Minerals, Vol. 5 (Non-Silicates), pp. 323-338, Longmans, Green and Co. LTD. (1962).
2. D.R. Simpson, "Problems of the Composition and Structure of the Bone Minerals," Clin. Ortho. Relat. Res., 86, 260-286 (1972).
3. D.W. Holcomb and R.A.Young, "Thermal Decomposition of Human Tooth Enamel," Calcif. Tissue Int., 31, 189-201 (1980).
4. Present authors, in preparation.
5. W.H. Waggaman, *Phosphoric Acid, Phosphates and Phosphatic Fertilizers,* 2nd ed., p. 3, Reinhold Publishing Corp., New York (1952).
6. A.D.F. Toy, The Chemistry of PHOSPHORUS, in *Inorganic Chemistry,* Vol. 3, Pergamon Press (1973).
7. A. Daubrée, "Expériences sur la production artficielle de l'apatite, de la topaze, et de quelques autres métaux fruoriféres," Compt. Rend. Acad. Sci. Paris, Vol. 32, p. 625 (1851).
8. D. McConnell, Apatite—Its Crystal Chemistry, Mineralogy, Utilization, and Geologic and Biologic Occurrences, Springer-Verlag (1973).
9. D.M. Roy, L.E. Drafall, and R. Roy, Crystal Chemistry, Crystal Growth, and Phase Equilibria of Apatites, Academic Press, Inc. (1978).
10. J.C. Elliott, "The Problems of the Composition and Structure of the Mineral Components of the Hard Tissues," Clin. Ortho. Relat. Res., 93,313-345 (1973).
11. R.A. Young, "Biological Apatite vs Hydroxyapatite at the Atomic Level," Clin. Ortho. Relat. Res., 113,249-262 (1975).
12. E.P. Egan, Jr., Z.T. Wakefield, and K.L. Elmore, "Low-Temperature Heat Capacity and Entropy of Hydroxyapatite," J. Am. Chem. Soc., 72, 5579-5580 (1951).
13. V.A. Palkin, T.A. Kuzina, V.P. Orlovskii, Zh.A. Ezhova, G.V. Rodicheva, and G.E. Sukhanova, "The Thermodynamic Properties of $Ca_{10}(PO_4)_6(OH)_2$," Russ. J. Inorg. Chem., 36[12], 1718-1720 (1991).
14. M. Aning, D.O. Welch, and B.S.H. Royce, "The Surface Energy of Fluorapatite," Phys. Lett., 37A[3], 253-254 (1971).

15. H.S. Yoon, and R.E. Newnham, "Elastic Properties of Fluorapatite," Am. Miner., 54, 1193-1197 (1969).
16. V.M. Bhatnagar, "The Melting Points of Synthetic Apatites," Miner. Mag., 37, [288], 527-528 (1969).
17. H.B. Van Rees, M. Mengeot, and E. Kostiner, "Monoclinic-Hexagonal Transition in Hydroxyapatite and Deuterohydroxyapatite Single Crystals," Mat. Res. Bull., 8, 1307-1310 (1973).
18. J.C. Trombe, and G. Montel, "Some Features of the Incorporation of Oxygen in Different Oxidation States in the Apatitic Lattice—I, On the Existence of Calcium and Strontium Oxyapatites," J. Inorg. Nucl. Chem., 40, 15-21 (1978).
19. P.Ducheyne, T. Kokubo and C.A. Van Blitterswijk, eds., Bone-bonding Biomaterials, Rees Healthcare Communications (1992).
20. H. Aoki, Science and Medical Applications of Hydroxyapatite, Japanese Association of Apatite Science; JAAS (1991).
21. L.L. Hench, "Bioceramics: From Concept to Clinic," J. Am. Ceram. Soc., 74[7], 1487-1510 (1991).
22. W.J.Dowson, "Hydrothermal Synthesis of Advanced Ceramic Powders," Am. Ceram. Soc. Bull., 67, 1673-1678 (1988).
23. M. Yoshimura, "Ceramic Powders Prepared by Hydrothermal Method," Electronic Ceramics (in Jpn.), 104,4-9 (1991).
24. E.B. Jaffe, "Abstracts of the Literature on Synthesis of Apatites and Some Related Phosphates," U.S. Geol. Surv., Circular 135, 78 pages (1951).
25. J.W. McCauley and R. Roy, Am. Miner., 59, 947-963 (1974).
26. P.D. Johnson, J. Electrochem. Soc., 108, 159-162 (1961).
27. J.S. Prener, "The Growth and Crystallographic Properties of Calcium Fluor- and Chlorapatite Crystals," J. Electrochem. Soc., 114[1], 77-83 (1967).
28. Y. Masuda, K. Matsubara, and S. Sakka, "Synthesis of Hydroxyapatite from Metal Alkoxides through Sol-Gel Technique," J. Ceram. Soc. Jpn., (in Jpn.) 98 [11] 1255-1266 (1990).
29. T. Brendel, A. Engel, and C. Russel, "Hydroxyapatite Coating by a Polymeric Route," J. Mater. Sci: Mater. Med., 3, 175-179 (1992).
30. G. Spegia, Acad. Sci. Torino Att., 40, 254 (1905).
31. G.W. Morey and P. Niggli, J. Am. Chem. Soc., 35, 1086 (1913).
32. S. Somiya (ed.), Proceedings of the First International Symposium on Hydrothermal Reactions, March 22-26, 1982, Tokyo Institute of Technology, Japan, Gakujyutsu Bunken Fukyu-Kai (1983).
33. E.U. Franck, "Supercritical Water," Endeavour, 27, 55-59 (1968).
34. S. Náray-Szabo, "The Structure of Apatite $(CaF)Ca_4(PO_4)_3$," Zeit. Krist., 75, 387-398 (1930).
35. M. Mehmel, "Uber die Struktur des Apatits," Zeit. Krist., 75, 323-331 (1930).
36. S.B. Hendricks, M.E. Jefferson, and V.M. Mosley,"The Crystal Structures of Some Natural and Synthetic Apatite-like Substances," Zeit. Krist., Vol.81, p. 352 (1932).
37. C.A. Beevers, and D.B. McIntyre, "The Atomic Structure of Fluoro-apatite and Its Relation to That of Tooth and Bone Material," Miner. Mag., 27, 254-257 (1946).

38. A.S. Posner, A. Perloff, and A.F. Diorio, "Refinement of the Hydroxyapatite Structure," Acta Cryst., 11,308-309 (1958).
39. M.I. Kay, R.A. Young and A. S. Posner, "Crystal Structure of Hydroxyapatite," Nature, 204, 1050-1052 (1964).
40. K. Sudarsanan, P.E. Mackie, and R.A. Young, "Comparison of Synthetic and Mineral Fluorapatite, $Ca_5(PO_4)_3F$, in Crystallographic Detail," Mater.Res.Bull., 7, 1331-1338 (1973).
41. J.C. Elliott, P.E. Mackie, and R.A. Young, "Monoclinic Hydroxyapatite," Science, 180, 1055-1057 (1973).
42. J.M. Hughes, M. Cameron, K.D. Crowley, "Structural Variations in Natural F,OH, and Cl apatites," Am. Miner., 74, 870-876 (1989).
43. A.T. Sänger and W.F. Kufs, "Structural Disorder in Hydroxyapatite," Zeit. Krist., 199, 123-148 (1992).
44. J.R. Farver, and B.J. Giletti, "Oxygen and Strontium Diffusion Kinetics in Apatite and Potential Applications to Thermal History Determination," Geochim. Cosmochim.Acta, 53, 1621-1631 (1989).
45. A. Shemesh, Y. Kolodny, and B. Luz, "Isotope Geochemistry of Oxygen and Carbon in Phosphate and Carbonate of Phosphorite Francolite," Geochim. Cosmochim. Acta, 52, 2565-2572 (1988).
46. J.R. Van Wazer, Phosphorus and Its Compounds, Vol.1. Chemistry, Wiley-Interscience, New York (1958).
47. (a) P.W. Brown, "Phase Relationships in the Ternary System $CaO-P_2O_5-H_2O$ at 25 °C," J. Am. Ceram. Soc., 75[1] 17-22 (1992).
(b) P.W. Brown, N. Hocker, and S. Hoyle, "Variations in Solution Chemistry During the Low-Temperature Formation of Hydroxyapatite," J. Am. Ceram. Soc., 74[8] 1848-1854 (1991).
(c) P.W. Brown, and M. Fulmer, "The Kinetics of Hydroxyapatite Formation at Low Temperature," J. Am. Ceram. Soc., 74[5]:934-940 (1991).
48. H.C.W. Skinner, "Studies in the Basic Mineralizing System, $CaO-P_2O_5-H_2O$," Calcif. Tiss. Res., 14, 3-14 (1974).
49. S.S. Feng, and T.J. Rockett, "The System $CaO-P_2O_5-H_2O$ at 200°C," J. Amer. Ceram. Soc., 62, [11-12], 619-620 (1979).
50. R A. Young, and D.W. Holcomb, "Variability of Hydroxyapatite Preparation," Calc. Tissue Int., 34, S17-S32 (1982).
51. G.W. Morey and E. Ingerson, Econ. Geol.,32, 607-761 (1937).
52. W. Rathje, Deut. Chem. Ges.74, 342 (1941).
53. E. Hayek, J. Lechtleitner, W. Bohler, Angew. Chem.,67, 326 (1955).
54. A. Perloff, A.S.Posner, "Preparation of Pure Hydroxyapatite Crystals," Science, Vol.124,583-584 (1956).
55. H. Jullmann and R. Mosebach, "Zur Synthese,Licht- und Doppelbrechung des Hydroxylapatits," Naturforsch, 21b,493-494 (1966).
56. J. F. Kirn and H. Leidheiser, Jr., "Progress in Efforts to Grow Large Single Crystals of Hydroxyapatite," J. Cryst. Growth, 2,111-112(1968).
57. D.M. Roy,"Crystal Growth of Hydroxyapatite," Mat. Res. Bull.6,1337-1340(1971).
58. M. Mengeot, M.L.Harvill and O.R.Gilliam, "Hydrothermal Growth of Calcium hydroxyapatite Single Crystals," J. Cryst. Growth,19,199-203(1973).)
59. W. Eysel and D.M. Roy, "Hydrothermal Flux Growth of Hydroxyapatites by Temperature Oscillation," J. Cryst. Growth, 20,245-250(1973).

60. (a) H. Aoki, K. Kato, and M. Shiba, "Synthesis of Hydroxyapatite under Hydrothermal Conditions, I : Kinetic Analysis of the Reaction Process from Monetite into Hydroxyapatite," J. Dent. Apparatus and Materials, 13 [27], pp.170-176 (1972).
(b) H. Aoki, and K. Kato, "Synthesis of Hydroxyapatite under Hydrothermal Conditions, II : Effects of pH and Temperature," J. Dent. Apparatus and Materials, (in Jpn.) 14[29], 36-39 (1973).
61. J. Arends, J. Schuthof, W.H.Van Der Linden, P. Bennema and P.J. Van Den Berg, "Preparation of Pure Hydroxyapatite Single Crystals by Hydrothermal Recrystallyzation". J. Cryst. Growth, 46,213-220 (1979).
62. M. Hata, and F. Marumo, "Synthesis and superstructure of $(Ca,M)_5(PO_4)_3OH$ (M=Mn, Fe, Co, Ni, Cu, Hg)," Miner. J., 11,7, 317-330 (1983).
63. G. Vereecke and J.Lemaître, "Caluculation of The Solubility Diagram in The System $Ca(OH)_2$-H_3PO_4-KOH-HNO_3-CO_2-H_2O," J. Cryst. Growth, 104, 820-832 (1990).
64. (a) H. Aoki, K. Kato, M. Shibata, and A. Naganuma, "Thermal Transition of Calcium Phosphates and Observation by a Scanning Electron Microscope," Rep. of Inst. Med. Dent. Eng., (in Jpn.) 6, 50-61 (1972).
(b) H. Aoki, K. Kato, and E. Yasuda, "Application of Synthetic Hydroxyapatite to Medical Use," Proc.23rd Conf. Jpn. Assoc. Dent. Eng., pp. 20 (1972).
65. M. Jarcho, C.H. Bolen, M.B. Thomas, J. Bobick, J.F. Kay, and R.H. Doremus, "Hydroxyapatite Synthesis and Characterization in Dense Polycrystalline Form," J. Mater. Sci., 11, 2027-2035 (1976).
66. G. De With, H.J.A. Van Dijk, U. Hattu, K. Prijs, "Preparation , Microstructure and Mechanical Properties of Dense Polycrystalline Hydroxyapatite," J. Mater. Sci., 16, 1592-1598 (1981).
67. K. Ioku, M. Yoshimura, and S. Somiya, "Hydrothermal Synthesis of Ultrafine Hydroxyapatite Single Crystals," Nippon Kagaku Kaishi, (in Jpn.) 1565-1570 (1988).
68. K. Ioku, M. Yoshimura, and S. Somiya, "Post-sintering of Apatite Ceramics from Fine Powders Synthesized under Hydrothermal Conditions," J. Ceram. Soc. Japan, (in Jpn.) 96, 109-110 (1988).
69. K. Ioku, S. Somiya, M. Yoshimura, "Dense/porous Layered Apatite Ceramics Prepared by HIP Post-sintering," J. Mater. Sci. Lett, 8, 1203-1204 (1989).
70. K. Ioku, M. Yoshimura, and S. Somiya, "Microstructure and Mechanical Properties of Hydroxyapatite Ceramics with Zirconia Dispersion Prepared by Post-sintering," Biomaterials, 11, 57-61 (1990).
71. K. Ioku, S. Somiya, and M. Yoshimura, "Hydroxyapatite Ceramics with Tetragonal Zirconia Particle Dispersion Prepared by HIP Post-sintering," J. Ceram. Soc. Jpn, Int. Edition, 13-20 (1991).
72. K. Ioku, T. Noma, N. Ishizawa, and M. Yoshimura, "Hydrothermal Synthesis and Sintering of Hydroxyapatite Powders Dispersed with Si_3N_4 Whiskers," J. Ceram. Soc. Jpn, Int. Edition, 48-53 (1990).
73. T. Kai, K. Ioku, M. Nishioka, K. Yanagisawa, and N. Yamasaki, "Sintering of Apatite Compacts Prepared by Hydrothermal Hot-Pressing," Transactions of the 5th Symposium on Apatite, (in Jpn.) pp. 61-63 (1989).

74. T. Kai, K. Ioku, M. Nishioka, K. Yanagisawa, and N. Yamasaki, "Dense Non-stoichiometric Hydroxyapatite with and without Carbonate Ion Prepared by Hydrothermal Hot-Pressing," Transactions of the 6th Symposium on Apatite, (in Jpn.), pp.5-6 (1990).
75. S.R. Kim, K. Hirota, F. Okamura, Y. Hasegawa and S.J. Park, "Densification of Calcium-Deficient Hydroxyapatite by Hot Isostatic Pressing," J. Ceram. Soc. Jpn., (in Jpn.), 98[3] 257-263 (1990).
76. T. Noma, N. Shoji, S. Wada, and T. Suzuki, "Sintering of Hydroxyapatite Powders with SiC Platelets Dispersion," J. Ceram. Soc. Jpn., (in Jpn.) 100, 1175-1178 (1992).
77. M. Takagi, M. Mochida, N. Uchida, K. Saito, and K. Uematsu, "Filter Cake Forming and Hot Isostatic Pressing for TZP-dispersed Hydroxyapatite Composite," J. Mat. Sci. Mat. Med., 3, 199-203 (1992).
78. T. Kawasaki, "Hydroxyapatite as a Liquid Chromatographic Packing," J. Chromatography, 544, 147-184 (1991).
79. H. Monma, S. Ueno, and T. Kanazawa, "Properties of Hydroxyapatite Prepared by the Hydrolysis of Tricalcium phosphate," J. Chem. Tech. Biotechnol., 31, 15-24 (1981).
80. H. Monma and T. Kamiya, "Preparation of Hydroxyapatite by the Hydrolysis of Brushite," J. Mater. Sci., 22, 4247-4250 (1987).
81. N. Christiansen and R.E.Riman, "Bioceramics—A Future through Microstructural and Chemical Design," Proc.5th Scandinavian Sympo. Mater.Sci., New Materials and Processes, May 22-23, 1989, pp. 209-220.
82. A. Mortier, J. Lemaitre, L. Rodrique and P. Rouxhet, "Synthesis and Thermal Behavior of Well-crystallized Calcium-deficient Phosphate Apatite," J. Solid State Chem., 78, 215-219 (1989).
83. (a) M. Kinoshita, A. Kishioka, H. Hayashi, and S. Itatani, "Preparation of Fibrous Calcium Phosphates by Homogeneous Precipitation Method and Their Thermal Changes," Gypsum & Lime (in Jpn.), 219, 23-31 (1989).
(b) M. Kinoshita, K. Itatani, S. Nakamura, and A. Kishioka, "Preparation and Morphology of Carbonate-Containing Hydroxyapatite by Homogeneous Precipitation and Hydrothermal Methods," Gypsum & Lime (in Jpn.), 227, 19-27 (1990).
84. K. Kamiya, T. Yoko, K. Tanaka, and Y. Fujiyama, "Growth of Fibrous Hydroxyapatite in the Gel System," J. Mater. Sci., 24, 827-832 (1989).
85. M. Yoshimura, H. Suda, K. Okamoto, and K. Ioku, "Hydrothermal Synthesis of Needle-like Aapatite Crystals," Nippon-Kagaku-Kaishi (in Jpn.), 10, 3101-3106 (1991).
86. H. Suda, N. Asaoka, and M. Yoshimura, "Preparation and Characterization of Hydroxyapatite Whiskers by Hydrothermal Method," pp. 31-34, in Bioceramics, Vol. 5, Proceedings of the 5th Int. Symp. Ceram. Medicine, T. Yamamuro, T. Kokubo, and T. Nakamura (eds.), Kobunshi Kankokai, Inc., (1992).
87. Present author, "Hydrothermal Synthesis of Biocompatible Whisker," submitted.
88. F. Nagata, Y. Yokogawa, M. Toriyama, Y. Kawamoto, T. Suzuki, K. Nishizawa, and H. Nagae, "Hydrothermal Synthesis of Plate-like Hydroxyapatite Crystals," submitted to Proc. of IUMRS-ICAM-93; 3rd IUMRS Int. Conf. Advanced Mater, Tokyo, Japan, 1993.
89. Present authors, in preparation.

90. K. de Groot, "Medical Applications of Calciumphosphate Bioceramics," J. Ceram. Soc. Jpn, 99[10] 943-953 (1991).
91. A. Hasegawa, T. Kameyama, A. Motoe, M. Ueda, K. Akashi, and K. Fukuda, "Coating of Hydroxyapatite on Zirconia Utilizing a Radio-Frequency Thermal Plasma Process," J. Ceram. Soc. Jpn. (in Jpn.), 100[4], 377-381 (1992).
92. M. Higashikata, O. Hayashi, M. Yoshizawa, Y. Ukegawa, Y. Kuroyama, Y. Tsutsumi, M. Akao, A. Aoki, and H. Tagai, "Characterization of Hydroxyapatite Coating Obtained by Hydrothermal Transformation of Plasma Sprayed a-Tricalcium Phosphate," 145-150, in Apatite Vol.1, Proc. First Int. Symp. Apatite, H. Aoki, M. Akao, N. Nagai, and T. Tsuji (eds.), Mishima, Japan, July 1991.
93. T. Miyazaki and Y. Ibe, "Deposition of Hydroxyapatite onto Titanium Using the Spark Discharge in Electrolyte," 155-158, , in Apatite, Vol.1, Proc. First Int. Symp. Apatite, H. Aoki, M. Akao, N. Nagai, and T. Tsuji (eds.), Mishima, Japan, July 1991.
94. K. Kawanura, Y. Fujishiro, H. Yabuki, T. Sato, and A. Okuwaki, "Synthesis of Phosphates Utilizing the Dissociation and Decomposition of Metal-EDTA Complex under Hydrothermal Conditions," Abst. Ann. Meet. Chem. Soc. Jpn., No. D508 (1990).
95. M. Nagai, K. Yamashita, and T. Umegaki, "Electrophoresis-deposited Composite Films of Hydroxyapatite and Zirconia," pp. 167-172 in Phosphorus Research Bulletin Vol. 1; Proc. Int. Symp. Inorg. Phosphate Mater. '91, T. Kanazawa, Y. Abe and T. Umegaki (eds.), Tokyo, Japan, July 24-26, 1991, Jpn. Assn. Inorg. Phosphorus Chem., Nihon Printing Co., Ltd. (1991).
96. (a) T. Kokubo, "Surface Chemistry of Bioactive Glass-Ceramics," J. Noncryst. Solids, 120,138-151 (1990).
    (b) Y. Abe, T. Kokubo, and T. Yamamuro, "Apatite Coating on Ceramics, Metals and Polymers Utilizing a Biological Process," J. Mater. Sci.: Mater. Med., 1, 233-238 (1990).
    (c) P. Li, C. Ohtsuki, T. Kokubo, K. Nakanishi, and N. Soga, T. Nakamura, T. Yamamuro, "Apatite Formation Induced by Silica Gel in a Simulated Body Fluid," J. Am. Ceram. Soc., 75[8], 2094-2097 (1992).
97. H. Ishizawa, M. Fujino, and M. Ogino, "Formation and Evaluation of Titanium Anodic Oxide Film Containing Ca and P," pp.43-47, in Bioceramics Vol. 5; Proc. of the 5th Intl. Symp. on Ceramics in Medicine, T. Yamamuro, T. Kokubo, T. Nakamura (eds.), Kyoto, Japan, November 1992, Kobunshi Kankokai (1992).
98. S. Ban and S. Maruno, "Electrochemical Synthesis of Calcium Phosphates in a Simulated Body Fluid," pp. 49-56, in Bioceramics, Vol.5 ; Proc. of the 5th Intl. Symp. on Ceramics in Medicine, T. Yamamuro, T. Kokubo, T. Nakamura (eds.), Kyoto Japan, November 1992. Kobunshi Kankokai, (1992).
99. H. Monma, "Electrochemical Deposition of Calcium-Deficient Apatite on Stainless Steel Substrate," J. Ceram. Soc. Jpn. (in Jpn.), 101[7], 737-739 (1993).
100. (a) M. Yoshimura, S-E. Yoo, M. Hayashi, and N. Ishizawa, Jpn. J. Appl. Phys., "Preparation of $BaTiO_3$ Thin film by Hydrothermal Electrochemical Method," 28 [11], 2007-2009 (1989).

(b) S-E. Yoo, M. Hayashi, N. Ishizawa, and M. Yoshimura, "Preparation of $SrTiO_3$ Thin Film on Ti Metal Substrate by Hydrothermal Electrochemical Method," J. Am. Ceram. Soc., 73 [8], 2561-2563 (1990).
(c) N. Ishizawa, H. Banno, M. Hayashi, S-E. Yoo, and M. Yoshimura, "$BaTiO_3$ and $SrTiO_3$ Polycrystalline Thin Film on Flexible Polymer Film Substrate by Hydrothermal Method," Jpn. J. Appl. Phys., 29 [11] 2467-2472 (1990).

101. G. Jander, H. Spandau, and C.C. Addison (eds.), Chemie in nichtwäßrigen iönisiereuden Losungsmitteln, Friedr. Vieweg & Sohn, Braunschweig (1966-1971).
102. L.F. Audrieth and J. Kleinberg, Non-Aqueous Solvents, John Wiley & Sons, New York (1953).
103. T.C. Waddington (ed.), Non-Aqueous Solvent Systems, Academic Press, London (1965).
104. S. Somiya, G. Sudoh, M. Tanaka, and Y. Fukaya, "Reaction Products of Si_3N_4 in Ammonia Solution at High Temperature under High Pressure," Report of Res. Lab. Eng. Mater., Tokyo Institute of Technology, 4, 5-10 (1979).
105. E. Lerner, R. Azoury, and S. Sarig, "Rapid Precipitation of Apatite from Ethanol-Water Solution," J. Cryst. Growth, 97, 725-730 (1989).
106. H. Otsu, H. Kominami, M. Inoue, and T. Inui, "Synthesis of Hydroxyapatite by Glycothermal Method," Abstr. Ann. Mtg. Ceram. Soc. Jpn., Tokyo, pp.137, 1991.

FORMATION AND DISSOLUTION MECHANISMS OF CALCIUM PHOSPHATES IN AQUEOUS SYSTEMS

George H. Nancollas and Jingwu Zhang*
Chemistry Department
State University of New York at Buffalo
Buffalo, NY 14214

INTRODUCTION

The elucidation of the mechanisms of precipitation in solutions containing calcium and phosphate ions provides a challenge to the chemist not only because of the need to calculate the activities of ionic species in the solution phase but also because of the numerous calcium and phosphate phases that may be involved in the crystallization reactions. At least 5 sparingly soluble crystalline phases have been characterized, including dicalcium phosphate dihydrate (DCPD, $CaHPO_4 \cdot 2H_2O$), dicalcium phosphate (DCPA, $CaHPO_4$), tricalcium phosphates (α and β TCP, $Ca_3(PO_4)_2$), octacalcium phosphate (OCP, $Ca_4H(PO_4)_3 \cdot 2.5H_2O$) and calcium hydroxyapatite (HAP, $Ca_5(OH)(PO_4)_3$).[1] Typical solubility isotherms as a function of pH are given in Fig. 1. Although the thermodynamically most stable phase is HAP, it is now generally accepted that the other phases, including defect apatites may participate in the overall precipitation process.[2-4] In the spontaneous precipitation of calcium phosphate in highly supersaturated solutions, the formation of apatite is usually preceded by the precipitation of one or more precursor phases including amorphous calcium phosphate (ACP) in which no long range order can be detected by X-ray diffraction studies.[5] The composition of this phase appears to depend upon the precipitation conditions and its formation may be followed by the nucleation of OCP which serves as a template for HAP growth.[6] In biological mineralization and demineralization, DCPD, OCP and HAP have been shown to be actively involved.[7] It can be seen in Fig. 1 that as the acidity of the solution is increased, OCP or DCPD may be the appropriate precursor phase in accordance with Ostwald's Rule of Stages which states that the least stable salt with the highest solubility will always form first in a sequential precipitation reaction.

The calcium phosphate phase that forms during mineralization depends upon the relative supersaturation with respect to the particular phase.

$$\sigma = (IP^{1/\nu} - K_{so}{}^{1/\nu})K_{so}{}^{-1/\nu}\ 1/\nu = S - 1 \qquad (1)$$

In equation 1, ν is the number of ions per formula unit of precipitating phase.

---

* Present Address: Dept. de Chimie Minerale, Analytique et Appliquee, Geneva, Switzerland.

0-8493-4750-5/94/$0.00 + $.50

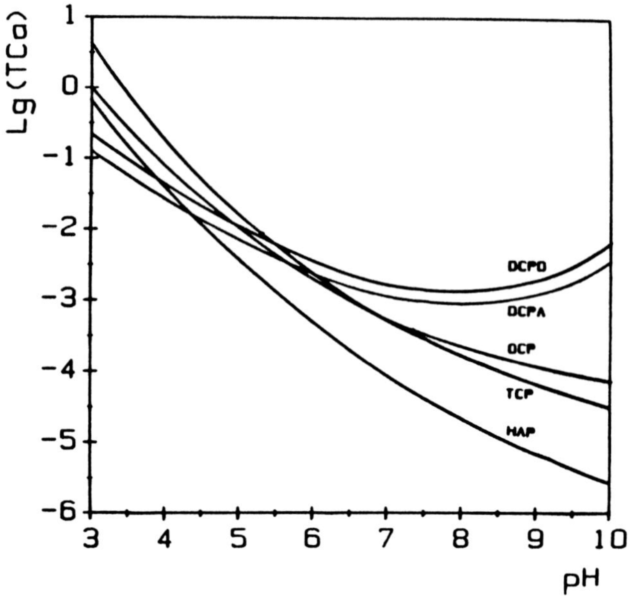

Figure 1. Solubility isotherms of calcium phosphate phases. Logarithmic products of total molar calcium concentration plotted against pH of the saturated solutions. (Equimolar calcium and phosphate; ionic strength 0.10 $molL^{-1}$.)

The ion products, IP, may be calculated using Eq. 2-4.

$$IP_{DCPD} = [Ca^{2+}][HPO_4^{2-}]y_2^2 \quad (2)$$

$$IP_{OCP} = [Ca^{2+}]^4[H^+][PO_4^{3-}]^3y_1y_2^4y_3^3 \quad (3)$$

$$IP_{HAP} = [Ca^{2+}]^5[PO_4^{3-}]^3[OH^-]y_1y_2^5y_3^3 \quad (4)$$

y_x is the activity coefficient of an x-valent species and can be calculated by using an extended form of the Debye Hückel equation such as that proposed by Davies.[7] In Eq. 1, S is the supersaturation ratio that can be used to calculate the Gibbs free energy of transfer, ΔG from the supersaturated solutions to an assumed saturated layer at the crystal surface as given by Eq. 5.

$$-\Delta G = RT \ln S \quad (5)$$

Since ion pair formation involves both calcium and phosphate ions, effectively decreasing their concentrations, the degree of supersaturation must be calculated in terms of the concentrations of free ionic species. This can be achieved using electroneutrality, mass balance and equilibrium constant relationships by successive approximations for the ionic strength.[8]

The sensitivity of thermodynamic driving force to pH and ionic strength is illustrated in Table 1.

TABLE 1

Influence of pH and ionic strength, I, on calcium phosphates relative supersaturation: Total molar concentrations; calcium = 5.8×10^{-3} mol L^{-1}, phosphate = 18.0×10^{-3} mol L^{-1}.

pH:	5.5	6.5	6.0	6.0
I mol L^{-1}:	0.15	0.15	0.15	0.05
σ_{HAP}	3.3	19.0	8.7	10.3
σ_{OCP}	0.7	4.4	2.2	2.6

It can be seen that at constant total molar concentrations of calcium and phosphate ions, the relative supersaturations with respect to each of the calcium phosphate phases depends markedly upon the pH of the solution. In addition, when calcium, phosphate and hydrogen ion concentrations are held constant, the relative supersaturations depend upon the ionic strength of the solution, maintained by the addition of inert electrolyte. This is especially important in biomineralization systems since both the pH and ionic strengths may change markedly in regions of pathological de- or remineralization. In the light of these factors that emphasize the complexity of calcium phosphate solution chemistry, it is quite clear that the common usage of the term "hydroxyapatite" to describe calcium phosphate precipitates formed under a wide variety of conditions is entirely misleading. Moreover not only must the thermodynamic driving force be taken into account in constructing models for the formation of the various calcium phosphate phases, but kinetic events may be even more important in determining which phase will be observed under a given set of conditions. In this paper, we explore some of the methods that have been used to investigate the kinetics of precipitation of calcium phosphates and the mechanisms of mineralization and demineralization of the various phases.

METHODS

Since the introduction of seeded growth techniques, kinetics studies of mineralization have been possible using methods such as free drift, pH-stat and constant composition (CC). In the pH-stat method, although changes in pH were avoided by using a glass electrode and potentiostat to control base addition, the concentration of lattice ions decreased during the reaction resulting in the possible sequential formation of multiple phases. These problems were avoided in the constant composition and, later, the dual constant composition (DCC) methods[9,10] in which the concentrations of lattice ions were maintained by titration with solutions containing calcium, phosphate and hydroxide ions as well as background electrolyte, from coupled burets. Adjustment of titrant solution stoichiometry to match the precipitated phases enabled the activities of all ionic species to be maintained constant even during extended reaction periods. By limiting reaction conditions to known points on the solubility diagram (Fig. 1), sufficient amounts of grown solid phases could be formed even at very low supersaturation for reliable solid phase characterization. Recently, it has been shown that the molar ratios of lattice ions in the solutions may also markedly influence the rates of mineralization and demineralization.[11]

Changes in surface activity, as the number of spiral dislocations decreases, may also reduce the rates of reaction even though the degrees of under and supersaturation are maintained constant.[12]

MECHANISMS OF GROWTH AND DISSOLUTION

Since crystal growth and dissolution are usually considered to be equivalent processes, most theoretical models and parameters used to describe the growth process may be applied to dissolution. The mechanisms for sparingly soluble electrolyte crystals can be divided broadly into two categories: dislocation and surface nucleation. Both may include volume diffusion as a limiting case. For the former, two comprehensive models have been proposed depending upon the role of surface diffusion.[13-15] In the direct detachment model, the lattice ions, detached from the crystal steps, immediately enter the solution phase, and diffuse to the bulk. Conversely, for crystal growth the lattice ions enter the kink sites directly. In the indirect detachment model, after detachment, the ions may move away from the step by surface diffusion before they desorb from the surface and diffuse into the bulk solution phase. In the corresponding growth process, surface diffusion is involved in transporting the ions to the kink sites.

As indicated above, one of the advantages of the constant composition methodology is the ability to grow and dissolve relatively large amounts of solid phase while maintaining the thermodynamic driving force constant. Since in general terms, the rate of growth or dissolution, J, can be written (Eq. 6),

$$J = kF\,(m/m_0)G(\sigma) \tag{6}$$

in terms of an effective rate constant, k, and as functions F and G of surface properties and solution concentration, the CC procedure maintains G (s) constant and enables studies to be made of changes in the surface activity. In Eq. 6, m_0 and m are the masses of the crystals initially and at time t, respectively. Since the total effective surface area of a crystal suspension at time t may be empirically related to the initial value, S_0, by writing $S_o\ (m/m_0)^p$, the crystal shape factor may also be included in the empirical rate equation. For isotropic three dimensional growth, $p = 2/3$, while p values of 0 and 1/2 indicate that growth occurs exclusively in one and two directions, respectively. Again, the advantage of the CC method is the ability to investigate not only influence of changes in the thermodynamic driving force, but also actual surface properties of the seed materials.

GROWTH

Despite complications due to the formation of defect apatites, under well defined supersaturation conditions, it is possible to grow pure DCPD or OCP on seed crystals of these phases. The growth rate of DCPD both at 25° and 37°C follows a parabolic rate law (Eq. 7).

$$j \propto \sigma^2 \tag{7}$$

This parabolic rate expression has also been observed for a number of sparingly soluble salts with effective orders of 2 over large ranges of supersaturation. This suggests that the concentration of active kink sites on the crystal surfaces is a function of supersaturation. In terms of this model, crystal growth occurs through the addition of ions mainly at the kink positions and thus it is very important to know the density of kink sites. Traditionally kink density is calculated using a thermodynamic approach which is valid only at equilibrium. Since crystal growth and dissolution processes are typical non-equilibrium situations, however, Christoffersen[16] developed a new model for deriving dissolution rates in which kink formation was considered as an essential process for step movement. Recently, a kinetic approach to derive kink density under non-equilibrium conditions has been developed by considering the elementary events leading to both kink formation and annihilation.[17] In terms of this model, the integration rate is in very good agreement with the empirical parabolic rate law (Eq. 7).

It is now well established that the crystal growth of the most important calcium phosphate phases, DCPD, OCP and HAP is controlled by surface processes. Constant composition studies show a wide range of growth rate with the thermodynamically less stable phases having much larger values than HAP. Although DCPD growth can be described in terms of a spiral growth, the effective order, $n \approx 4$ for OCP growth in the range $0.45<\sigma<1.05$ suggests a polynucleation mechanism.[18] At higher driving forces ($1.11<\sigma<1.69$), the rate of reaction is proportional to the supersaturation and is sensitive to changes in stirring speed. Thus it appears that the reaction at higher driving forces may be diffusion controlled. Moreover, it has been found that at very low driving forces ($\sigma<0.6$), OCP growth kinetics can be interpreted in terms of an integration controlled spiral growth mechanism.[19] In the light of these results, three supersaturation regions may be identified for OCP growth (i) at very low supersaturations the reactions follow a spiral dislocation mechanism, (ii) at intermediate supersaturation a polynucleation mechanism dominates the rate while (iii) at even higher driving forces the surface reactions become so fast that the transport of ions from bulk solution to the surface may become rate determining. It is interesting that even simple ions such as magnesium significantly influence the order of apparent stabilities. Thus for OCP, the addition of magnesium follows a Langmuir-type adsorption isotherm with modest rate inhibition. However this ion markedly inhibits HAP crystal growth while having little influence on the growth of DCPD.[17] The ability to control the supersaturations using the constant composition method also enables the growth of defect apatites of stoichiometry intermediate between OCP and HAP to be studied over a range of pH.[20]

MECHANISM OF DISSOLUTION

The observation that normal growth rates of many crystal surfaces decrease with time at sustained supersaturation has received considerable attention. In the case of salts such as sodium chlorate and potassium dihydrogen phosphate, it was suggested that the observed decrease in crystal growth could be related to a reduction in the number of defects on the crystal faces. A similar observed decrease in the growth rate along the z-axis of ammonium dihydrogen phosphate crystallites was attributed to the accumulation of inhibitor in the adsorption layer resulting in a change in supersaturation at the crystal surface.[21] It was postulated that the gradual adsorption of impurities reduced the two dimensional nucleation rate and that complete termination of growth would be achieved when the coverage was sufficiently large so as to prevent the formation of critical surface nuclei.

In the case of gypsum crystal growth, it was suggested that the decrease in rate was attributed to surface step bunching.[22] Although such a phenomenon involving either surface annealing or kink site inhibition could intuitively lead readily to the idea of crystal growth rate reduction, it was shown that the rate deceleration phenomenon was also displayed during the dissolution of sparingly soluble salts. Thus the dissolution rate of HAP microcrystals decreased with time and it was suggested that this could be attributed to increased smoothness of the crystal surface.[23]

More recently, studies of the dissolution kinetics of DCPD and OCP have been made using the CC method.[12] The rates of reaction were sensitive to changes in fluid dynamics (stirring speeds) only at higher undersaturations, becoming insensitive to stirring effects at lower undersaturations. This suggests that the rates are controlled by a combined mechanism of volume diffusion and surface processes and the latter dominate at lower undersaturations. For DCPD, the effective order of dissolution, $n = 1.4\pm0.1$ suggests a spiral dissolution mechanism. Calculations of activation energy barriers for the direct and indirect detachment models discussed above, suggest that the indirect detachment model with the ions leaving the surface only after diffusing along the surface from the kink sites is most appropriate for both DCPD and OCP.

Mathematically, the rate reduction is described by introducing a surface activity parameter, ρ, into Eq. 6 to yield Eq. 8.

$$J = k\,\rho\,F(m/m_0)G(\sigma) \tag{8}$$

Since CC experiments are made at constant undersaturation, changes in the surface activity factor (ρ at time t and ρ_0 initially) could be related to the corresponding rates of reactions by Eq. 9

$$\rho/\rho_0 = (J/J_0)\,(m/m_0)^{-2/3} \tag{9}$$

for isotropic three dimensional dissolution. Calculated surface activity parameters as a function of time show marked reductions with extent of dissolution for both OCP and DCPD. Moreover the surface activity decreased more rapidly at lower undersaturation. Studies involving changes in reagent purity confirmed that although they had a small effect on the rates of these surface controlled dissolution reactions, the marked decrease with extent of reaction could not be attributed to inhibition by these foreign ions.

Since dissolution of DCPD and OCP follow spiral mechanisms in which screw dislocations play an essential role, as the crystals dissolve the dislocation line will move closer to the edge of the crystallites with the eventual possibility of being dissolved away from the surface. Thus if a crystal surface contains three cooperative dislocations, they can send out three times as many spiral steps per unit area as a single dislocation. If one such dislocation is dissolved away, the apparent rate of dissolution will be reduced by 33%. If the surface contains only one dislocation, once it is removed, spiral dissolution will be terminated. This has been observed for both DCPD and OCP despite the fact that the solutions remain appreciably undersaturated. Further dissolution of the phases can proceed from crystal edges or by surface nucleation which is normally much slower. At relatively low undersaturations, the dissolution rates of DCPD and OCP are controlled by a detachment and a surface diffusion process. In this case, the rate is directly proportional to the step density on the surface and will be expected to decrease upon removal of the dislocation. At very high undersaturations, however, the rate is controlled by desorption and volume diffusion and does not depend as strongly upon surface topography. This explains why the rate decreases more rapidly at lower driving forces. For DCPD, the participation of volume diffusion at higher driving forces is more marked than in the case of OCP which remains surface controlled over a larger region of undersaturation.

In the case of HAP dissolution, there is little doubt that the reaction follows a polynucleation mechanism[23] with effective orders of reaction varying markedly with undersaturation.

CONCLUSION

Although numerous studies of calcium phosphate precipitation often refer to the exclusive formation of hydroxyapatite, it is clear that there are very few cases in which such a simplistic approach is justified. In almost all cases, the overall precipitation or dissolution reaction involves the formation of transient phases ranging from poorly characterized ACP's and defect apatites through the well characterized DCPD, TCP and OCP. Since the overall process involves both the formation and dissolution of such phases, an understanding of the mechanisms of these reactions is essential. In this paper we have discussed some of the more recent studies in which attempts have been made to elucidate the important steps involved in the reactions. Although thermodynamic driving forces provide unequivocal information as to whether a reaction is possible, kinetic effects may be very much more important in explaining the appearance or non-appearance of particular calcium phosphate phases during precipitation reactions. This is especially true in biomineralization processes in which the presence of other foreign ions and molecules can markedly change the growth and dissolution rates of selective calcium phosphate phases. In general, the thermodynamically more stable phases are more sensitive to the influence of such foreign substances. It is clear that factors such as the activity ratios of the lattice ions in the reacting solutions and changes in surface properties of the growing phases may be even more important considerations than those based simply on classical thermodynamic principles.

Acknowledgements: We thank the National Institutes of Health for a grant (DE03223) in support of this work.

REFERENCES

1. Nancollas, G. H., *In Vitro studies of calcium phosphate crystallization in Biomineralization. Chemical and Biochemical Perspectives*, Mann, S., Webb, J. and Williams, R.J.P., Eds., VCH Verlagsgesellschaft, Weinheim, 157, 1989.
2. Brown, W. E., Smith, J. P., Lehr, J. R. and Frazier, A. W., Crystal structure of octacalcium phosphate, Nature 196, 1048, 1962.
3. Francis, M. D. and Webb, N. C., Hydroxyapatite formation from hydrated calcium monohydrogen phosphate precursor, Calcified Tissue Res. 6, 335, 1971.
4. Nancollas, G. H., Phase transformation during precipitation of calcium salts, in *Biological Mineralization and Demineralization*, Nancollas, G. H., Ed., Springer-Verlag, New York, 79, 1982.
5. Betts, F., Blumenthal, N. C. and Posner, A. S., Bone mineralization, J. Crystal Growth 53, 63, 1981.
6. Brown, W. E., Schroeder, L. W. and Ferris, J. S., Interlayering of crystalline OCP and HAP, J. Phys. Chem. 83, 1385, 1979.
7. Davies, C. W., Ion association, London, Butterworths, 34, 1962.
8. Nancollas, G. H., Interaction in electrolyte solutions, Elsevier, Amsterdam, 1966, chap. 3.
9. Tomson, M. B., Nancollas, G. H., Mineralization kinetics: A constant composition approach, Science 200, 1059, 1978.
10. Ebrahimpour, A., Zhang, A., Nancollas, G. H., Dual constant composition method and its application to studies of phase transformation and crystallization of mixed phases, J. Crystal Growth 113, 83, 1991.
11. Zhang, J., Nancollas, G. H., Influence of calcium/sulfate molar ratio on the growth rate of calcium sulfate dihydrate at constant supersaturation, J. Crystal Growth 118, 287, 1992.
12. Zhang, J., Nancollas, G. H., Dissolution deceleration of calcium phosphate crystals at constant undersaturation, J. Crystal Growth 123, 251, 1992.
13. Chernov, A. A., The spiral growth of crystals, Soviet Phys. Uspekhi, 5, 116, 1961.
14. Gilmer, G. H., Ghez, R. and Cabrera, N., An analysis of combined surface and volume diffusion processes in crystal growth, J. Crystal Growth, 8, 79, 1971.
15. van der Eerden, J. P., The advance velocity of steps under the influence of volume and surface diffusion, by direct and indirect incorporation of growth units, J. Crystal Growth, 56, 174, 1982.
16. Christoffersen, J. and Christoffersen, M.R., A revised theory for the growth of crystals by surface nucleation, J. Crystal Growth, 1992.
17. Zhang, J. and Nancollas, G. H., Kink densities along a crystal surface step at low temperatures and under non equilibrium conditions, J. Crystal Growth 106, 181, 1990.
18. Heughebaert, J. C. and Nancollas, G. H., The kinetics of crystallization of octacalcium phosphate, J. Phys. Chem. 88, 2478, 1984.
19. Lundager Madsen, H. E., Calcium phosphate crystallization III. Overall growth kinetics of tetracalcium monohydrogen phosphate, Acta Chem. Scand., A36, 239, 1982.

20. Zawacki, S. J., Heughebaert, J. C. and Nancollas, G. H., The growth of non-stoichiometric apatite from aqueous solution at 37°C. II. Effect of pH upon the precipitated phase., J. Coll. Interface Sci., 135, 33, 1990.
21. Davey, R. J. and Mullin, J. W., J. Crystal Growth 23, 89, 1974.
22. van Rosmalen, Daudey, P. J. and Marchée, W. G. J., An analysis of growth experiments of gypsum crystals in suspension., J. Crystal Growth 52, 801, 1981.
23. Budz, J. A. and Nancollas, G. H., The mechanism of dissolution of hydroxyapatite and carbonated apatite in acidic solution., J. Crystal Growth 91, 490, 1988.

PATHOLOGICAL CRYSTALLIZATION OF CALCIUM OXALATE AND CALCIUM PHOSPHATE

Saeed R. Khan and Raymond L. Hackett
Department of Pathology
College of Medicine
University of Florida
Gainesville, FL 32611

INTRODUCTION

Crystallization and deposition of calcium salts are common phenomena (1). Generally the processes are physiologically necessary for the well being of the individual. But occasionally they are abnormal and pathological with devastating consequences causing a wide variety of diseases and disorders including urinary stones, dental calculus, salivary stones, biliary stones, crystal deposition in joints, various forms of ectopic calcification, and failure of catheters and bioprosthetic devices (2). While calcium phosphate deposition can be either physiological or pathological, calcium oxalate deposition is typically pathological. In spite of these differences, a number of similarities exist between the normal and abnormal crystallization processes; for example, both types of crystallization require existence of supersaturation, occur in the presence of nucleating substrates and are influenced positively as well as negatively by a variety of modulators. In addition, all products of crystallization are comprised of a crystalline phase and a non-crystalline phase, usually called matrix. A consensus is developing that both types of crystallization mechanisms involve cellular membranes, specifically their phospholipids which play an important initiating role (3). Using the example of urinary stones we will discuss here the role of membranes in crystallization of calcium phosphate (CaP) and calcium oxalate (CaOx).

Urinary stone formation or urolithiasis is a common urological disorder which afflicts 10% to 12% of the Western and Westernized populations (4). Stones can form anywhere in the urinary tract, kidneys, ureters or bladder but the ones formed in the kidneys are most destructive (5). The kidney is composed of an outer cortex and an inner medulla which terminates in the papilla. Urine leaves the kidney at the papillary tip. The functional unit of a kidney is called the nephron, a tubular structure which is lined by a continuous layer of cells, the tubular epithelium. Formation of stones in kidneys, particularly in their tubular lumina, is called nephrolithiasis. We have studied the structure of urinary stones by various microscopic and biochemical techniques and are investigating the mechanisms involved in formation of urinary stones by *in vitro* and *in vivo* procedures.

0-8493-4750-5/94/$0.00 + $.50

STRUCTURE OF CALCIFIC URINARY STONES

Urinary stones consist of two major components, crystals and matrix, the former accounting for up to 98% of the stone weight (6). CaOx and CaP are the two most common calcific crystals and usually occur together with CaOx constituting the bulk of the crystalline components in over 90% of the calcific stones. CaP, even though ubiquitous, is often present in very small quantities, comprising only 3 to 5% of the stone weight. Smaller CaP crystals typically appear as fillers between the larger CaOx crystals. All three forms of CaOx; calcium oxalate monohydrate (COM), calcium oxalate dihydrate (COD) and calcium oxalate trihydrate (COT) are found in the urinary stones. COM is encountered frequently while COT is rare. COD and COT being thermodynamically unstable require stabilizers for their existence and eventually transform into COM. Urine is normally supersaturated with respect to all three hydrates of CaOx and initial precipitation of COT is kinetically favored. Thus COT may play a key role in CaOx stone formation.

In most stones (7), CaP is usually present as apatite, sometimes as brushite (calcium hydrogen phosphate dihydrate) and on rare occasions as whitlockite (β-tri-calcium phosphate). Apatite occurs in two forms, hydroxylapatite (HAP) and carbonate apatite (CAP), both with varying degrees of ionic substitutions. HAP is present in stones formed in sterile urine while CAP is a major constituent of stones associated with infection.

In order to study matrix by microscopic techniques stones are demineralized (8,9) by treatment with ethylenediaminetetraacetic acid (EDTA). Demineralization of calcific stones causes a dissolution of crystals and formation of crystal ghosts preserving the architectural integrity of stones. Electron microscopic examination of crystals reveals that crystal ghosts are limited by a thin organic coat. Intercrystalline spaces are filled with loosely organized fibrils, amorphous material, membranous cellular degradation products and red cells, all of which contribute to the organic matrix of the stone. Histochemically, stone matrix is periodic acid schiff, colloidal iron (10) and alcian blue positive indicating the presence of neutral and acidic mucosubstances. Toluidine blue staining suggests the presence of sulfated acidic mucosubstances (11). The matrix is also sudan black positive (12), indicating the presence of phospholipids. Biochemically stone matrix consists of approximately 65% proteins, 15% carbohydrates and 11% lipids (6). Stones with calcific crystals contain as much as 10 times more phospholipids than organic stones such as uric acid (12).

URINARY STONE FORMATION

Stone formation proceeds in three stages (1) crystallization, (2) crystal retention, and (3) stone growth. Crystallization involves nucleation, growth and aggregation of crystals. But crystallization alone results in only crystalluria i.e. excretion of crystals in the urine. Urinary stone formation on the other hand begins when these crystals are retained within the urinary tract. Human urine is normally supersaturated with respect to calcium salts but the degree of urinary supersaturation is not sufficient for homogeneous nucleation of crystals. Thus crystal nucleation within the urine must be heterogeneous.

CALCIUM OXALATE CRYSTALLIZATION *IN VIVO*

To understand the mechanisms involved in CaOx crystallization and stone formation we studied CaOx crystal deposition in kidneys of male rats. Normal rats, like normal humans, do not form kidney stones. Induction of hyperoxaluria is essential (13). Acute hyperoxaluria causes rapid deposition while a chronic hyperoxaluria induces delayed deposition of CaOx crystals in the kidneys. Acute hyperoxaluria was induced by intraperitoneal administration of sodium oxalate which resulted in the appearance of CaOx crystals in the rat renal tubules within 15 minutes. Crystals appeared first in the proximal tubules and then in the rest of the nephron. Initially crystals were restricted to the tubular lumina but later were also seen in the interstitium. Crystallization was associated with injury to renal epithelium lining the proximal tubules (14) and was manifested by an increase in urinary enzymes of proximal tubular origin (15) and shedding of the proximal tubular brush border membrane as well as the entire cells into the urine. Membrane shedding frequently preceded the appearance of crystals in renal tubular lumen and crystals were invariably found associated with vesicular, membranous and fibrillar material (Fig. 1). Cytochemical staining suggested that calcium complexation with brush border membrane started the process of CaOx crystal formation (14).

Chronic hyperoxaluria was induced by administration of ethylene glycol, a precursor of oxalate, in drinking water at a concentration of 0.25% or 0.75%. Ethylene glycol was administered alone or in association with subcutaneous injections of gentamicin sulphate that results in membranuria of proximal tubular cellular origin. Administration of ethylene glycol for 24 days at 0.25%, produced mild hyperoxaluria but did not cause crystalluria or deposition of crystals in the renal tubules. It was however associated with an increase in urinary excretion of N-acetyl-β-glucosaminidase indicating injury to the proximal tubular epithelial cells (15). But when rats on 0.25% ethylene glycol were exposed to gentamicin sulfate they developed CaOx crystalluria by day 4 of the combined protocol (16). Crystals isolated from the urine were found attached to a membranous material. Apparently mild hyperoxaluria itself was not enough to induce crystallization and imposition of membranuria was necessary for crystal formation. Rats receiving only 0.75% ethylene glycol generally developed CaOx nephrolithiasis after 2 weeks. Crystals were preferentially located in the collecting ducts of the renal papilla and were found mixed with amorphous, fibrillar and membranous cellular degradation products.

CALCIUM OXALATE CRYSTALLIZATION *IN VITRO*

All our animal studies indicated an intimate relationship between cellular membrane and crystallization of calcific crystals. To determine the role of membranes in crystal nucleation we isolated brush border membrane of the rat renal proximal tubules and incubated them at 37°C in metastable solutions of low CaOx relative supersaturation of 6, 10 or 12. Calcium oxalate relative supersaturation of mammalian urine can reach 25 (17). We used two crystallization techniques; 1) conventional solution depletion technique in which concentration of calcium and oxalate ions were allowed to decrease during

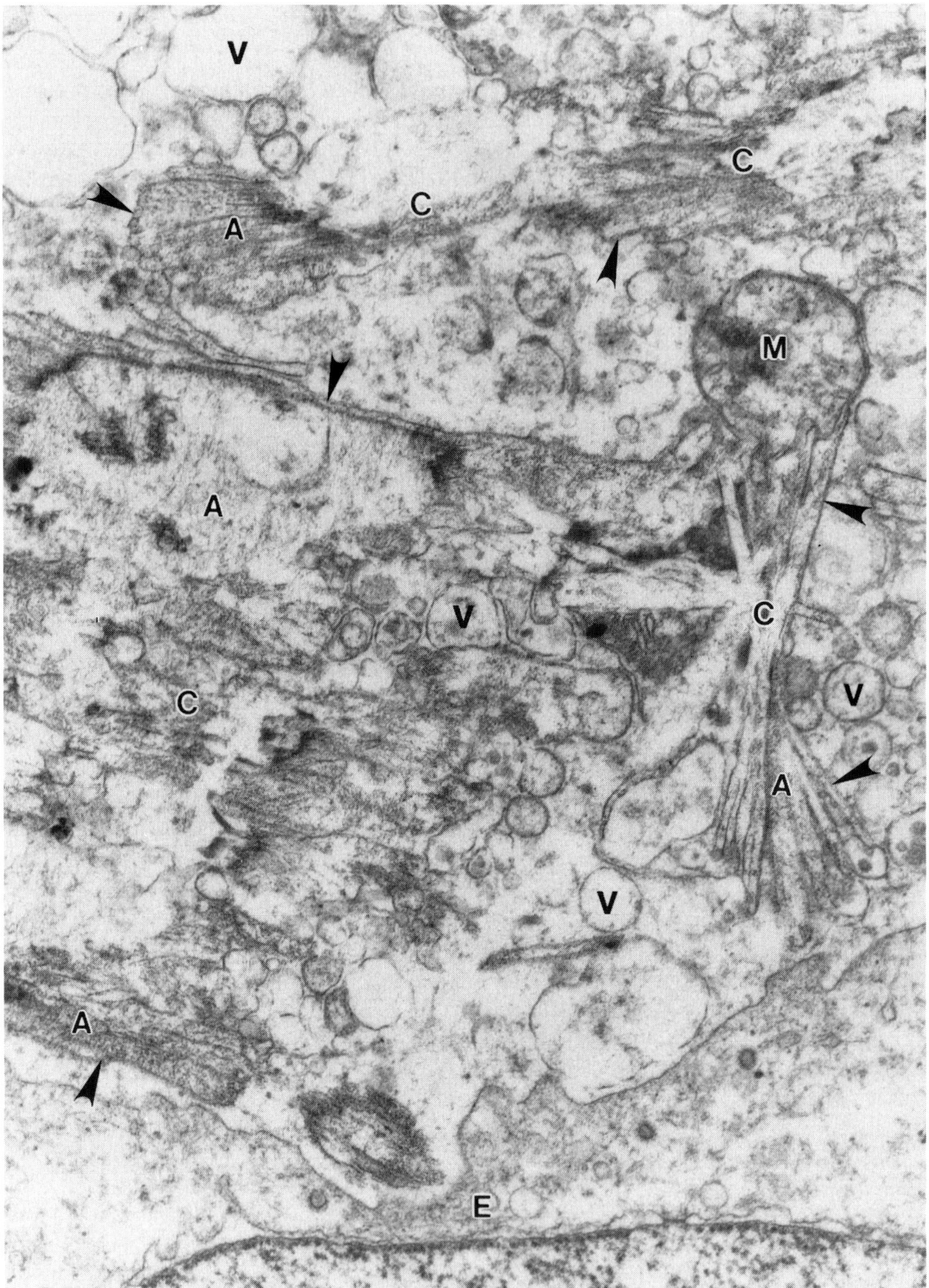

Figure 1. Ghosts of calcium oxalate crystals (C) in the lumen of a rat renal tubule following intraperitoneal injection of sodium oxalate. Ghosts are limited by electron dense membranes (arrowheads), contain amorphous material (A) inside and are intimately associated with cellular degradation products including membrane bound vesicles (V) and a mitochondrion (M). An epithelial cell (E) is present nearby (X27,000).

the precipitation; and 2) constant composition technique where concentrations of calcium and oxalate ions were maintained constant during the precipitation. In depletion experiments addition of brush border membrane vesicles caused precipitation of calcium oxalate from a solution of RSS 6 (18), which would otherwise not support crystallization. In the constant composition experiments, addition of the membrane vesicles reduced the nucleation lag time from 127±4 minutes to 32±17 minutes in case of a solution of RSS 10, and from 22±14 minutes to 7.8±3 minutes in case of a solution of RSS 12. In both types of crystallization experiments, crystals were seen in close contact with the membrane vesicles. They may have actually started inside the vesicles. Newly formed crystals were thin and plate-like with serrated edges. Crystals isolated long time after the commencement of crystal nucleation were well formed, typically monoclinic in habit with sharp edges. They were identified by x-ray diffraction as calcium oxalate monohydrate.

CALCIUM PHOSPHATE CRYSTALLIZATION *IN VIVO*

Calcium phosphate nephrolithiasis can be induced in rats by dietary manipulations (19). Weanling female rats fed a semi-purified AIN76 diet for 18 days developed CaP calculi in their tubules. These calculi were detectable by light microscopy on day 12 and were located intraluminally at the corticomedullary junction. Ultrastructural changes seen in proximal tubules prior to the intraluminal deposition included increased intracellular calcium, complexation of calcium with the brush border membrane, and vesiculation and shedding of the brush border. These vesicles were later seen inside the intraluminal calculi.

CRYSTAL RETENTION

As discussed earlier, crystal formation is only one stage in the development of stone disease and in most people the process does not proceed any further. Individual crystals remain small and free and are uneventfully eliminated. Only when crystals are retained within the urinary system do they become stone nuclei with a chance to grow and eventually develop into urinary calculi. An analysis of supersaturations prevalent in the urine, anatomical dimensions of the urinary tract and the rate of urinary flow through them, indicates that crystal growth rate in the urine is not fast enough for their individual retention (20). However, they can aggregate and form a large enough unit that is not expelled (21). Evidence that crystal aggregation plays such a role is obtained by morphological examination of renal tubules in experimentally induced calcium oxalate urolithiasis in rats, by study of human crystalluria particles and by examination of nuclei of human urinary stones. Crystals of calcium oxalate are almost always present as aggregates in the renal tubules and often appear to totally obstruct the tubular lumen. Human urinary stone formers excrete larger and more aggregated crystals than the normal individuals (22) and nuclei of the majority of calcific human urinary stones contain aggregates of crystals (6,7). Thus, crystal aggregation, the most rapid and effective mechanism of mass accretion, appears to play an important initiating role in stone formation. Of the various forces by which aggregates are held together, van der Waal forces and viscous binding forces appear to be most involved in aggregation of urinary crystals (22). Viscous binding results from inter-particle bridging by a polymeric material such as matrix mucoproteins. One end of the polymer molecule attaches to the surface of one crystal and the other end to the surface of another crystal. This particle to particle apposition is then followed by the formation of solid bridges.

In vivo studies indicate that crystals can also be retained by adhering to the damaged epithelium and their exposed basal lamina (23). Urinary stones with eccentric nuclei growing on the papillary tips clearly demonstrate the importance of crystal attachment to the stone development (24,25).

STONE GROWTH

Once crystals are retained and a nucleus is established, stones increase in size by crystal growth and aggregation as well as nucleation of new crystals on the surface of the existing stone. Crystal growth and nucleation of new crystals on stone surfaces can occur at relatively low supersaturations while nucleation of crystals in the urine to eventually aggregate with the growing stones would require higher supersaturations. In the case of very low supersaturation a stone may stay small and reside in the urinary tract for a long time. Since urine can be supersaturated for a variety of salts and urinary supersaturation may change a number of times during the life of a stone, crystals that aggregate with the growing stone and nucleate on their surfaces may be different from the crystals that constituted the original stone nucleus. Thus a stone containing more than one type of crystal indicates periodic supersaturation of urine with respect to the salts of the constituent crystals. It has been suggested that stones with mixed crystalline composition are formed by epitaxy, a process in which a substrate induces crystal nucleation because the atomic arrangement at its surface is chemically and structurally compatible with the new crystal. But a close examination of atomic structures of a variety of crystals that occur together in the urinary stones has led investigators to conclude that epitaxy can not play a major role in stone formation (26). However, it is possible for a urinary macromolecule adsorbed on a crystal surface to act as a substrate for epitaxial nucleation of other crystals. A number of macromolecules and cellular degradation products present in the urine are incorporated in the growing stone and become a part of the stone matrix. Stones also undergo a process of maturation during which unstable crystals of higher hydrate may transform into more stable low hydrate forms.

DISCUSSION AND CONCLUSIONS

Pathological calcification can be subdivided into two major categories: 1. metastatic calcification which occurs in undamaged tissue and is associated with elevated serum levels of calcium and 2. dystrophic calcification which occurs in injured tissue but normal serum levels of calcium (2). In normal circumstances free calcium concentration in the cytosol is approximately 10^{-7}M, while extracellular calcium is approximately 10^{-3}M. This concentration gradient across the membranes is largely maintained by intracellular buffering and energy requiring processes which extrude calcium into the extracellular space or into mitochondria. Calcium enters the cells by diffusion but is removed from the cells by an energy requiring adenosine 5'-triphosphate (ATP) dependent pump. In metastatic calcification more calcium from the serum enters the cell through diffusion and is ejected back or segregated into the mitochondria where it is deposited as calcium phosphate. Continuous deposition of calcium phosphate in the mitochondria results in reduced ATP production. Consequently the cellular capacity to expel calcium declines and the amount of intracellular calcium increases. Eventually preformed mineral in the mitochondria can provide a nidus for further calcification of the cell, subsequently advancing into the extracellular space.

Dystrophic calcification starts in cells that are already damaged. Cellular membranes are non-functional and calcium pumps are non-operative. Thus calcium levels within and without the cell are the same. In these circumstances cells and cell membrane derived vesicles develop localized areas of high ionic concentration and supersaturation resulting in the deposition of crystals. Moreover phospholipid distribution in the cellular membranes is asymmetrical. Inner side of the membrane has more acidic phospholipids such as phosphatidylserine which have strong affinity for calcium. Thus injury to the membrane results in increased cytosolic calcium which can form complexes with the acidic phospholipids available on the inner surface of the membranes, thus initiating the process of crystallization.

According to current concepts initial calcium phosphate deposition in a number of calcific diseases occurs in association with cellular membranes which are present at the calcification sites either as limiting membrane of the so called matrix vesicles (27) or as cellular degradation products. For example, in medial sclerosis of the large arteries and in calcific disease of the aortic valve, electron microscopic studies have established that extracellular vesicles serve as initial sites of apatite deposition (28,29). The same is true of atherosclerotic plaque formation. Calcification of tumors is also associated with membranes, for example intracellular membrane vesicles appear to nucleate the apatite of the psammoma bodies in ovarian tumors. When human meningiomas were cultured *in vitro*, psammoma bodies arose in association with extracellular vesicles. Extracellular vesicles derived from degenerating neoplastic cells were also shown to be involved in neoplastic calcinosis. In tympanosclerosis of the middle ear, matrix vesicles derived from fibroblastic cells were the initial site of apatite deposition. Calcification during apatitic osteoarthritis and calcifying tendonitis is also shown to be matrix vesicle mediated. During placental calcification hydroxyapatite precipitates in association with extracellular membranous vesicles (30). Calcification of bioprosthetic heart vales fabricated from porcine aortic valves or bovine pericardium, a main cause of their functional failure is also membrane mediated (31). Initial nuclei of calcification are associated with cellular membrane fragments derived from the pig cusp cells in case of porcine heart valves and from connective tissue cells in case of bovine pericardium. Calcification of intrauterine devices also appears to be initiated by cellular membranous material that is deposited on the devices during their exposure to the uterine fluid (32). Dental plaque and calculus formation is yet another example of calcification initiated by cellular membrane (33). Membranes of microorganisms present in the dental plaque nucleate hydroxyapatite and thus initiate the calculus formation.

One of the main reasons for cellular membranes to act as specific nucleators of calcium phosphate is suggested to be the presence of lipids and particularly the acidic phospholipids therein (3, 34, 35). Lipids have been demonstrated both histochemically and biochemically at physiological as well as pathological calcification sites. Although lipids account for a relatively small portion of the organic matrix, 7-14% of bone, 2-6% of dentin, 12-22% of newly mineralized enamel, 9.6% of submandibular salivary gland calculi and 10.2% of supragingival calculi, they have been isolated from matrices of all types of mineralized tissues. In vitro, membranes, acidic phospholipids, and lipid extracts from various calcified tissues have been shown to initiate the formation of calcium phosphate from metastable solutions.

Two major membrane-associated lipidic elements which have been shown to be involved in mineralization are proteolipids and calcium-phospholipid-phosphate complexes (CPLX). Calcium-acidic phospholipid-phosphate complexes were first isolated from calcifying tumors and were believed to be associated with the initiation of calcification in these tumors. Such complexes have since been isolated from both normal and pathological calcification sites including bovine dentin, rat, rabbit, bovine and human bone, healing fracture callus, mineralization front of human articular cartilage, human atherosclerotic aortas, and salivary stones. Moreover, CPLX have also been isolated from matrix vesicles, the membrane bound extracellular structures found at sites of new calcification. These complexes have been shown to cause hydroxyapatite deposition both in vitro and in vivo. Recent studies have established a relationship between proteolipids and CPLX formation. Calcifiable proteolipids may be involved in organizing the membrane phosphatidylserine in proper conformation for the formation of complexes during the initial interactions of calcium, phosphate and acidic phospholipids. In addition, proteolipids may also act as ionophores promoting proton transport.

In this brief review of some of our work and those of others relating to calcium oxalate and calcium phosphate crystallization we have provided evidence that calcific nephrolithiasis is a process of dystrophic calcification. Formation and deposition of calcific crystals in the urinary tract is associated with and may be preceded by shedding of the renal epithelial brush border membrane vesicles into the tubular lumen. Both types of crystals are formed in close contact with the cellular membrane. Brush border membrane vesicles isolated from the rat renal cortex are capable of inducing calcium oxalate crystal nucleation *in vitro* from a metastable solution of calcium oxalate of a low relative supersaturation. In addition, membranous cellular degradation products are common in the urinary stones and phospholipids constitute a substantial portion of the urinary stone matrix.

ACKNOWLEDGMENTS

Supported in part by NIH grants #RO1 DK414345 and PO1 DK20586.

REFERENCES

1. Lowenstam, H.A. and Weiner, S., Mineralization by organisms and the evolution of biomineralization. in *Biomineralization and Biological Metal Accumulation*, Westbrook, P. and DeJong, E.W., Eds., D. Reidel Publishing Company, Dodrecht, Holland, 1983, 191.
2. Anderson, H.C., Calcific Diseases, *Arch. Path. and Lab. Med.*, 107, 341, 1983.

3. Boskey, A.L., Phospholipids and calcification, in *Calcified Tissue*, Hukins, D.W.L., Ed, CRC Press, Boca Raton, Florida, 1989, 215.
4. Sirekowsky, R., Finlayson, B., Landes, R., Finlayson, C.D. and Sirekowsky, N., The frequency of urolithiasis in hospital discharge diagnoses in the United States, *Investigative Urology*, 15, 438, 1978.
5. Finlayson, B., Renal lithiasis in review, *Urolo. Clin. North Am.*, 1, 181, 1974.
6. Khan, S.R., Structure and development of Calcific Urinary Stones, in *Calcification in Biological Systems*, Bonnuci, E, Ed., CRC Press, Boca Raton, Florida, 1992, 345.
7. Otnes, B., Urinary stone analysis, methods, materials and value, *Scand. J. Urol. Nephrol., Suppl. 71, 1, 1983.*
8. Khan, S.R., Finlayson, B. and Hackett, R.L., Agar-embedded urinary stones: a technique useful for studying microscopic architecture, *J. Urol.*, 130, 992, 1983.
9. Khan, S.R. and Hackett, R.L., Microstructure of decalcified human calcium oxalate urinary stones, *Scanning Electron Microsc.*, 2, 925, 1984.
10. Khan, S.R. and Hackett, R.L., Histochemistry of colloidal iron stained crystal associated material in urinary stones and experimentally induced intrarenal deposits in rats, *Scanning Electron Microsc.* 2, 761, 1986.
11. Watanabe, T., Histochemical studies on mucosubstances in urinary stones, *Tohoku J. Exp. Med.*, 107, 345, 1972.
12. Khan, S.R., Shevock, P.N. and Hackett, R.L., Presence of lipids in urinary stones, *Calcif. Tissue Intl.*, 42, 91, 1988.
13. Khan, S.R., Pathogenesis of oxalate urolithiasis: Lessons from experimental studies with rats, *Am. J. Kid. Dis.*, 17, 398, 1991.
14. Dykstra, M.J. and Hackett, R.L., Ultrastructural events in early calcium oxalate crystal formation in rats, *Kid. Intl. 15, 640, 1979.*
15. Khan, S.R., Shevock, P.N. and Hackett, R.L., Urinary enzymes and calcium oxalate urolithiasis, *J. Urol.*, 142, 846, 1989.
16. Hackett, R.L., Shevock, P.N. and Khan, S.R., Cell injury associated calcium oxalate crystalluria, *J. Urol.*, 144, 1535, 1990.
17. Finlayson, B., Physicochemical aspects of urolithiasis, *Kid. Intl. 13, 334, 1978.*
18. Khan, S.R., Shevock, P.N. and Hackett, R.L., Membrane associated crystallization of calcium oxalate in vitro, *Calcif. Intl.*, 46, 116, 1989.
19. Nguyen, H.T. and Woodard, J.C., Intranephronic calculosis in rats, *Am. J. Pathol.*, 100, 39, 1980.
20. Finlayson, B., The expectation of free or fixed particles in urinary stone disease, *Invest. Urol.*, 15, 442, 1978.
21. Khan, S.R. and Hackett, R.L., Retention of calcium oxalate crystals in renal tubules, *Scanning Microscopy*, 5, 707, 1991.
22. Robertson, W.G. and Peacock, M., Pathogenesis of urolithiasis, in *Urolithiasis, Etiology, Diagnosis,* Schneider, H.-J., Ed., Springer-Verlag, Berlin, 1985, 185.
23. Khan, S.R., Finlayson, B. and Hackett, R.L., Experimental calcium oxalate nephrolithiasis in rat, role of renal papilla, *Am. J. Pathol.*, 107, 59, 1982.
24. Randall, A., The origin and growth of renal calculi, *Ann. Surg.*, 105, 1009, 1937.

25. Cifuentes-Delatte, L., Minon-Cifuentes, J. and Medina, J.A., New studies on papillary calculi, *J. Urol.*, 137, 1024, 1987.
26. Mandel, N.S. and Mandel, G.S., Epitaxis between stone forming crystals at the atomic level, in *Urolithiasis: Clinical and Basic Research*, Smith, L.H., Robertson, W.G. and Finlayson, B., Eds., Plenum Press, New York, 1981, 469.
27. Sela, J., Schwartz, Z., Swain, L.D. and Boyan, B.D., The role of matrix vesicles in calcification, in *Calcification in Biological Systems*, Bonnuci, E, Ed., CRC Press, Boca Raton, Florida, 1992, 73.
28. Kim, K.M., Calcification of matrix vesicles in human aortic valve and aortic media, *Fed. Proc.*, 25, 156, 1976.
29. Kim, K.M., Calcification in aging canine aortic valve, *Scanning Electron Microsc.*, 3, 1151, 1986.
30. Varma, V.A. and Kim, K.M., Placental calcification, *Scanning Electron Microsc.*, 4, 1567, 1985.
31. Schoen, F.J., Harasaki, H., Kim, K.M., Anderson, H.C. and Levy, R.J., Biomaterial-associated calcification: pathology, mechanisms, and strategies for prevention, *J. Biomed. Mat. Res.*, 22, 11, 1988.
32. Khan, S.R. and Wilkinson, E.J., Scanning electron microscopy, x-ray diffraction, and electron microprobe analysis of calcific deposits on intrauterine contraceptive devices, *Human Pathol.*, 16, 732, 1985.
33. Boyan B.D., Swain, L.D. and Everett, M.M., Mechanisms of microbial mineralization, in *Calcification in Biological Systems*, Bonnuci, E, Ed., CRC Press, Boca Raton, Florida, 1992, 129.
34. Boskey, A.L., Current concepts of the physiology and biochemistry of calcification, *Clin. Orthop. Rel. Res.*, 157, 225, 1981.
35. Boskey, A.L., Mineral-matrix interactions in bone and cartilage, *Clin. Orthop. Rel. Res.* 281, 244, 1992.

CHARACTERIZATION OF MINERAL PHASES IN CARDIOVASCULAR CALCIFICATION

Branko B. Tomazic
ADAHF Paffenbarger Research Center
National Institute of Standards and Technology
Gaithersburg, MD 20899

I. INTRODUCTION

The hardening of arteries is commonly understood as a deposition of cholesterol in the pathways of the cardiovascular system. An additional significant complication is pathologic calcification. The latter complication is quite often overlooked in spite of the fact that it takes place in both blood vessels[1] and heart tissues.[2] Cardiovascular bioprostheses, when used for a prolonged time, also host calcific deposits that may severely limit the longevity and performance of the bioprostheses.[3-6]

The formation of cardiovascular calcific deposits (CD) needs to be viewed in the context of the larger picture of biomineralization that encompasses the formation of other types of biominerals that constitute bones and teeth. There is an impressive amount of scientific information on chemistry and mechanisms of formation of biominerals or biological calcium phosphates in bodies of vertebrates. Application of this knowledge can help the understanding of the special case of formation of pathologic biomineral in cardiovascular system.

Pathologic cardiovascular calcification is a complex process governed by many biochemical factors, including proteins,[7] proteolipids,[8] phospholipids,[9] and cholesterol.[10] Urist[7] described the aorta as a site that calcifies more readily than other soft tissues. His explanation for this greater frequency takes into account many biogenic factors, such as enzymes, abnormal cell function, inflammation and altered hydrostatic forces. All these factors may greatly affect the surface activity of noncollagenous tissue matrix protein, the postulated site for the formation of tissue-Ca^{2+} complexes. These complex species are responsible for initiating the "triphasic mechanism" of localization/formation of calcium mineral deposits.[7] Boskey[11] provides a comprehensive review of the role of organelles and macromolecules in calcification. Phosphatidylserine, a lipid component of the cell membrane, has also been proposed to form a 1:1 Ca^{2+}-phospholipid complex, a possible precursor to pathologic mineral nucleus formation.[9] The study of co-crystallization of cholesterol and calcium phosphate *in vitro*[12] supports a proposition that cholesterol has an important role in aorta calcification *in vivo*.[10] However, a comparative evaluation of the significance and role of these factors has not been accomplished; therefore, the exact mechanism of cardiovascular calcification is not completely known.

0-8493-4750-5/94/$0.00 + $.50

This review chapter provides compositional information on the inorganic component of cardiovascular CD. More extensive knowledge of the reactivity of different calcium phosphate phases can provide essential information on the mechanism of formation of pathologic cardiovascular CD and, in this way, help to identify the precursor(s). The combined physicochemical information, supported by solubility measurements, suggests octacalcium phosphate (OCP), $Ca_4H(PO_4)_3 \cdot 2.5\ H_2O$, as a precursor in the formation of cardiovascular CD.[6] The results of comparative *in vitro* and *in vivo* mineralization of bovine pericardium provided additional support that OCP may be a valid precursor in the formation of bioapatites.[13] Subtle differences in chemical composition elucidate the nature of the maturation process, which may be understood as a time-dependent hydrolytic transformation of precursor(s). Objective and comprehensive information on the mechanism of pathologic calcification is essential for achieving control and suppression of the process at the outset in blood vessels, tissues and bioprostheses.

The topic of this review has been addressed through different approaches and researchers, as referenced in text. The major emphasis of the present review is on the author's research, part of which has been reported.[6,13]

II. MATERIALS

The following types of cardiovascular CD were examined and characterized: (1) atherosclerotic deposits retrieved from the intima layer of calcified thoracic and abdominal aortas from post-autopsy of human subjects, 40-80 years of age; the aortas were classified as grade IV (14); (2) bioprosthetic total artificial heart (TAH) calcification (isolated from polyurethane ventricular assist devices of TAH) implanted into experimental animals, provided by Hershey Medical Center, Hershey, PA); (3) bioprosthetic heart valve deposits (isolated from surgically retrieved porcine valve bioprostheses serving patients from 2-13 years and provided by Brigham and Women's Hospital, Boston, MA); (4) aortic and mitral valve CD formed under conditions of a) aortic stenosis, b) senile aortic stenosis, c) rheumatic aortic stenosis, or d) rheumatic mitral stenosis (isolated from surgically retrieved heart valves from four groups of 10 patients, age group 51-84 years, and provided by Mayo Clinic, Rochester, MN). (5) In addition to pathologic cardiovascular CD, the deposits formed in bovine pericardium (BP) segments were critically examined in order to compare calcification that occurs under *in vitro* (BP segments immersed into supersaturated calcium phosphate medium) and *in vivo* (BP segments subcutaneously implanted in rats) conditions.

III. METHODS*

The methods used include isolation and purification of CD to become reference materials for detailed physicochemical characterization, involving

* Certain commercial materials and equipment are identified in this paper to specify the experimental procedure. In no instance does such identification imply recommendation or endorsment by the National Institute of Standards and Technology or ADA Health Foundation or that the materials or equipment identified are necessarily the best available for the purpose.

chemical analyses of major and minor constituents, structural and morphological description and solubility properties.

A. ISOLATION OF CD MATERIALS

1. Atherosclerotic Calcific Deposits

The aortas were refrigerated (-30°C) after autopsy. Isolation included thawing, dissection and removal of mineral deposits from adjoining tissue, and careful processing as described.[6] After separation, cryogenic grinding and deproteination, the CD materials were stored in a refrigerator until further use. This approach was applied to other types of examined CD. The amounts of native CD isolated from the intima layer of abdominal or thoracic aortas varied from 1 to 30 g, dry weight.

2. Bioprosthetic TAH Calcific Deposits

The removal of CD from ventricular assist devices and further processing outlined above, was reported.[6] The amounts of TAH CD were up to 2 g, dry weight native biomineral.

3. Bioprosthetic Heart Valve Calcific Deposits

After surgical explantation, the porcine valves (PV) were rinsed with saline solution and stored in neutral phosphate-buffered 10% formalin, which does not *change the calcium content* in calcified tissue.[15] Later, CD were removed from bioprostheses and carefully processed.[16] The amounts of native CD isolated from a PV varied from 0.1 to 0.8 g, dry weight.

4. Aortic and Mitral Heart Valve Calcific Deposits

The same separation and buffered formalin solution storage procedure used in 3 was used for surgically-retrieved aortic and mitral heart valves. The amounts of retrieved native CD varied from 0.2 to 3.5 g/valve, dry weight.

5. Bovine Pericardium Calcific Deposits

In vitro and *in vivo* mineralization of glutaraldehyde-treated BP and the recovery and processing of segments have been described in detail.[13] A fraction of the segment was used for histologic characterization.

B. PURIFICATION OF CALCIFIC DEPOSITS

An important objective of the present work was to isolate the inorganic component of CD, preferably without structural or compositional alteration of biominerals. Hydrazine[17] and hypochlorite treatments[18] were applied and critically evaluated for deproteination of biominerals .[19]

C. CHEMICAL AND STRUCTURAL CHARACTERIZATION OF CALCIFIC DEPOSITS

The listed methods were utilized to obtain comprehensive information on chemical composition of major and minor constituents of CD,[1] structural and phase information,[2] molecular and bonding information,[3] morphology, refractive properties and spatially resolved x-ray microanalysis[4] and physicochemical solubility properties.[5]

1. Chemical Analysis

Weighed amounts of CD were dissolved, and Ca, Na, Mg contents were determined by atomic absorption spectroscopy (AA). Phosphate content was determined spectrophotometrically (20); the fraction of HPO_4^{2-} was determined from the difference in absorbance of molybdo-vanadate-phosphate complex between hydrolyzed and nonhydrolyzed samples.[6,19,21] Carbonate analysis was performed by a modified Conway microdiffusion method.[22] The fluoride content of deproteinated atherosclerotic CD was determined by an ion-selective fluoride electrode.[23]

2. X-ray Diffraction

Native and deproteinated CD were characterized by x-ray diffraction (XRD).[6] The powder patterns were compared with JCPDS[24] for selected calcium phosphate phases. The crystallinity of the apatite phase was evaluated separately by measurement of the width at half maximum intensity ($\beta_{1/2}$) of the (002) diffraction peak.[17]

3. Fourier Transform Infrared Spectroscopy (FTIR)

FTIR spectroscopy of native and deproteinated CD was performed with a Nicolet 7000 FTIR spectrometer, and 100 FTIR scans were performed over a 400-4000 cm^{-1} range.

4. Scanning Electron Microscopic, Electron Microprobe and Optical Microscopic Analysis

The morphology and chemical composition of atherosclerotic CD were examined with a Cambridge 250 Mark II scanning electron microscope (SEM), equipped with a Princeton Gamma-Tech energy dispersive x-ray analyzer (EDX) system.[6] Deproteinated pieces of CD were placed on a carbon stub, gold plated and scanned by standard SEM preparation and observation procedures. Ca, P, Na, and Mg concentrations were determined with FRAME C correction procedures.[25] The morphology of native and deproteinated bioprosthetic heart valve CD was examined with a JEOL JSM-5200 or JEOL JSM-6400 scanning electron microscope.[19]

A Leitz Ortholux polarizing microscope was used to examine optical properties of atherosclerotic and bioprosthetic deposits. Measurements of average refractive indices, *n*, of microcrystalline materials were performed by the immersion method.[26]

5. Solubility Measurements

Solubility is one of the most important physicochemical characteristics of pathological cardiovascular CD materials. It provides information on the nature of the biomineral in the deposits and on the mechanism of its formation. The same criteria apply to the determination of the solubilities of other biominerals like bone and teeth, that has been extensively studied and reported.[27]

The solubilities of deproteinated CD were determined by equilibrating samples of finely ground biominerals with dilute solutions of phosphoric acid. The details of the equilibration procedures are described elsewhere.[6] The solution data were used to calculate solubilities expressed as ion activity products (IAP) for the representative calcium-phosphate phases: hydroxyapatite (HAP), $Ca_5(PO_4)_3OH$, octacalcium phosphate (OCP), $Ca_4H(PO_4)_3 \cdot 2.5\ H_2O$, tricalcium phosphate (TCP), $Ca_3(PO_4)_2$, and dicalcium phosphate dihydrate (DCPD), $CaHPO_4 \cdot 2H_2O$. The pIAP for the above calcium phosphate phases are defined as:

$$pIAP_{DCPD} = -\log (Ca^{2+})(HPO_4^{2-}) \quad (1)$$

$$pIAP_{OCP} = -\log (Ca^{2+})^4 (PO_4^{3-})^3 (H^+) \quad (2)$$

$$pIAP_{TCP} = -\log (Ca^{2+})^3 (PO_4^{3-})^2 \quad (3)$$

$$pIAP_{HAP} = - \log (Ca^{2+})^5 (PO_4^{3-})^3 (OH^-) \quad (4)$$

(parentheses represent ionic activities).

IAP values were calculated with a computer program that calculates ion activity coefficients and takes into account $Ca\text{-}PO_4$ complex ion equilibria (28), as well as $Ca\text{-}CO_3$ complex formation (29) when systems were equilibrated under the flow of a CO_2/N_2 gas mixture. The solubility properties of CD are presented by chemical potential plots (CPP), which are useful in multicomponent systems (27). CPP were derived by plotting $-\log (Ca^{2+})(OH^-)^2$ against $-\log (H^+)^3(PO_4^{3-})$ values, yielding a straight line with a slope of $- 1/x = a$, where x corresponds to the Ca/P molar ratio of salt(s), which control the equilibrium condition. The term $K_{XZ} = b$ is the intercept of CPP that is the constant specific to the applicable calcium phosphate salt. The x values for HAP, TCP, OCP and DCPD are 1.66, 1.5, 1.33 and 1.0 respectively, and the corresponding CPPs are provided to indicate the relative solubilities of CD in comparison with stoichiometric calcium phosphate compounds. This can give some indication of the physicochemical identity of any particular CD.

C. RESULTS

1. Chemical Composition of Calcified Deposits

The deproteination procedures efficiently removed the organic fraction from CD materials. After hydrazine or hypochlorite treatment, the organic fraction of 20-30 wt% was reduced to less than 1-2 wt%.[6,19] The deproteinated CD became suitable for structural (FTIR), micro-Raman and solubility characterization. The chemical compositions of multisite cardiovascular CD are shown in Table I, along with the composition of experimentally formed CD.

The quantitative chemical composition data on the large number of specimens isolated from different sites of the cardiovascular system show that the CD are calcium phosphates that contain several inorganic components such as carbonate, acidic phosphate, sodium, magnesium and fluoride. The presence of these chemical species in other bioapatites has been well documented and extensively reviewed.[30] All CD materials, regardless of the site of their formation, contain an appreciable fraction of carbonate (Table I). When the fraction of carbonate is expressed as weight %, amounts of 6.99±0.59% (n=10) for aortic and 6.91±0.39% (n=3) for TAH bioprosthetic, hydrazine-deproteinated CD, were observed. After equilibration in dilute hydrochloric acid (20 mg CD/ml 0.01 $m\cdot L^{-1}$ HCl), the carbonate content decreased to approximately 4.7%, and remained practically constant during and after 10 repeated equilibrations. This finding indicates that a fraction of carbonate is loosely bound, perhaps at the surface of CD, while the larger fraction is incorporated in the inorganic lattice of CD. Independent analysis of 7 aortic CD showed a content of 1221±409 ppm of fluoride (1221±409 μg F/g CD) and a Ca/F ratio of 131±34. A similar fluoride content was found in TAH CD. For comparison, the fluoride content in fluoroapatite is 37700 ppm and the Ca/F ratio is 5. The data presented in Table I make it possible to compare the average composition of three types of hydrazine deproteinated CD:

Table 1.
Chemical Composition Multisite Calcific Deposits
(all compositions are expresed as molar ratios).

Sample	(n)	Ca/P	Na/P	Mg/P	CO_3/P	HPO_4/P
AN	(5)	1.74	N.A.	N.A.	0.197	0.024
		0.03	-			0.007
A*	(10)	1.73	0.063	0.043	0.244	N.A.
S.D.		0.06	0.006	0.007	0.024	
TAH N	(4)	1.74	0.061	0.056	0.221	0.021
S.D.		0.08	0.037	0.007	0.082	0.008
TAH*	(3)	1.75	0.047	0.048	0.238	N.A.
S.D.		0.08	0.020	0.003	0.017	
C.A.	(2)	1.71	0.087	0.040	0.201	N.A.
MC	(1)	1.56	0.267	0.042	N.A.	0.092
MC*	(1)	1.61	0.217	0.039	N.A.	0.067
PVBN	(10)	1.30	0.245	0.031	N.A.	0.110
S.D.		0.12	0.159	0.006	-	0.014
PVB*	(8)	1.43	0.241	0.046	0.198	0.082
S.D.		0.07	0.089	0.012	0.042	0.043
PVB**	(9)	1.63	0.101	0.031	N.A.	0.005
S.D.		0.02	0.038	0.005	-	
in vitro	(6)	1.25	N.A.	N.A.	N.A.	0.080
S.D.		0.06	-	-	-	-
in vivo$_1$	(10)	1.26	N.A.	N.A.	N.A.	N.A.
		0.20				
in vivo$_2$	(6)	1.71	N.A.	N.A.	N.A.	N.A.
		0.04				

Abbreviations: A = aortic CD, TAH = total artificial heart CD, C.A. = carotid artery CD, MC = myocardium CD, PVB = porcine valve bioprosthetic CD, in vitro = CD, 16 hour reaction product,[13] *in vivo*$_1$ = CD, formed in subcutaneous implant, 14 days residence time in rat, *in vivo*$_2$ = CD, formed in subcutaneous implant, 49 days residence time in rat,[13] N = native CD, * = hydrazine treated CD, ** = hypochlorite treated CD, n = number of specimens, S.D. = standard deviation, N.A. = not analyzed. [Portion of data shown in Table I was reported in (6), (13) and (16)].

atherosclerotic CD:

$$Ca_{8.66}Mg_{0.22}Na_{0.32}H_{0.15}(PO_4)_5(CO_3)_{1.22}(OH,F,Cl)_{0.80} \quad (5)$$

TAH CD:

$$Ca_{8.73}Mg_{0.24}Na_{0.24}H_{0.14}(PO_4)_5(CO_3)_{1.20}(OH,F,Cl)_{0.90} \quad (6)$$

PVB CD:

$$Ca_{7.15}Mg_{0.23}Na_{1.21}H_{0.41}(PO_4)_5(CO_3)_{0.98}(OH,F,Cl)_{-0.6} \quad (7)$$

These compositions approximate the compositions of substituted, HAP-like materials as proposed by Kuhl and Nebergall:[31]

$$Ca_{10-x-y}(PO_4)_{6-x}(HPO_4,CO_3)_x(OH)_{2-x-2y} \quad (8)$$

This empirical formula is useful for comparing the composition of biological minerals regardless of their structural properties, that usually are derived from instrumental characterization. It is evident that the products (5) and (6) are very similar in chemical composition. The (OH,F,Cl) term was derived by the charge balance condition $\Sigma n_i z_i = 0$, where n (0.8 and 0.9, respectively) represents the ionic fraction with charge z. Since $n > 0$, these compounds are basic calcium phosphates. Product (7) appears to be substantially different in chemical composition and with $n < 0$, which represents a more acidic calcium phosphate substrate. This is in agreement with experimental evidence that this material (7) contains a high fraction of acidic phosphate. Even with these adjustments, the nature of the residual cationic imbalance ($n = -0.6$) is not clear.

The high HPO_4 content in heart valve bioprosthetic CD (11%) is somewhat reduced after hydrazine treatment (8%) and is practically eliminated after hypochlorite treatment (19). This indicates that acidic phosphate is loosely bound in the structure of biological apatites as a consequence of the proposed special structural site and coordination requirements.[33] The average HPO_4 content in 31 native heart valve CDs is 4.9±0.8% and decreases after hydrazine deproteination to 3.0±0.8%. As shown by the Neuman-Keuls multiple comparison test,[32] the average values of HPO_4 contents are not significantly different among the four described pathologic conditions. The lower level of acidic phosphate in natural valves vs. bioprosthetic valves CD indicates more mature biomineral. Depending on a patient's age (51-84 y), natural valve CD may have a considerably longer lifetime than a bioprosthetic CD (2-13 y), a fact which is in agreement with XRD data (Fig. 1).

2. Structural Properties of Calcific Deposits

The XRD pattern of hydrazine deproteinated aortic CD is characteristic of microcrystalline apatite (6). The CD pattern does not show the presence of α-TCP (2010 and 220 β-TCP reflections are absent), DCPD (020 and 141 DCPD reflections are absent), or OCP (100 reflection is absent) in detectable amounts. A systematic analysis of the XRD patterns of 16 different samples of aortic CD reveals an average 0.5% decrease in the *a*-axis, resulting in a 1% shrinkage of the HAP unit cell volume (6). Fig. 1 shows the XRD patterns of five cardiovascular CD, labeled B-F, compared to the XRD pattern of bone, labeled A. All of the patterns are apatitic with no indication of DCPD or β-TCP. However the general profile of the patterns reveals considerable differences in crystal development. The crystallinity of each particular CD, B-F, is uniquely influenced by the composition and character of the tissue growth medium, the age of CD and the relative exposure to blood flow. Materials that have shorter tissue residence times such as TAH CD and bioprosthetic heart valve CD appear to be less crystalline than those with longer tissue residence times such as aortic or heart valve CD. The most crystalline materials are heart valve CD. This may be attributed to donor age; crystal maturation may also have been enhanced by continuous valve movement during the lifetime of the CD. CD isolated from rheumatic mitral valves shows the poorest crystal development (i.e., largest $\beta_{1/2}$ = 0.37°2Θ), perhaps because this CD was embedded in bulky soft tissue, which prevented the mechanical stress that may be a major factor in the time-dependent transformation and maturation of CD crystals. Three other heart valve CDs do not show significant differences in $\beta_{1/2}$ values (0.29-0.32° 2Θ). However, the aortic CD and bioprosthetic CD $\beta_{1/2}$ values of 0.39-0.41^{o} and 0.36-0.47°, respectively, are significantly different ($p \leq 0.05$) and indicate more poorly crystalline material (19). The bone value, $\beta_{1/2}$= 0.42°,[19] is comparable to that of the bioprosthetic TAH CD.

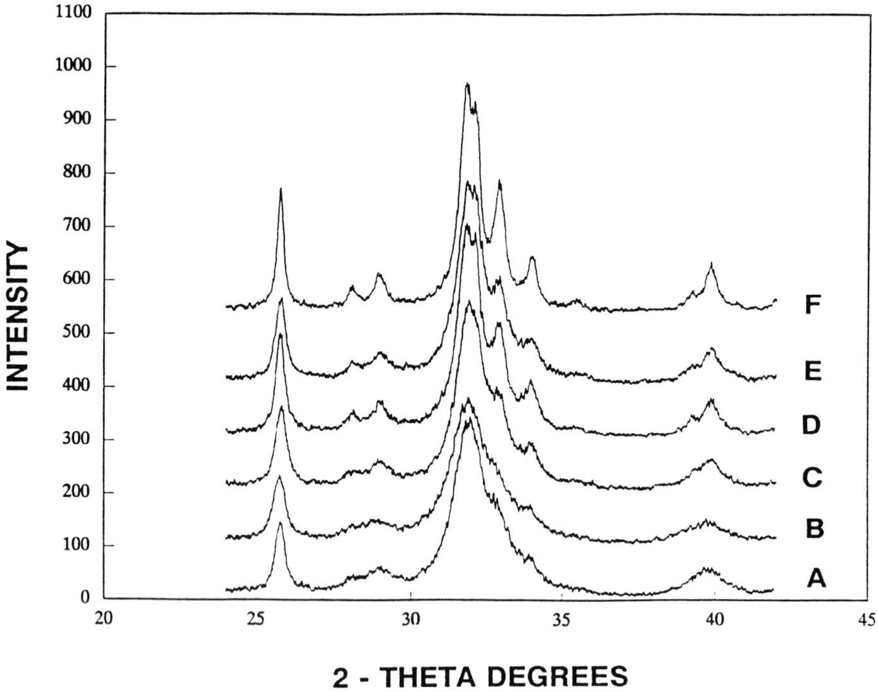

Figure 1. XRD pattern of five cardiovascular deposits, labeled as: B (TAH CD), C (PV CD), D (aortic CD), E (miocardium CD), F (mitral valve CD). Bone pattern labeled A.

FTIR spectroscopy confirms the analytical carbonate results for multisite CD (Table I). FTIR spectra of deproteinated aortic and TAH bioprosthetic CD are shown in Fig. 2. The most important finding is the presence of 872 cm^{-1}, 1421 cm^{-1}, 1448 cm^{-1} and 1470 cm^{-1} bands, which indicate carbonate substituting for phosphate in the apatitic structure, forming "B" type carbonated apatite.[35,36] The complete absence of a 1545 cm^{-1} band indicates the absence of "A" type carbonated apatite, where carbonate substitutes for the hydroxyl ion.[37] The 631 cm^{-1} librational and 3570 cm^{-1} stretching modes for OH^- in HAP and the 910 cm^{-1} mode for OCP[38] are absent in the infrared spectra of all the examined CD.

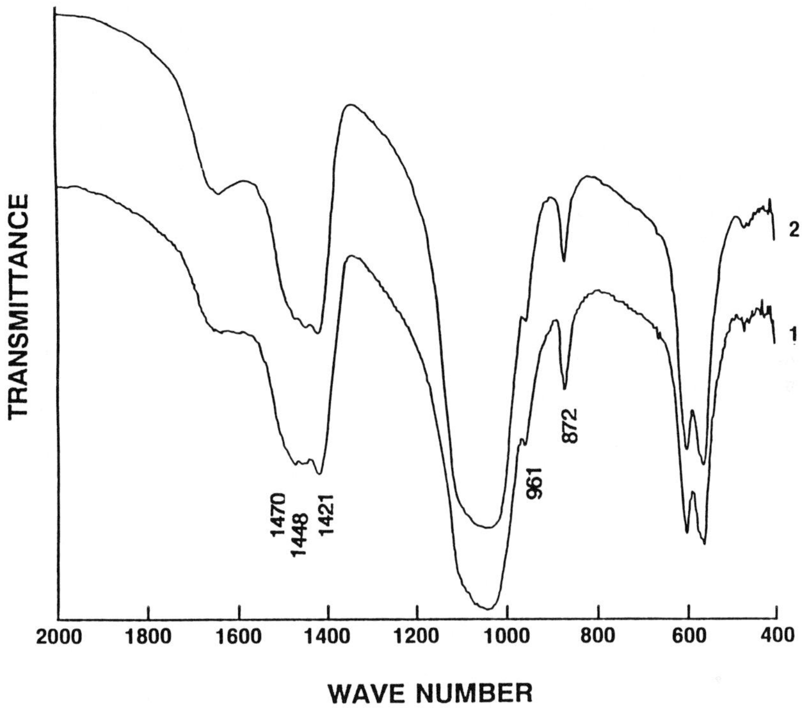

Figure 2. FTIR spectra of deproteinated aortic (1) and TAH bioprosthetic (2) CD (previously reported in Ref. 6).

3. Microscopic Properties of Calcific Deposits

Scanning electron micrographs of native, hydrazine- and hypochlorite-purified porcine valve bioprosthetic CD are shown in Fig. 3 a-c. The smooth particles of native CD that contained organic matrix (a) displayed their rough surfaces after hydrazine treatment that removed smooth organic "filler" (b); however the original size of the particles apparently did not change. Following hypochlorite treatment, which was performed under ultrasonic conditions, the texture of CD changed to finely dispersed material [50-200 nm particle size, shown in (c). This fragmentation behavior was common for all examined CD.

Fig. 3 d-e shows some interesting characteristics of hydrazine-treated aortic CD. The morphological heterogeneity contained in the same CD specimen reveals smooth spherical particles (d), spongy surfaces of irregularly shaped particles (e) and, most abundantly, an appearance that resembles a layer-type scale (f). These three shapes were the most common morphologies seen, but other shapes and combinations of shapes were present, as previously reported (39). The observed heterogeneity of CD is additionally confirmed by electron

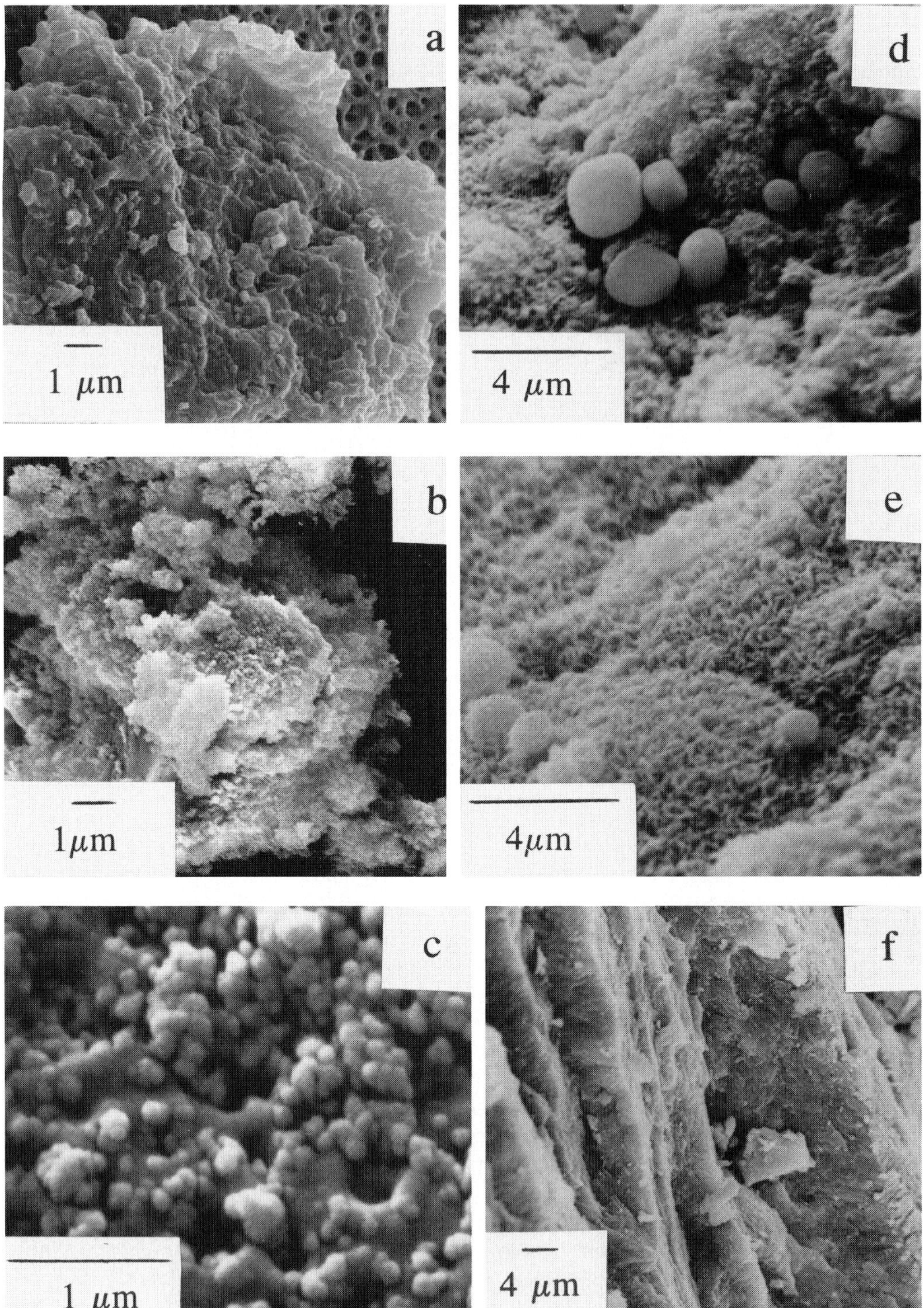

Figure 3. SEM micrographs of native (a), hydrazine-(b) and hypochlorite-purified (c) porcine valve bioprosthetic CD. SEM micrographs of hydrazine-treated aortic CD (d-f).

probe analysis: an average Ca/P ratio of the smooth spheres of 1.56, spongy surfaces 1.68, and smooth layer-type scales 1.79, respectively, have been reported previously (6).

Optical microscopic examination of deproteinated CD materials provided additional qualitative information. The optical characteristics of CD materials provide supporting information on the absence of traceable amounts of β-TCP or HAP, since their refractive indices, ranging from 1.620-1.645 (40), are considerably higher than indices for CD that range from 1.550-1.585 (6,16). The latter indices are close to the well-established values for OCP, which range from 1.576-1.585 (41). The lower value n = 1.55 would indicate DCPD (42); however, the XRD patterns ruled out this compound as a fraction of the CD complex mixture. An aortic deposit had n = 1.549-1.550 and an apatitic XRD pattern. After heating at 550°C, n increased to 1.585-1.60, close to the value for carbonated apatites (43,44), and became n = 1.64 after heating to 1100°C, indicating the formation of HAP after high temperature release of carbonate, which takes place in the temperature range 700-800°C.[6]

4. Solubilities of Calcific Deposits

Due to the complexity of the composition of CD materials, the task of defining their solubility is not straightforward. A typical approach to obtain solubility information on heterogeneous cardiovascular CD is repeated equilibrations in the system: CD - 10^{-3} mol/L H_3PO_4 (20g/L) – 5%CO_2. After each 30 min equilibration, the solution is analyzed and the CD residue resuspended in fresh solvent. The results of eight independent equilibrations on deproteinated aortic CD are summarized in Fig. 4. The equilibrations leach a major fraction of the sodium and magnesium from CD, and the initial high ΔCa/ΔP dissolution ratio indicates the kinetic complication of the dissolution process accompanied by a simultaneous reprecipitation that consumes an excess of solution phosphate. Consequently, the dissolution can be viewed as a surface reaction, controlled rate process.[16,45] After 30 min, the pH of the solution is stable, this condition indicates a steady state condition. The calculated average pIAP values and standard deviation (S.D.) for DCPD, OCP, TCP and HAP, and corresponding thermodynamic solubility product values, pK_{sp}, are listed in Table 2: these data show that the solubility of aortic deposit approximates the solubility of OCP or β-TCP.

Figure 4 shows the $pIAP_{OCP}$ trend to the $K_{sp}OCP$ suggesting that the fraction of CD that dissolves during the first four equilibrations is more soluble than OCP. A simple calculation shows that this fraction is approximately 3% by weight of the total CD. The remaining material following four more equilibrations appears to be slightly less soluble than OCP. The average $pIAP_{OCP}$ of 48.49±0.45 is remarkably close to the thermodynamic solubility product of OCP (46). The kinetics of dissolution of deproteinated TAH CD is shown in Fig. 5. As dissolution progresses, the $pIAP_{OCP}$ decreases to the value of 49.1 after 200 min, an equilibrium value close to the thermodynamic solubility of OCP. During the entire equilibration sequence, the ΔCa/ΔP dissolution ratio held constant at the value of 1.327±0.031, approximating OCP stoichiometry. A similar dissolution trend was apparent in the course of dissolution of deproteinated aortic CD, but the dissolution ΔCa/ΔP ratio was higher at 1.577±0.086. On the basis of these data one can conclude that steady-state equilibrium can be reached within three hours. This information establishes criteria for producing chemical potential plot diagrams for cardiovascular CD materials.

Table 2.
Average pIAP Values Obtained from Eight Equilibrations of Deproteinated Aortic Calcific Deposit. Conditions: CD(20 g/L) - 10^{-3}mol/L H_3PO_4 - 5% CO_2, 30 min, 25°C.

Compound	pIAP	S.D.	K_{sp}	Condition	%	Ref
OCP	48.49	0.45	48.6	SS	0.2	46
β-TCP	29.23	0.41	28.91	US	-0.1	47
HAP	53.18	0.77	58.55	SS	9.2	28
DCPD	6.92	0.05	6.60	US	-4.8	48

Abbr. % = $[(pK_{sp} - p\,IAP)/pK_{sp}] \times 100$
SS = supersaturated; % > 0
US = undersaturated; % < 0

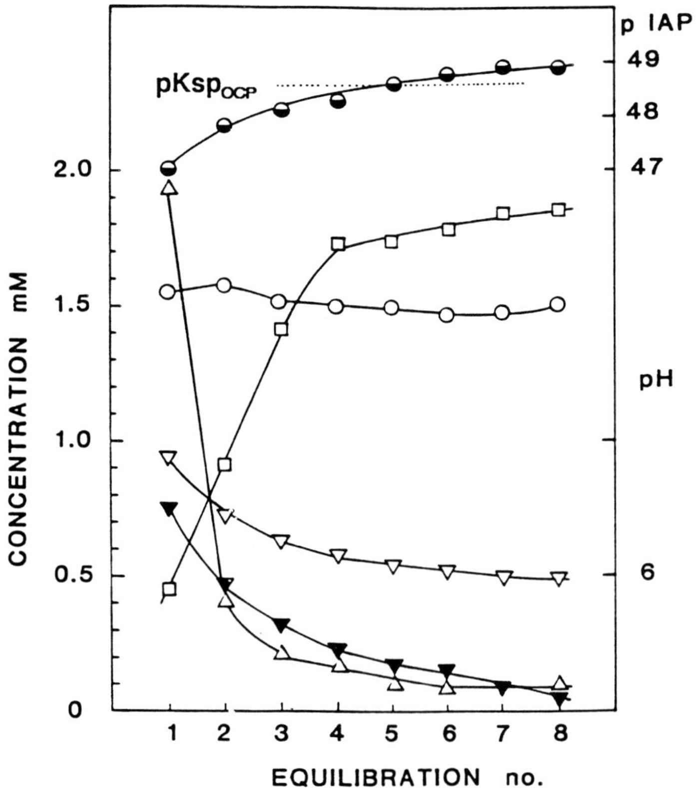

Figure 4. Repeated equilibration of deproteinated aortic CD; concentration data: (Δ Na, ▾ Mg, ○ Ca, □ P, ▿ pH) and solubility data [● ($pIAP_{OCP}$)] [previously reported in (45)].

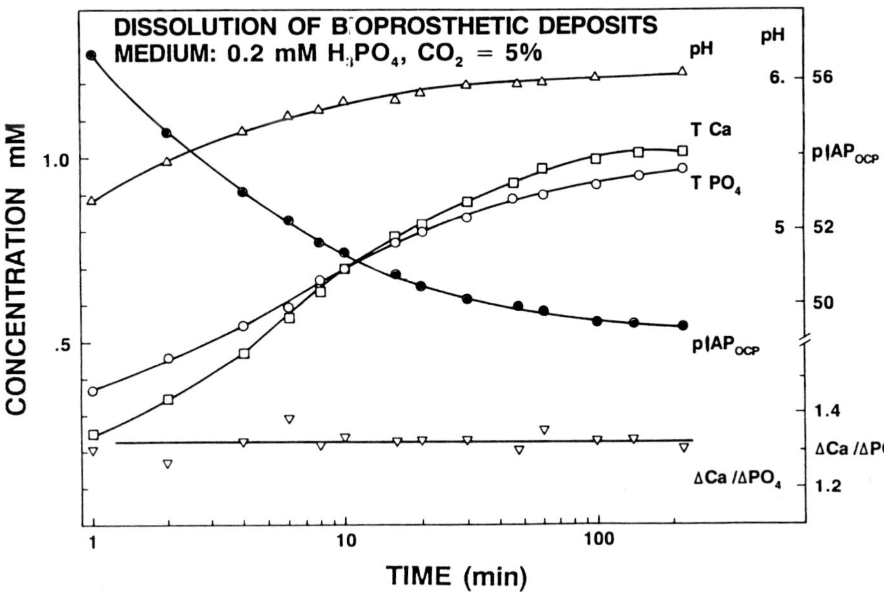

Figure 5. Dissolution of deproteinated TAH CD, concentration data: (□ Ca, O P, Δ pH, ∇ ΔCa/ΔP) and solubility data ● ($pIAP_{OCP}$).

Table 3 represents the solubility data for multisite CD materials. It lists average pIAP values and their S.D. values corresponding to two defined calcium phosphate phases and statistically related CD groups and regression parameters of chemical potential plots.

As shown in Table 3, CD materials equilibrated 6 hours under 5% CO_2 flow show significantly higher solubility than the materials equilibrated 8 days under N_2 flow. The average pIAP values, S.D. and 95% confidence limits for 6-hour equilibrations are 49.46±0.20; 49.30-49.63 (OCP data) and 54.41±0.47; 54.02-54.81 (HAP data). The average pIAP values, S.D. and 95% confidence limits for 8 day equilibrations are 50.31±0.22; 50.04-50.57 (OCP data) and 53.81±0.52; 53.16-54.45 (HAP data). The 6-hour and 8-day pIAP data are significantly different ($p<0.05$). These differences indicate an intrinsic heterogeneity in CD mineral. After the condition of steady-state is attained, as illustrated in Fig. 5, the solution is markedly supersaturated with respect to HAP. However, due to the CO_2 flow, the solution pH is relatively low and as experimentally shown, does not increase. Therefore, the steady-state condition is lasting. The meaning of "steady-state" can be illustrated for the simple case of OCP dissolution and reprecipitation into HAP (equation 9):

$$5Ca_4H(PO_4)_3+4H_2O \rightleftarrows 20Ca^{2+}+9H^+$$

$$+15PO_4^{3-} \underset{\text{low pH}}{\overset{\text{high pH}}{\rightleftarrows}} 4Ca_5(PO_4)_3OH+3H_3PO_4 \qquad (9)$$

Table 3.
Solubility Data and Chemical Potential Plot Parameters for
Deproteinated Cardiovascular Calcific Deposits.

CD	Ca/P	t	CO_2%	$pIAP_{OCP}$	S.D.	$pIAP_{HAP}$	S.D.	a	b	$n^{\&}$	
A4-6	1.77	8d	0	50.46	0.19	53.84	0.44	1.44	54.96	8	#
A11-I	1.73	8d	0	50.54	0.45	54.50	0.94	1.46	55.30	5	#
A7-3	1.73	8d	0	50.11	0.57	53.20	1.10	1.41	54.27	8	#
TAH1s	1.67	8d	0	50.38	0.39	54.08	1.05	1.41	54.57	7	#
TAH6c	1.74	8d	0	50.05	0.36	53.42	1.07	1.39	53.85	8	#
A7-2	1.78	6h	1	49.23	0.53	53.61	0.62	1.47	53.60	6	#
A7-2*	1.78	6h	1	49.46	0.38	54.46	0.55	1.44	54.80	6	##
A7-2	1.78	6h	5	49.53	0.99	54.44	0.90	1.66	58.78	6	##
A7-2*	1.78	6h	5	50.61	0.57	55.93	0.40	1.67	59.51	5	##@
A7-2	1.78	6h	33	49.39	0.28	54.46	0.11	1.56	56.98	6	##
A7-2*	1.78	6h	33	49.58	0.13	55.06	0.29	1.43	54.67	5	##
PV	1.62	6h	5	49.20	0.37	54.14	0.48	1.49	55.56	5	##
A10-0%	1.65	6h	5	49.51	0.33	54.14	0.45	1.37	53.47	5	##
A10-20%	1.64	6h	5	49.57	0.29	54.76	0.81	1.33	52.93	5	
A10-80%	1.62	6h	5	50.79	0.39	56.42	0.32	1.53	57.12	5	

No significant difference in solubilities (p>0.1) after 8 d equilibrations. ## No significant difference in solubilities (p>0.1) after 6 h equilibrations. @ Solubility data for A7-2* significantly different from other ## systems. ...**Significant difference in solubilities (p<0.05) between # and ## systems.**

Abbreviations: Ca/P = molar ratio in CD; t = equilibration time; CO_2% = fraction in N_2/CO_2 gas flow; pIAP = average value from $n^{\&}$ independent equilibrations with corresponding standard deviation, S.D.; a = (-1/x) = slope (r ≥ 0.98) and b = intercept of chemical potential plot. A = aortic CD; TAH = TAH CD from c = calve or s = sheep application;
PV = porcine valve bioprosthetic CD. A7-2* = redissolution data; A10-X% : aortic CD, partially (X%) dissolved.

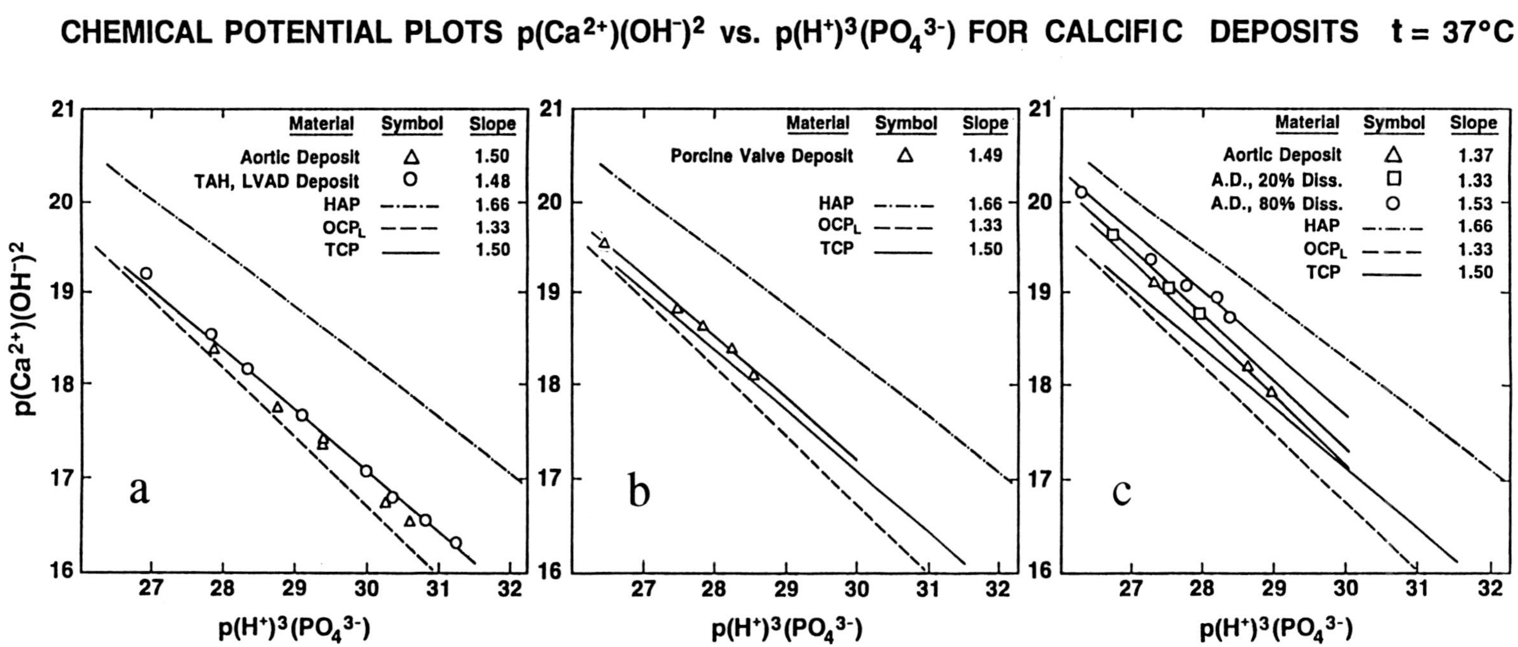

Figure 6. Chemical potential plots data obtained through equilibration of aortic and TAH CD (a), PV CD (b) and fractionally dissolved aortic CD (c).

Such a condition could arise over prolonged equilibration times. In the case of dissolution of CD under N_2 flow, the pH continues to rise due to slow release of carbonate from dissolving mineral. As a result, the HAP supersaturation increases and precipitation commences.[6] Since the apatitic product formed is more basic, the resulting solubility after a prolonged time is lower, as is documented by increased pIAP values seen in the eight-day group. This process is equivalent to the solution-mediated hydrolysis of OCP and results in the formation of OCP hydrolyzate, OCPH.[34,49] The present finding is important inasmuch as it provides indirect evidence that the majority of pathologic biomineral formed in the cardiovascular system may mature through the process of hydrolytic transformation. On the basis of pIAP values, CD solubilities are slightly lower than the solubility of OCP but markedly higher than HAP. Thirteen equilibrated systems represented by 80 independent readings, produced an average $pIAP_{OCP}= 49.89\pm0.67$ and $pIAP_{HAP}= 54.14\pm0.99$, to be compared to $pK_{spOCP}= 48.65$ and $pK_{spHAP} = 58.65$. The information from the Table 3 is graphically presented in Fig. 6. As shown in Fig. 6a, the aortic and TAH CD display very comparable solubilities, approximating the solubility of OCP and β-TCP. Their CPP are located below the HAP isotherm, indicating that these materials are markedly more soluble than HAP: these data are in agreement with listed pIAP values. The average slope (-1/x) of CPP varies from 1.4-1.5. This low value rules out HAP as the material that controls the dissolution equilibrium of CD. CPP is located slightly above the OCP isotherm; this means that CD materials are slightly less soluble than OCP. Similar results for the solubility of deproteinated PV bioprosthetic CD are illustrated in Fig. 6b. The $pIAP_{OCP}$ of porcine valve CD, determined on the basis of 57 independent equilibrations is 49.74–0.34,[16] was one p unit higher than pK_{spOCP}[46] but almost identical to the $pIAP_{OCP}$ (49.78–0.30) for octacalcium phosphate hydrolyzate.[49] Figure 6c demonstrates the solubility heterogeneity of deproteinated aortic deposits that underwent partial dissolution (0, 20 and 80%). The resulting CPP show that the remaining partially dissolved CD have a significantly different solubility. Even the remaining CD after 80% dissolution is significantly more soluble than HAP. A final slope of CPP, 1.53, indicates that the material that determines the solubility in the remaining 20% is more basic than the starting material (-1/x = 1.37).

D. DISCUSSION

The formation of calcific deposits in the cardiovascular system is a very complex phenomenon that cannot be easily monitored or changed. Some medical professionals consider the presence of CD as a final, irreparable stage of severe cardiovascular pathology. From the physicochemical and biophysical perspective such a view may not be justified. At least three areas of applied research effort appear to be recognized: (1) Investigation of the mechanisms of nucleation and growth of CD *in vitro* and *in vivo*. (2) Investigations of the inhibition of cardiovascular CD formation in media approximating or involving real cardiovascular fluids. (3) Investigation of practical ways for elimination of CD *in vivo* by chemical means such as solvent (acid) dissolution or complexation (EDTA). Information from these and related investigations could lead to the practical control of the formation and elimination of cardiovascular DC and possibly reduce the frequency of costly invasive surgical treatments to replace natural or bioprosthetic heart valves.

In addressing item (1), the first question should be: What is the role of mineral precursors in cardiovascular CD? In spite of considerable effort, this question has not been answered successfully. Since a precursor by definition is an initially formed species, implying small transient quantities, an accurate assignment of its role is very difficult. In the simplest case, considering inorganic constituents only, amorphous calcium phosphate (ACP) may be a good precursor candidate because the formation of this material is kinetically favored and not affected by the presence of many inhibitors. The presence of ACP has been documented as a constituent of bone[17,51] and human aortic valve CD.[50] Another attractive candidate as a precursor to bioapatite *in vivo* is OCP, which has been experimentally confirmed in rat enamel.[52] A close structural relationship between OCP and HAP supports this precursor hypothesis.[41] Meyer and Eanes have provided thermodynamic data to show that the transition of freshly precipitated ACP into apatite involves OCP.[53,54] An intermediate stage occurs in the transition in which the suspension maintains a condition of thermodynamic equilibrium with OCP; this suggestion that the ACP precursor transforms first into this unstable crystalline precursor as described by the equation:

$$4\,Ca_3(PO_4)_2 + 3H^+ + PO_4^{3-} + 2.5\,H_2O \rightleftarrows 3\,Ca_4H(PO_4)_3 \cdot 2.5\,H_2O \qquad (10)$$

In the absence of inhibitors, the product of equation 13 is unstable and may transform into octacalcium phosphate hydrolyzate, OCPH,[34,49] another intermediate product to the final HAP phase *in vitro*. An OCP precursor has been independently confirmed experimentally in the early stages of calcium phosphate precipitation in serum.[55] The serum components helped to stabilize the OCP precursor for up to 20 days prior to its hydrolytic transformation into an apatitic product. Recently, Markovic et al. were able to prepare and characterize a series of OCP-carboxylates, OCPC, compounds related to OCP that incorporate carboxylates involved in the Krebs cycle, namely pyruvate, malate, fumarate, succinate, α-ketoglutarate and citrate.[56] This result offers the prospect that in addition to OCP[52,55] and ACP,[17,50,51] OCPC may perform the precursor function in the formation of bioapatites, including cardiovascular CD.

Kim has pointed out the importance of tissue factors in calcification and, in particular, considered surfaces of collagen, elastin, phospholipids, glycosoamino- glycans, matrix vesicle and mitochondria membranes to be especially important in cardiovascular calcification.[57] A variety of different functional groups on these surfaces, particularly membranes, may define the nucleation sites for the forming complexes that may become the nidi of calcification[57] in accord with Urist's triphasic model.[7] Since at point of our understanding the precursor complexes do not have an ordered structure, it is very hard to prove their identity by structural analysis. The initial nucleation of CD precursors may be the consequence of cell injury. In healthy tissues, the ratio between extracellular and intracellular fluid calcium concentrations exceeds 10,000. This situation, however, changes when the cell is injured and the Ca/Na ionic pump fails, leading to the unimpeded accumulation of calcium in the cell.[58] From the high concentration of intracellular orthophosphate and the large excess of ATP that can supply additional orthophosphate, together with the possible lack of natural inhibitors in intracellular fluid, rapid nucleation, i.e., formation of precursors, especially on available cell membrane fragments may take place. Because of lower surface tension of hydrated precursor, ACP or OCP most likely forms preferentially to anhydrous HAP under these *in vivo* conditions.[59,60]

The present review provides an overview of many of the properties of CD isolated from different sites in the cardiovascular system. An important and generally accepted finding is that all isolated minerals are microcrystalline and apatitic, free of coexisting calcium phosphate phases such as DCPD or β-TCP. The difference in crystallinity demonstrated in Fig. 1 indicates the dynamic nature of CD formation and supports a mechanism suggested by independent *in vitro* studies.[13,49] The differences between pattern B (TAH CD) and F (heart valve CD) clearly show that the "young" CD that has formed on a polyurethane surface, although largely apatitic, contains an amorphous fraction, as evidenced by the broad band in the range 27-30°2Θ. On the other hand, pattern F shows a well aged apatitic product that formed in the valve of a 73-year-old patient. This contrast suggests that the precursor is a less crystalline, possibly amorphous, fraction. This result supports the electron diffraction (ED) evidence of Kim[50] for the coexistence of ACP and HAP in human aortic valve. This was the first visualization of ACP in nonskeletal human tissue. ED also provided evidence of the presence of OCP in aortic valve.[61] The heterogeneous nature of CD material is also supported by the morphological heterogeneity of aortic CD, as illustrated in Figs. 6 d-f.

An important observation follows from the comparison of *in vitro* and *in vivo* histology data.[13] The chemical composition of CDs is comparable, but morphologies are different and highly dependent on the site of formation. *In vitro* products form only on the surface and show microcrystalline morphology that is different from the product *in vivo* that forms under the surface of bovine pericardium implant. The lack of an endothelium layer on bioprosthetic implant may be responsible for relatively fast progression of mineralization of tissue-derived bioprostheses, compared to natural valves in human. This *in vivo* evidence would support the advancement of cell technologies that provide the reconstitution of the endothelial layer on commercial tissue-derived bioprostheses. The *in vitro* tests are simple and inexpensive, but *in vivo* tests are more objective.

The solubilities of CD materials also provide important information on the formation and maturation of pathologic bioapatites. The data in Table III and Fig. 6 suggest that OCP and possibly even more soluble materials may be precursors in cardiovascular CD. Such heterogeneity establishes CD formation as a dynamic, time-dependent process that involves nucleation, growth and transformation. This hypothesis has been supported by independent *in vitro* experimental evidence that the hydrolytic transformation of OCP to apatite[34,49] produced products that are structurally, compositionally and physicochemically comparable to *in vivo*-formed cardiovascular CD materials.[6,13,61]

Overall microscopic examination of CD materials provides information on the heterogeneity of bioapatites isolated from different sites of the cardiovascular system and indicates no evidence of HAP or β-TCP even as a minor phase component. The refractive indices data also point to OCP as an important precursor candidate. However, the presence of fractions that have n values ranging from 1.55-1.56 indicates the coexistence of another precursor;

based on morphology and XRD data this precursor is not DCPD, but possibly an amorphous phase in agreement with solubility data provided in Fig. 4. The presence of HPO_4^{2-} in CD materials chemically supports the OCP precursor hypothesis. Interestingly, the fraction of acidic phosphate decreases with the aging of the CD; that is evidence for continuous hydrolytic transformation of CD. The relative ease of removal of HPO_4^{2-} from CD matrices by hypochlorite treatment[19] is the evidence that this ion resides in specific interlayers on the boundary between OCP and HAP[33] where coordinative binding of Ca^{2+} to HPO_4^{2-} is weaker than to PO_4^{3-}.

Comprehensive information about the basic properties of multisite cardiovascular CD may lead to more appropriate strategies for its prevention. Already, pioneering successful efforts in controlling and inhibiting of the calcification of heart valve bioprosthesis by biphosphonates is a very appealing approach.[62] Application of specific metal ions such as Mg^{2+} that inhibit hydrolytic transformation of precursors also has a very significant potential.[63] Levy et al.[64] have shown that preincubation of bioprosthetic implants with Al^{3+} and Fe^{3+} has a pronounced retarding effect in the progression of calcification. Encouraged by ***in vivo*** findings, the authors suggested that the control of alkaline phosphatase, an important cofactor in the mechanism of bioprosthetic valve mineralization by inorganic ions, may open new venues in anticalcification treatments.[64] The application of synergistic mixtures that would both prevent mineral augmentation and control enzymatic factors appears to be one of the most promising strategies for efficient pretreatment of bioprostheses.

E. CONCLUSION

The literature indicates that the proliferation of cardiovascular calcific deposits is a complicated, dynamic process and that an understanding of the reaction mechanism from its early nucleation stage to the formation of mature deposits still requires extensive basic and applied research. A significant contribution to solving this problem is derived from scientific information about the processes that govern the formation of biominerals contained in bones and teeth of vertebrates. The essential mineral, thought to be calcium phosphate, is an extremely reactive medium that, in course of its formation, experiences a variety of interactions, followed by incorporation of organic and inorganic constituents that produce an extremely complex matrix of the final biomineral. While the essential condition for the successful solution of the problem is the coordinated effort by diversified specialists applying different methods, the solubility of biominerals appears to be a very promising tool. Solubility data may indirectly lead to a proper interpretation of the processes in the early stages and elucidate the nature of bioapatite precursor(s). It is reasonable to conclude that the whole spectrum of precursors may be involved, including amorphous calcium phosphate, octacalcium phosphate and various complexes involving calcium, phosphate and biogenic species. The present data indicate that octacalcium phosphate, which undergoes hydrolytic transformation, appears to be a valid candidate for the transient precursor role in the formation of pathological biomineral.

ACKNOWLEDGMENT

The author gratefully acknowledges the late W. E. Brown for his inspiring leadership. Special thanks are due to E. D. Eanes, NIDR/NIST, C. M. Carey, ADA/NIST and E. S. Etz, NIST, for critically reviewing and discussing the manuscript.

This investigation was supported, in part, by USPHS Research Grant HL30035 to the American Dental Association Health Foundation from the National Institutes of Health–National Heart, Lung, Blood Institute and is part of the dental research program conducted by the National Institute of Standards and Technology in cooperation with the American Dental Association Health Foundation.

REFERENCES

1. Fleckenstein, A., Frey, M., Thimm, F. and Fleckenstein-GrHn, G., Excessive mural calcium overload - a predominant casual factor in the development of stenosing coronary plaques in humans, *Cardiovascular Drugs and Therapy*, 4, 1005, 1990.
2. Passik, C. S., Ackermann, D. M., Pluth, J. R. and Edwards, M. D., Temporal changes in the causes of aortic stenosis: a surgical pathologic study of 646 cases, *Mayo Clin. Proc.*, 62, 119, 1987.
3. Schoen, F. J., Fernandez, J., Gonzales-Lavin, L. and Cernianu, A., Causes of failure and pathologic findings in surgically removed Ionescu-Shiley standard bovine pericardial heart valve bioprostheses: Emphasis on progressive structural deterioration, *Circulation*, 76, 618, 1987.
4. Schoen, F. J., Cardiac valve prostheses: Review of clinical status and contemporary biometarials issues, *J. Biomed. Mat. Res.: Applied Biomaterials*, 21, 91, 1987.
5. Pierce, W. S., Donachy, J. H. and Rosenberg, G., Calcification inside artificial hearts: Inhibition with warfarin-sodium, *Science*, 208, 601, 1980.
6. Tomazic, B. B., Brown, W. E., Queral, L. A. and Sadovnik, M., Physicochemical characterization of cardiovascular calcified deposits, *Atherosclerosis*, 69, 5, 1988.
7. Urist, M. R., Biologic initiators of calcification, in *Biological Mineralization*, Zipkin , I., Ed., John Wiley & Sons, New York 1973.
8. Ennever, J., Vogel, J. J. and Riggan, L. J., Calcification by proteolipid from atherosclerotic aorta, *Atherosclerosis*, 35, 209, 1980.
9. Dmitrovsky, E. and Boskey, A. L., Calcium-acidic phospholipid-phosphate complexes in human atherosclerotic aortas, *Calc. Tiss. Int.*, 37, 121, 1985.
10. Sarig, S., Hirsch, D., Azoury, R., Weiss, T. A., Katz, I. and Kruth, H. S., Apatite - cholesterol agglomeration in human atherosclerotic lesions, *Cells and Materials*, 2, 339, 1992.
11. Boskey, A. L., Current concepts of the physiology and biochemistry of calcification, *Clin. Orthoped.*, 157, 225, 1981.
12. Hirsch, D., Azoury, R. and Sarig, S., Co-crystallization of cholesterol and calcium phosphate as related to atherosclerosis, *J. Crystal Growth*, 104, 759, 1990.

13. Tomazic, B. B., Siew, C. and Brown, W. E., A comparative study of bovine pericardium mineralization: a basic and practical approach, *Cells and Materials*, 1, 231, 1991.
14. McGill Jr., H. C., Introduction to the geographic pathology of atherosclerosis, *Lab. Invest.*, 19, 465, 1968.
15. Schoen, F. J., Kujovich, J. L., Webb, C. L. and Levy, R. J., Chemically determined mineral content of explanted porcine valve bioprostheses: correlation with radiographic assessment of calcification and clinical data, *Circulation*, 76, 1061, 1987.
16. Tomazic, B. B., Brown, W. E. and Schoen, F. J., Physicochemical properties of calcific deposits isolated from porcine bioprosthetic valves removed from patients following 2-13 years function, *J. Biomed. Mater. Res.*, in press.
17. Termine, J. P., Eanes, E. D., Greenfield, D. J., Nylen, M. U. and Harper, R. A., Hydrazine-deproteinated bone mineral, *Calcif. Tiss. Res.*, 12, 73, 1973.
18. Weiner, S. and Price, P. A., Disaggregation of bone into crystals, *Calcif. Tiss. Int.*, 39, 365, 1986.
19. Tomazic, B. B., Brown, W. E. and Eanes, E. D., A critical evaluation of the purification of biominerals by hypochlorite treatment, *J. Biomed. Mat. Res.*, 27, 217, 1993.
20. *Standard Methods for Examination of Water and Wastewater*, 15th ed., Greenberg, T. M., Connors, J. J., Jenkins, D. and Franson, M. A. H., Eds., Prepared and published jointly by American Public Health Association, American Water Works Association, Water Polution Federation, Washington, DC, 1981, pp. 415.
21. Gee, A. and Dietz, V. R. J., Pyrophosphate formation upon ignition of precipitated basic calcium phosphates, *J. Am. Chem. Soc.*, 77, 2961, 1955.
22. Conway, E. J., Microdiffusion Analysis and Volumetric Error, C. Lockwood, London, 1962, pp. 201.
23. Vogel, G. L., Carey, C. M. , Chow, L. C. and Brown, W. E., Micro-electrode technique for the analysis of oral fluids, *J. Dent. Res.*, 66, 1691, 1987.
24. *Powder Diffraction File (1986)*, Swarthmore, PA 19801 USA: International Center for Diffraction Data, Card No.9-432 (HAP), No. 26-1056 (OCP), No. 9-169 (β-TCP), No. 11-293 (DCPD), No. 21-145 (Dahlite) and No. 19-272 (Carbonate apatite).
25. Myklebust, R. L., Fiori, C. E and Heinrich, K. F. J., FRAME C: A compact procedure for quantitative energy-dispersive electron probe X-ray analysis, *National Bureau of Standards Technical Note 1106*, U. S. Government Printing Office, Washington, DC, 1979.
26. Bloss, F. J, An Introduction to the Methods of Optical Crystalography, Holt, Rinehart and Winston, Inc., Philadelphia, 1961.
27. MacGregor, J. and Brown, W. E., Blood:bone equilibrium in calcium homeostasis, *Nature*, 205, 359, 1965.
28. McDowell, H., Gregory, T. M. and Brown, W. E., Solubility of $Ca_5(PO_4)_3OH$ in the system: $Ca(OH)_2$-H_3PO_4-H_2O at 5°, 15°, 25° and 37°C, *J. Res. Natl. Bur. Stand.*, 81A, 273, 1977.
29. Plummer, L. N. and Busenberg, E., The solubilities of calcite, aragonite and vaterite in CO_2-H_2O solutions between 0° and 90°C, and an evaluation of the aqueous model for the system $CaCO_3$-CO_2-H_2O, *Geochim. Cosmochim. Acta*, 46, 1011, 1982.

30. Daculsi, J., Pou.zat, J., P*ru, L., Maugars, Y. and LeGeros, R. Z., Ectopic calcifications, in *Calcification in Biological Systems*, Bonucci E., Ed., CRC Press, Boca Raton, 1992, chap. 15.
31. Kuhl, G. and Nebergall, W. H., Hydrogen phosphate and carbonate apatite, *Z. Anorg. Allg. Chem.*, 324, 313, 1963.
32. Wall, F. J., Statistical Data Analysis Handbook, McGraw Hill Company, New York, 1968.
33. Mathew, M., Brown, W. E., Schroeder, L.W. and Dickens. B., Crystal structure of octacalcium bis(hydrogenphosphate) tetrakis(phosphate) pentahydrate, *J. Crystal. Spectr. Res.*, 18, 250, 1988.
34. Tomazic, B. B., Tung, M.S, Gregory, T. M. and Brown W. E., Mechanism of hydrolysis of octacalcium phosphate, *Scanning Microsc.*, 3, 119, 1989.
35. Zapanta-LeGeros, R., Effect of carbonate on the lattice parameters of apatite, *Nature*, 206, 403, 1965.
36. LeGeros, R. Z., Crystallographic Studies of the Carbonate Subsitution in the Apatite Structure, *Ph.D. Thesis, New York University*, 1967.
37. Elliot, J. C., The problems of the composition and structure of the mineral components of the hard tissue, *Clin. Orthoped.*, 953, 313, 1973.
38. Fowler, B. O., Moreno, E. C., and Brown, W. E., Infrared spectra of hydroxyapatite, octacalcium phosphate and pyrolyzed octacalcium phosphate, *Arch. Oral. Biol.*, 11, 477, 1966.
39. Schmid, K., McSharry, W.O., Pameijer, C. H. and Binette, J. P., Chemical and physicochemical studies on the mineral deposits of the human atherosclerotic aorta, *Atherosclerosis*, 37, 199, 1980.
40. Palache, C., Berman, H. and Frondel, C., Dana's System of Mineralogy, Vol. II, 7-th Ed., John Willey and Sons, New York, 1944.
41. Brown, W. E., Smith, J. P., Lehr, J. R. and Frazier, A. W., Octacalcium phosphate and hydroxyapatite, *Nature*, 196, 1048, 1962.
42. Lehr, J. R., Brown, W. E., Frazier, A. W., Smith, J. P. and Trasher, R. D., Crystalographic Properties of Fertilizer Compounds, *Chemical Engineering Bulletin No. 6*, Tennessee Valey Authority, 1967, pp. 76.
43. Washington, H. S., Dahllite from St. Pauls Rocks (Atlantic), *The American Mineralogist*, 14, 369, 1929.
44. Kerr, P. F., Optical Mineralogy, Mac Graw Hill, New York, 1962, pp. 268.
45. Tomazic, B. B., Etz, E. S. and Brown, W. E., Nature and properties of cardiovascular deposits, *Scanning Microsc.*, 1, 95, 1987.
46. Tung, M., Eidelman, N., Sieck, B. and Brown, W. E., Octacalcium phosphate solubility product from 4° to $37^{O}C$, *J. Res. Nat. Bur. Stand.*, 93, 613, 1988.
47. Gregory, T. M., Moreno, E. C., Patel, J. M. and Brown, W. E., Solubility of β-$Ca_3(PO_4)_2$ in the system $Ca(OH)_2$-H_3PO_4-H_2O at 5°, 15°, 25° and 37°C. *J. Res. Nat. Bur. Stand., (U.S.)* 78A (Phys. and Chem.) 6, 667, 1974.
48. Gregory, T. M., Moreno, E. C. and Brown, W. E., Solubility of $CaHPO_4 \cdot 2H_2O$ in the system $Ca(OH)_2$-H_3PO_4-H_2O at 5°, 15°, 25° and 37°C. *J. Res. Nat. Bur. Stand.*, 74A (Phys. and. Chem.) 461, 1974.
49. Tomazic, B. B., Mayer, Y. and Brown, W. E., Ion incorporation into octacalcium phosphate hydrolyzates, *J. Cryst. Growth.*, 108, 670, 1991.
50. Kim, K. M. and Trump, B. F., Amorphous calcium precipitation in human aortic valve, *Calcif. Tiss. Res.*, 18, 155, 1975.

51. Wuthier, R. E., Bisaz, S, Russell, R. G. G. and Fleisch, H., Relationship between pyrophosphate, amorphous calcium phosphate and other factors in the sequence of calcification in vivo, *Calcif. Tiss. Res.*, 10,198,1972.
52. Brown, W. E., Chow, L. C., Siew, C. and Gruninger, S., Acidic calcium phosphate precursors in formation of enamel mineral, in *Tooth Enamel IV*, Fearnhead, R. W. and Suga, S., Eds., Elsevier Science Publishers, Amsterdam, 1984, pp. 8-13.
53. Meyer, J. L. and Eanes, E. D., A thermodynamic analysis of the amorphous to the crystalline calcium phosphate transformation, *Calcif. Tiss. Res.*, 25, 59, 1978.
54. Meyer, J. L. and Eanes, E. D., A thermodynamic analysis of the secondary transition in the spontaneous precipitation of calcium phosphate, *Calcif. Tiss. Res.*, 25, 209, 1978.
55. Eidelman, N., Chow, L. C. and Brown, W. E., Calcium phosphate phase tranformation in serum, *Calcif. Tiss. Int*, 41, 18, 1987.
56. Markovic, M., Fowler, B. O., and Brown, W. E., Octacalcium phosphate carboxylates. I. Preparation and identification., *Chem. Mater.*, in press.
57. Kim, K. M., Pathological calcification, in *Pathobiology of Cell Membranes, vol. III.* Arstrilla, A. U. and Trump, B. F., Eds., Academic Press, New York, 1983, pp. 117-155.
58. Schoen, F. J., Harasaki, H., Kim, K. M., Anderson, H. C. and Levy, R. J., Biomaterial-associated calcification: Pathology, mechanisms, and strategies for prevention, *J. Biomed. Mater. Res.*, 22, 11, 1988.
59. Brown, W. E., Eidelman, N. and Tomazic, B., Octacalcium phosphate as a precursor in biomineral formation, *Adv. Dent. Res.*, 1, 306, 1987.
60. Eanes, D. E., Dynamics of calcium phosphate precipitation, in *Calcification in Biological Systems*, Bonucci E., Ed., CRC Press, Boca Raton, 1992, chap. 1.
61. H@hling, Fearnhead, R. W. and Lotter, G., The mineral components in aortic "calcification" studied by X-ray and electron diffraction combined with electron microscopy, *German Med. Mth.*, 13, 135, 1968.
62. Golomb, G., Dixon, M., Smith, M. S., Schoen, F. J. and Levy, R. J., Controlled-release drug delivery of diphosphonates to inhibit bioprosthetic heart valve calcification: release rate modulation with silicone matrices via drug solubility and membrane coating, *J. Pharm. Sci.*, 76, 271, 1987.
63. Tung, M. S., Tomazic, B. and Brown, W. E., The effects of magnesium and fluoride on the hydrolysis of octacalcium phosphate, *Arch. oral biol.*, 37, 585, 1992.
64. Levy, R. J., Schoen, F. J., Flowers, W. B. and Staelin S. T., Initiation of mineralization in bioprosthetic heart valves: Studies ol alkaline phosphatase activity and its inhbibition by $AlCl_3$ or $FeCl_3$ preincubations, *J. Biomed. Mat. Res.*, 25, 905, 1991.

CHEMISTRY AND STRUCTURE OF CALCIUM-CONTAINING COATINGS AND MODIFIED SURFACES FOR TITANIUM ALLOY ORTHOPEDIC PROSTHESES

M. Spector[1], J.G. Hanlon[1], and G.H. Nancollas[2]

[1]Brigham and Women's Hospital, Harvard Medical School,
Brockton/West Roxbury VAMC, Boston, MA., and
[2]State University of New York, Buffalo, NY.

INTRODUCTION

A major problem associated with the use of internal skeletal prostheses is the fixation of the device to bone [1]. Deficiencies in current methods of mechanical fixation ("bone cement" and bone ingrowth into porous coatings) limit the function and longevity of total joint replacement prostheses. Recent studies have indicated that bone will bond chemically as well as mechanically to coatings of a calcium phosphate substance, hydroxyapatite[2, 3, 4]. Plasma-spray (PS) techniques [5] are currently being employed to apply hydroxyapatite (HA) coatings to certain titanium (Ti) alloy orthopedic and dental implants. Histological evaluation of specimens retrieved from animal models and human subjects has revealed that bone forms directly on the surface of these coatings within a few weeks of implantation. The strength of attachment of the bone to the coating is much greater than that achieved with uncoated Ti alloy control specimens, providing evidence that the bonding is chemical as well as mechanical. However, investigations indicate that the strength of attachment of the PS coating to the metallic substrate degrades with time, leading to detachment of the coating[6]. Detachment of the PS coating can result in loosening of the prosthesis and abrasion of the fragments of the coating against the Ti alloy device. This wear process can lead to large amounts of metallic particulate debris that is capable of eliciting an inflammatory response with the production of agents that are known to stimulate bone resorption. This loss of bone stock, that can occur relatively rapidly, greatly complicates revision arthroplasty. A recent histological investigation of PS HA coated femoral stems [7], retrieved at autopsy, revealed that after only 5 months the coating was no longer present along as much as 20% of the perimeter of the device. These findings indicate that there is a need for coatings or surface treatments that allow for bone bonding, but that are more durable and have a higher strength and longer-lasting bond to the metallic substrate than current PS coatings.

The development of improved surfaces for bone bonding requires a deeper understanding of how the chemistry and crystalline structure of the calcium phosphate surface act as determinants of the biological processes underlying bone bonding. In working toward this goal, the objective of this investigation was to characterize the chemistry and crystalline structure of HA PS coatings and novel calcium-ion-implanted (CaII) Ti alloy surfaces. The characteristics of the Ti alloy surface exposed by dissolution of PS coatings were compared with the features of noncoated specimens.

0-8493-4750-5/94/$0.00 + $.50

MATERIALS AND METHODS

Ti alloy (6Al-4V) disks, 22 mm in diameter and 2.5 mm thick, and rods, 6 mm in diameter, were employed as substrates for PS HA coating and CaII. A generic PS HA coating was chosen as a control because it is the type that is currently used clinically and has been shown in numerous animal investigations to undergo bone bonding. The PS coatings were applied by Bio-Coat (Southfield, MI) and Biointerfaces (San Diego, CA) using the procedures currently employed commercially for the manufacture of coated joint replacement prostheses and endosseous dental implants. The nominal thickness of the coating was 35-50 μm. CaII was achieved using an accelerating voltage of 120 keV and a retained dose of $2.5 x 10^{17}$ atoms/cm^2. CaII has the advantage of employing considerably higher energies, than employed in PS, in directly implanting calcium ions into metallic surfaces. The result is more of a surface treatment than a defined coating. Therefore, this method might provide the highest attachment strength of the calcium-rich surface layer to the substratum metal. The CaII was performed at Implant Sciences, Wakefield, MA.

Near surface chemistry and crystalline structure were determined using x-ray photoelectron spectroscopy (XPS), secondary ion mass spectroscopy (SIMS), energy dispersive x-ray analysis (EDX), conventional and thin film x-ray diffraction (XRD and TFXRD), and scanning electron microscopy (SEM). XPS data were obtained before and after argon sputtering to remove the adsorbed carbon film. The depth profiles of calcium ions implanted into Ti alloy substrates and the thickness of the oxide layer on CaII and nontreated Ti alloy were determined using cesium sputtering in conjunction with SIMS. The surface chemistry and structure of the Ti alloy surface revealed by dissolving the PS HA coating *in vitro* were obtained in order to determine what effect the PS coating process had on the metal substrate. PS HA samples and noncoated Ti controls were soaked in EDTA solution for 72 hours in order to dissolve the coating. If the PS HA dissolved/resorbed *in vivo* would the Ti alloy surface revealed to the biological environment display the same "biocompatibility" as nontreated material?

Surface composition and chemistry (5-10 nm sampling depth) were evaluated with Perkin-Elmer and Surface Science Lab SSX-100 x-ray photoelectron spectrophotometers with a Al-Kα source. A gun flood of between 5-10 eV was used to minimize surface charging for the non-conductive ceramic coating. Survey scans, evaluating binding energies from 0-1000 eV, were used to access relative composition, while high resolution scans were done over relevant elemental peaks to access surface chemistry. High resolution scan analysis involved peak de-convolution, assignment of functionalities, and subsequent peak integration to evaluate relative chemistry. Bulk composition (1-2 μm sampling depth) and surface morphology were evaluated using a Joel 6-400 scanning electron microscope with a light element x-ray detector fitted with a diamond window to allow detection of carbon and oxygen.

The SIMS system (Vacuum Generators model IX70S) employed a cesium ion gun for depth profiling. Surveys included light sputtering of the surface to develop mass spectrums from 0-100 AMU. After initial peak consideration and assignment, depth profiles were carried out tracking the detection of Ti, TiO, and CaO with sputtering time. Estimates of the depth of sputtering were obtained for the calcium depth profiling using contact profilometry. This analysis was carried out with a Dektak II Contact Profilometer, with a 2.5 μm tip. The sample was placed on the profilometer analysis table, and the sputter pit located by use of a 10X objective and table X-Y translation. Multiple scans and slow speeds (lateral resolution of 0.1 μm) were used while varying the trace direction over the etch pit. Sputtering rates for the CaII and Ti alloy control specimens were similar. For the SIMS surface oxide analysis, the resultant sputter etch pits were of insufficient depth, relative to the existing surface profile, to allow for confident assessment of depth.

Crystallographic analysis was performed using XRD and TFXRD. PS HA and CaII samples were analyzed using a Rigaku X-ray powder diffractometer at 12kV and 200 mA. A step size of 0.01 2Θ/step with 1° divergence and scatter slits and a 0.15° receiving slit were used. Thin film X-ray diffraction was carried out with a fully automated Ru 200 Generator/Diffractometer with a thin film attachment. Scan conditions were 50 kV and 200 mA with 0.2° and 5° incident and scatter slits, respectively. Scans were done between 15 - 55 degrees 2Θ, at a step size of 0.01 degree 2Θ and a scan speed of 3 degrees 2Θ/minute. Theta was set to 1.5°, which was found to be an optimal position between detecting the surface-most features for the materials while retaining sufficient signal for peak detection and subsequent data analysis. Data analysis was performed using Rigaku software on a minicomputer. Analysis included subtraction of continuous and amorphous scattering by a linearization routine, and subsequent peak assignment and phase analysis by comparing sample diffraction peaks to the computer data base of the Joint Committee on Powder Diffraction Standards. Crystallite size was determined by measurement of the full width half maximum of the HA (002) and (111) peaks with subsequent size calculation using the Debye-Scherrer equation with a silicon powder (111) peak as the standard for instrument line broadening. Relative crystallinity was estimated by dividing the integrated areas for total peak scattering (after background subtraction) by the total scattering in the range of 2θ from 20 to 55°.

Surface roughness was determined using a Dektak II Contact Profilometer with a 2.5 μm diameter tip. Roughness (R_a) was calculated automatically by this device. Trace lengths varied from 300 to 3000 μm depending upon sample roughness.

RESULTS

Plasma-Sprayed Hydroxyapatite Coatings

The morphological features of the PS HA coatings applied by the two vendors were comparable, and similar to the surface features reported previously [8, 9, 10]. SEM revealed a rough surface, consistent with an R_a of about 4.5 (Table 1), comprised of many globular structures, 0.1-3 μm in diameter, protruding from an irregular, porous, smooth-surfaced substrate (Fig. 1). Plate-like structures with rounded corners could be found within the substrate and protruding from it.

The Ca:P ratio of 1.67 of the PS HA coating, determined by EDX (bulk compositional analysis), agreed with the stoichiometry of this substance (Table 1). Surface compositional analysis assayed by XPS yielded a Ca:P ratio of 1.27. This indicates that the surface (the outermost 5-10 nm) might be a calcium deficient HA. Surface chemistries of the PS HA coatings from the different vendors were comparable. XPS of all of the specimens revealed at least 30% carbon, present as ubiquitous contaminant. The noncoated grit blasted Ti alloy specimens demonstrated higher levels of aluminum at the surface, attributable to entrapped aluminum-oxide grit particles used for the grit blasting treatment (Table 1). This is commonly observed for orthopedic surfaces textured in this manner. The PS coatings of HA and the grit blasted Ti alloy specimens had comparable roughness as determined by profilometry (Table 1).

Most of the XRD and TFXRD peaks of the PS HA coating could be assigned to HA (Tables 2 and 3). Approximately 10% of the PS HA coating was noncrystalline, as

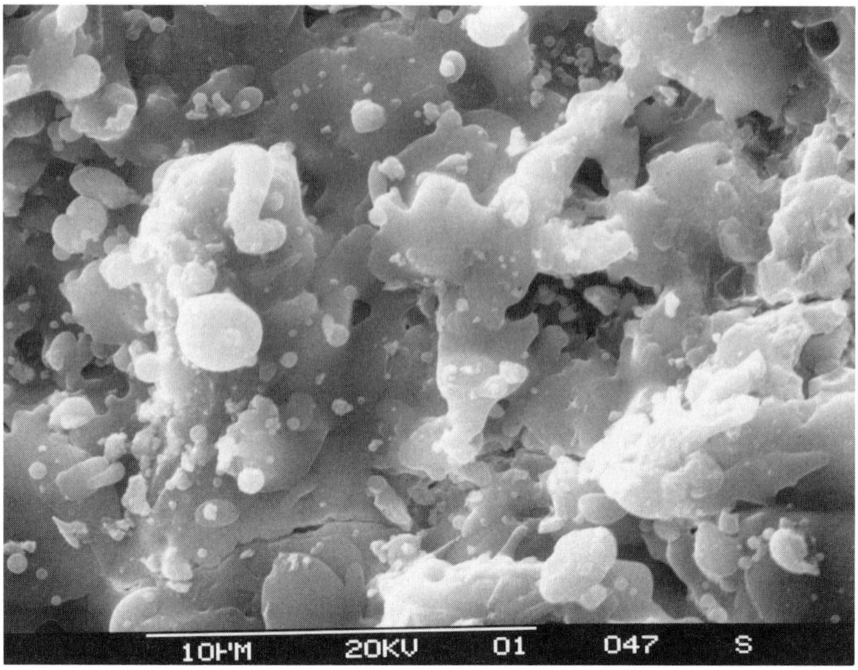

Fig. 1 Scanning electron micrograph of a plasma-sprayed hydroxyapatite surface.

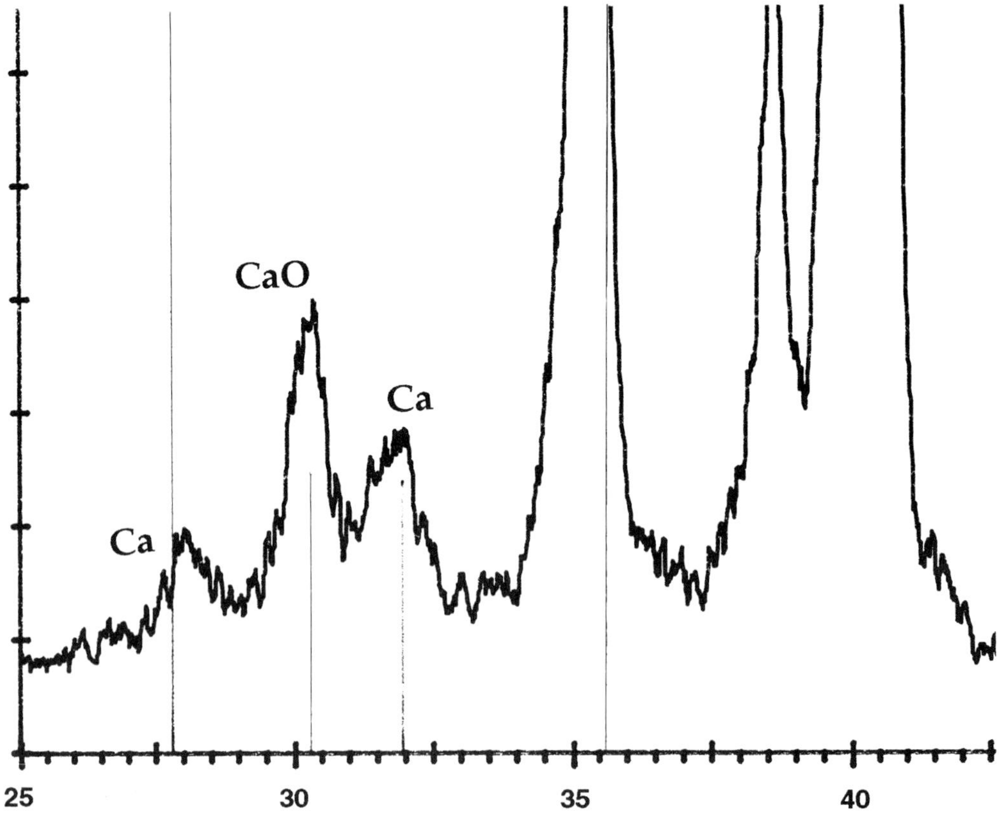

Fig. 2 XRD pattern of CaII sample displaying peaks assigned to calcium oxide (CaO) and elemental calcium (Ca). The other peaks are assignable to titanium (Ti) alloy.

Table 1
Composition and Chemistry of the Plasma-Sprayed Hydroxyapatite Coating and Calcium Ion-Implanted Surface

Ti Alloy Surface Treatment:	Roughness (Ra, μm)	Analysis §	Ti	Al	V	Ca	P	O	C	Surface Chem: Ti Binding	Surface Chem: Ca Binding
Ca - implanted	0.03 μm	Bulk	78	10	3	9	--	--	--	Ti: 0%	Ca: 40%
CaII(polished)		Surface	13	--	--	7	--	43	36	Ti-oxide:100%	Ca-oxide:60%
		Surf/Spt*	23	6	--	9	--	55	5		
Non-Implanted	0.04 μm	Bulk	86	10	4	--	--	--	--	Ti: 7%	nd†
Ti (polished)		Surface	21	6	--	--	--	26	43	Ti-oxide: 93%	
		Surf/Spt	37	18	2	--	--	38	--		
											Ca:P Ratio ††
Plasma Spray	4.43 μm	Bulk	--	--	--	24	14	62	--	nd	Bulk: 1.67
PS HA		Surface	--	--	--	14	10	48	24		Surface: 1.27
Grit Blasted	7.78 μm	Bulk	27	13	1	--	--	57	--	Ti: 7%	nd
Ti Control		Surface	13	18	--	1	--	38	37	Ti-oxide: 93%	

§: Bulk composition (at. %): Energy Dispersive X-ray, 0-2μm sampling depth.
Surface composition (at. %): X-ray Photoelectron Spectroscopy, 0-5nm sampling depth.
Trace surface detection of Na, Cl, N, and Si.

*: Sputtering of the surface was performed in the XPS with an argon beam to remove the adventitious carbon layer.

†: nd = not detected.

††: The stoichiometric ratio of Ca:P for hydroxyapatite ($Ca_{10}(PO_4)_6(OH)_2$) is 1.67.

Table 2
Crystallographic Analysis of the PS HA Coating and the CaII Surface and Ti Alloy Controls

Ti Alloy Surface Treatment	Structural Identification	Rel. Crystallinity Bulk†	Surface§	Crystallite Size nm Peak	Bulk	Surface
CaII polished	Ti - Alloy: 93% Ca: 2 Ca - oxiode: 6	96%	85	$(100)_{Ti}$:	103	44
Non - Implanted, polished control	Ti - Alloy: 100%	98	94	$(100)_{Ti}$:	103	66
PS HA (Bio-Coat)	HA: 99.3% TCP: 0.3 CaO: 0.3 b-Ca2P2O7: 0.2	89	91	$(002)_{HA}$:	101	182
Grit blasted control	Ti-Alloy: 77% Al-Oxide: 23	93	94	$(101)_{Ti}$:	57	28

†: Bulk analysis: Powder X-ray Diffraction (XRD), 0-10 μm sample depth.
§: Surface analysis: Thin Film X-ray Diffraction (TFXRD), 0-1μm sample depth

Table 3

Analysis of PS HA Coatings from Two Vendors

Vendor	Relative Phase Analysis	Crystallite Size (nm)		Relative Crystallinity
		(111)	(002)	
Bio-Coat	HA - 99.3% α+β-TCP - 0.3 β-$Ca_2P_2O_7$ - 0.2 CaO - 0.2	90	101	89.3±0.5% (n=2)
Bio-Interfaces	HA - 98.7% α+β-TCP - 0.5 β-$Ca_2P_2O_7$ - 0.4 CaO - 0.4	75	76	88.1±2.1% (n=3)

estimated by XRD. XRD revealed peaks of very low intensity consistent with α-and β-tricalcium phosphate, calcium pyrophosphate, and calcium oxide. Line broadening measurements revealed crystallite sizes of approximately 75 and 100 nm for the specimens obtained from the two vendors (Table 3). Differences in crystallite size and/or orientation between surface and bulk HA (Table 2) were reflected in the broader 002 peak obtained from XRD, compared to the 002 reflection in the TFXRD pattern. However, determination of crystallite size from line broadening in TFXRD is complicated by the difficulty of obtaining an assessment of the component of line broadening due to instrument factors. It was not possible to obtain a clearly distinguishable $K_{\alpha 1}$ peak from the silicon powder instrument calibration standard by TFXRD.

The roughness of the PS HA specimen was comparable to a literature value for this feature [11], but less than the particular grit blasted surface that was produced on the Ti alloy control. However, this difference should not have significantly affected results from chemical and crystallographic procedures. The fact that the roughnesses of PS HA coatings and noncoated controls can be adjusted to be comparable facilitates animal implantation studies designed to demonstrate that HA coatings achieve chemical as well as mechanical bonding.

Ti Alloy Underlying the PS HA Coating

XPS detected no significant difference in surface composition between the Ti alloy substrate underlying the PS HA coating and the grit blasted control surface (Table 4). The same alloying elements were detected on both specimens. Aluminum detection was high (>6%) for both groups and was probably due to the presence of entrapped aluminum-oxide grit particles. Calcium was detected on both the control and HA PS substrates in trace amounts (1% for both).

Table 4
Elemental Composition of the Ti Alloy Underlying the PS HA Coating (At. Wt. %)

	Ti Revealed by HA Dissolution	Ti Control
Ti	9	13
Al	16	18
Ca	1	1
O	40	38
C	33	27

High resolution scans of the Ti2*p* peak for both the control and HA PS substrates did not detect any clear difference in the relative binding (chemistry) for the Ti in the top 10 nm. For both samples approximately 80% of the Ti existed as TiO_2, 10% in the suboxide Ti_2O_3 and TiO region, with the remainder being metallically bonded Ti. TiO depth profile analysis for both groups did not detect any measurable difference between the depths of the oxides layers for the HA PS substrate sample and the control grit blast specimen.

C1*s* peak deconvolution analysis demonstrates that the carbon on the HA PS substrate was present in a different form than that upon the grit blasted control. Seventy percent of the carbon on the HA PS substrate surface existed as hydrocarbon ($(CH_2)_n$) while for the grit blast control only 48% existed in this form. This was a measurable difference in relative binding.

Calcium Ion-Implanted Surfaces

SEM revealed a smooth surface with features (polishing marks) similar to those of the non ion-implanted controls. The R_a of the CaII surface was comparable to the roughness of the nontreated surface. The calcium concentration at the surface of the CaII surface was found to be approximately 10% (at. wt.) by XPS and EDX. XPS revealed that the calcium near the surface was present principally as calcium oxide (60%). This was confirmed by XRD (Fig. 2) and SIMS. XRD also revealed the presence of elemental calcium in the samples. The intensities of the CaO and elemental calcium peaks, relative to Ti reflections, were greater in TFXRD than XRD. The absolute intensities of the Ti peaks were lower in the CaII samples than in the Ti control. Depth profiling by SIMS revealed a calcium peak, 125% of surface concentration, approximately 100 nm below the surface (Fig. 3) . SIMS analysis showed that the coincident calcium oxide and Ti oxide layers had equivalent thicknesses, 4 times greater than the thickness of the passivated Ti oxide layer on non ion-implanted Ti alloy controls.

DISCUSSION

The rational development of calcium-containing surfaces to serve as attachment vehicles for orthopedic prostheses requires an understanding of the correlation of certain chemical and structural features of the surface with biological response (*i.e.*, bone bonding). Publications dating back several years have described the use of PS HA coatings as attachment vehicles for orthopedic prostheses [2, 4, 5, 12]. While there have been a large number of animal studies and human trials there have been relatively few studies that have detailed the near-surface chemistry and crystalline structure of the PS coating. Our analysis of the surface chemistry of PS HA coatings from two sources has revealed a substance with a stoichiometry and crystallinity consistent with a predomination of the mineral, hydroxyapatite. Our finding of TCP, β-$Ca_2P_2O_7$, and CaO in trace amounts confirms a few previous studies employing XRD [8, 11]. This investigation demonstrated a difference in HA crystallite size in coatings applied by different vendors. A previous report [11] has documented crystallite sizes 2-20 fold smaller than those found in our study. This is a reflection of the different operating conditions employed during the PS process, effecting changes in the crystallinity and morphology of the starting HA powder as it is melted in the plasma and impacted on the metal substrate.

There was a noncrystalline phase present up to approximately 10 % and a significant atomic weight percent of carbon on the PS HA surface, present as a ubiquitous contaminant. Previous work [10] has attributed the noncrystalline phase to a supercooling of the molten HA particles, building up the coating on the metal substrate. Vacuum heating of the PS HA coating to 630°C led to crystallization of this amorphous phase.[10] The presence of a noncrystalline phase has an uncertain impact on clinical performance of the coated prosthesis, because of the likelihood that it is more soluble that HA. [13] These findings suggest that future investigations might continue to focus on post PS treatments in order to increase the percent crystallinity of the PS HA coating.

Studies in which the PS HA coating was dissolved from the Ti alloy substrate revealed that the chemistry and crystalline structure of the metal surface, thus revealed, had the characteristics of noncoated material. This indicates that removal of the PS HA coating *in vivo* should not yield a surface that would be any less "biocompatible" than a native Ti alloy prosthesis surface.

Ion-implantation investigation has demonstrated that a significant amount of calcium can be impregnated into the surface layer of Ti alloy. The question of whether calcium alone in the surface can result in bone bonding will require future investigations employing implants in animal models. Future studies will also have to address what effect the significant increase in thickness of the oxide layer on the CaII specimen will have on the mechanical integrity of the oxide. The biological importance of the carbon contamination on the surface of these and other implants remains uncertain. Sputtering of the surface layer removed most, but not all of the carbon, questioning how readily exchangeable the carbon at the surface will be once the device is implanted into the body.

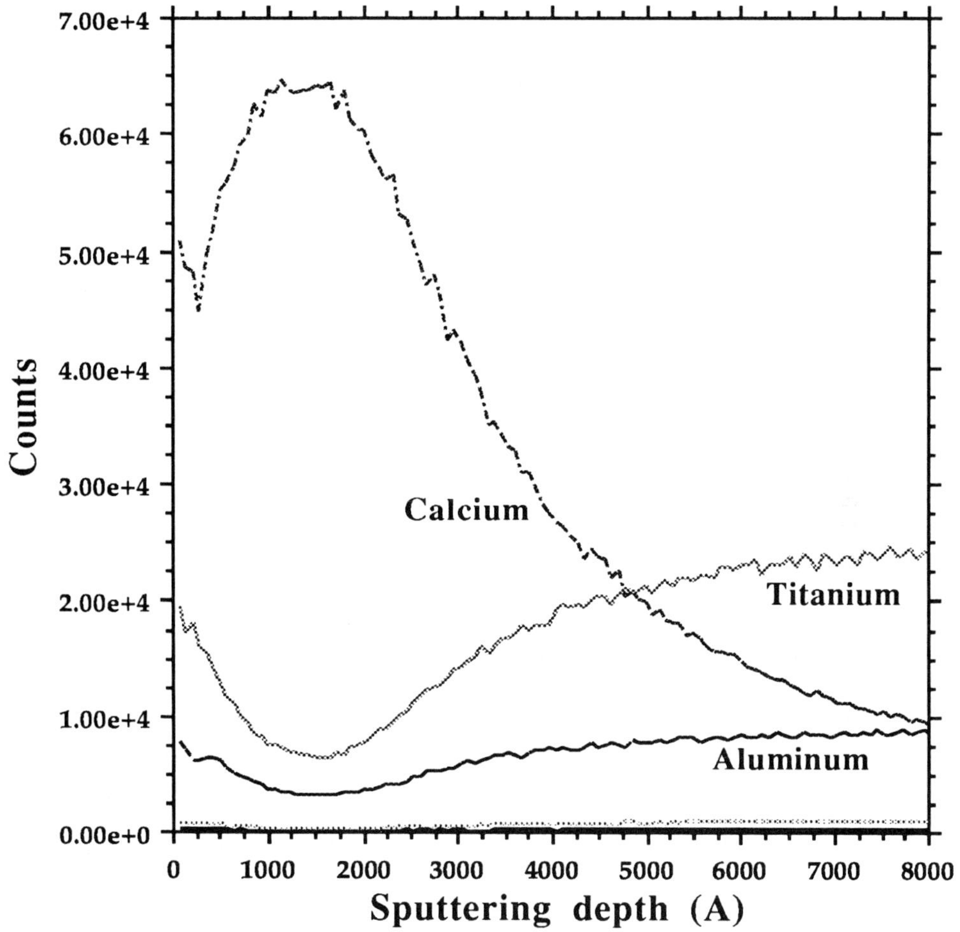

Fig. 3 SIMS elemental depth profile of a CaII specimen.

ACKNOWLEDGMENTS

We gratefully acknowledge support from NIH AR40427 and VA Rehabilitation R&D, and the assistance of the National ESCA and Surface Analysis Center for Biomedical Problems at the University of Washington in Seattle, WA. Discussions with B.D. Ratner of the University of Washington and J.R. Martin of the Massachusetts Institute of Technology were appreciated.

REFERENCES

1. Poss, R., Walker, P., Spector, M., Reilly, D. T., Robertson, D. D. and Sledge, C. B., Strategies for improving fixation of femoral components in total hip arthroplasty, *Clin Orthop* 1988, **235**, 181-194

2. Geesink, R. G. T., deGroot, K. and Klein, C., Chemical implant fixation using hydroxy-apatite coatings, *Clin. Orthop.* 1987, **225**, 147-170

3. Thomas, K. A., Cook, S. D., Haddad, R. J. J., Kay, J. F. and Jarcho, M., Biologic response to hydroxylapatite-coated titanium hips. A preliminary study in dogs, *J. Arthroplasty* 1989, **4**, 43-53

4. Geesink, R., de Groot, K. and Klein, C. P. A. T., Bonding of bone to apatite-coated hip implants, *J. Bone Jt. Surg.* 1988, **70-B**, 17-22

5. deGroot, K., Geesink, R., Klein, C. P. A. T. and Serekian, P., Plasma sprayed coatings of hydroxylapatite, *J. Biomed. Mater. Res.* 1987, **21**, 1375-1381

6. Dhert, W. J. A., Klein, C. P. A. T., Wolke, J. G. C., van der Velde, E. A. and de Groot, K., A mechanical investigation of fluorapatite, magnesiumwhitlockite, and hydroxylapatite plasma-sprayed coatings in goats, *J. Biomed. Mater. Res.* 1991, **25**, 1183-1200

7. Bauer, T. W., Geesink, R. C. T., Zimmerman, R. and McMahon, J. T., Hydroxyapatite-coated femoral stems: histological analysis of components retrieved at autopsy, *J. Bone Jt. Surg.* 1991, **73-A**, 1439-1452

8. Ellies, L. G., Nelson, D. G. A. and Featherstone, J. D. B., Crystallographic changes in calcium phosphates during plasma-spraying, *Biomat.* 1992, **13**, 313-316

9. Oguchi, H., Ishikawa, K., Ojima, S., Hirayama, Y., Seto, K. and Eguchi, G., Evaluation of a high-velocity flame-spraying technique for hydroxyapatite, *Biomat.* 1992, **13**, 471-477

10. Zyman, Z., Weng, J., Liu, X., Zhang, X. and Ma, Z., Amorphous phase and morphological structure of hydroxyapatite plasma coatings, *Biomat.* 1993, **14**, 225-228

11. Koch, B., Wolke, J. G. C. and deGroot, K., X-ray diffraction studies on plasma-sprayed calcium phosphate-coated implants, *J. Biomed. Mater. Res.* 1990, **24**, 655-667

12. Jansen, J. A., Waerden, J. P. C. M. v. d. and Wolke, J. G. C., Histologic investigation of the biologic behavior of different hydroxyapatite plasma-sprayed coatings in rabbits, *J. Biomed. Mater. Res.* 1993, **27**, 603-610

13. Hurson, S., Lacefield, W., Lucas, L., Ong, J., Whitehead, R. and Bumgardner, J., Effect of the crystallinity of plasma sprayed HA coatings on dissolution, The 19th Annual Meeting of the Society for Biomaterials, Birmingham, Alabama, 1993, pp.

FORMATION OF HYDROXYAPATITE IN CEMENT SYSTEMS

Laurence C. Chow, Shozo Takagi, and Kunio Ishikawa
National Institute of Standards and Technology
Gaithersburg, MD 20899

I. INTRODUCTION

Self-setting calcium phosphate cements (CPC) have been a subject of considerable interest in recent years. These materials contain only calcium phosphates, have neutral pH, and form hydroxyapatite (OHAp) as the end product. As a result, the cements were found to be highly biocompatible and osteoconductive. Since CPC also sets to a hard mass at the site of application, it has been shown in experimental studies to be highly useful in a wide range of dental and medical procedures.[1-10] Among the self-setting calcium phosphate cement systems, those cements that consist of tetracalcium phosphate (TTCP) and dicalcium phosphate anhydrous (DCPA) or dicalcium phosphate dihydrate (DCPD) form OHAp as the only reaction product.[11-13] The chemistry of reactions between TTCP and DCPA or DCPD have been studied extensively.[11-23] This paper reports the effects of several additional factors on the formation of OHAp in the TTCP + DCPA system. Also described is the formation of OHAp in new cement compositions comprising TTCP and a-tricalcium phosphate (α-TCP), octacalcium phosphate (OCP), amorphous calcium phosphate (ACP), or monocalcium phosphate monohydrate (MCPM).

II. METHODS AND MATERIALS

Tetracalcium phosphate was prepared by heating an equimolar mixture of calcium carbonate and DCPA to 1500° C for 6 h.[24] α-TCP was prepared by heating a mixture containing 2 moles of DCPA and 1 mole calcium carbonate to 1200° C for 6 h. OCP and ACP were prepared in aqueous systems following the methods of Tung[25] and Eanes,[26] respectively. MCPM, a commercially obtained reagent grade chemical, was used as received. The calcium phosphate materials were ground in a planetary ball mill to obtain the desired particles sizes.

The cement specimens were prepared by mixing for 30 seconds 0.3 grams of the CPC powder with 0.14 to 0.075 mL of a CPC liquid phase; the powder to liquid ratio (P/L) ranged from 2.0 to 4.0. The paste was packed into a stainless steel mold (6 mm D x 3 mm H) with a 20-Newton force (70 Newton/cm^2) applied by means of a plunger. The top and bottom surfaces of the mold were then covered with two glass plates held by a "c"-clamp and stored in a 37°C, 100% humidity box. Specimens were removed from the molds after 4 h, and were placed in water for 20 h. The diametral tensile strength (DTS) measurements

0-8493-4750-5/94/$0.00 + $.50

were then conducted on the 24-h specimens. The diameter and length of each specimen were measured with a micrometer. The sample was placed between steel platens that were covered with one thickness of wet filter paper, and crushed at a loading rate of 1 mm/min. The average DTS value was obtained from 5 specimens.

The extent of conversion of the CPC starting materials to OHAp was measured by powder X-ray diffraction (XRD). The specimens were prepared as described above. After the specimens were placed in the incubator for the prescribed time, they were frozen in liquid N_2 and then freezed dried. In this way, the process of CPC conversion to OHAp was stopped at the specific times. The freeze dried samples were ground to fine powders and characterized by XRD. The XRD patterns of the specimens were recorded with a diffractometer using graphite-monochromatized CuKa radiation (λ = 0.1540 nm) generated at 40 kV and 25 mA. The samples were scanned from 3 to 60 degrees 2θ in a continuous mode (1.0°/min, time constant 2 s) and peak intensities were recorded on a strip-chart recorder. The relative peak intensities of the 013 (29.2°) and 040 (29.8°) reflections for TTCP, the 110 (26.6°) reflection for DCPA, and the 002 (25.9°) reflection for OHAp were recorded a minimum of four times, and the averaged values were used to estimate the amount of CPC conversion to OHAp. The percent conversion (% Conv) of the TTCP + DCPA mixture to OHAp was calculated using the following equation:[12]

$$\% \text{ Conv} = \frac{\dfrac{OHAp_t}{OHAp_\infty} + \dfrac{1-(DCPA_t/DCPA_0) + 1-(TTCP_t/TTCP_0)}{2}}{2} \times 100 \qquad (1)$$

where $DCPA_0$ and $TTCP_0$ are the peak intensities of DCPA and TTCP, respectively, in the unreacted CPC, $OHAp_\infty$ is the peak intensity of OHAp in set CPC where no TTCP or DCPA residuals were observed, and $DCPA_t$, $TTCP_t$ and $OHAp_t$ are the peak intensities of the corresponding compounds in the specimen collected at time t after mixing.

III. OHAp FORMATION IN THE TTCP + DCPA SYSTEM

A. EFFECTS OF THE TTCP/DCPA RATIO.

Reactions that occur of an equimolar mixture of TTCP and DCPA or DCPD in water were shown[11-13] to form stoichiometric OHAp, following the reaction described by eqn. (2) or (3), respectively.

$$Ca_4(PO_4)_2O + CaHPO_4 \rightarrow Ca_5(PO_4)_3OH \qquad (2)$$

$$Ca_4(PO_4)_2O + CaHPO_4 \cdot 2H_2O \rightarrow Ca_5(PO_4)_3OH + 2H_2O \qquad (3)$$

Brown and Fulmer[17] reported that in an aqueous slurry reactions of 1 mole of TTCP with 2 moles of DCPA formed a calcium-deficient apatite with a Ca/P ratio of 1.5 as the only product following the reaction,

$$6\,Ca_4(PO_4)_2O + 12\,CaHPO_4 \rightarrow 4\,Ca_9(HPO_4)(PO_4)_5OH + 2H_2O \qquad (4)$$

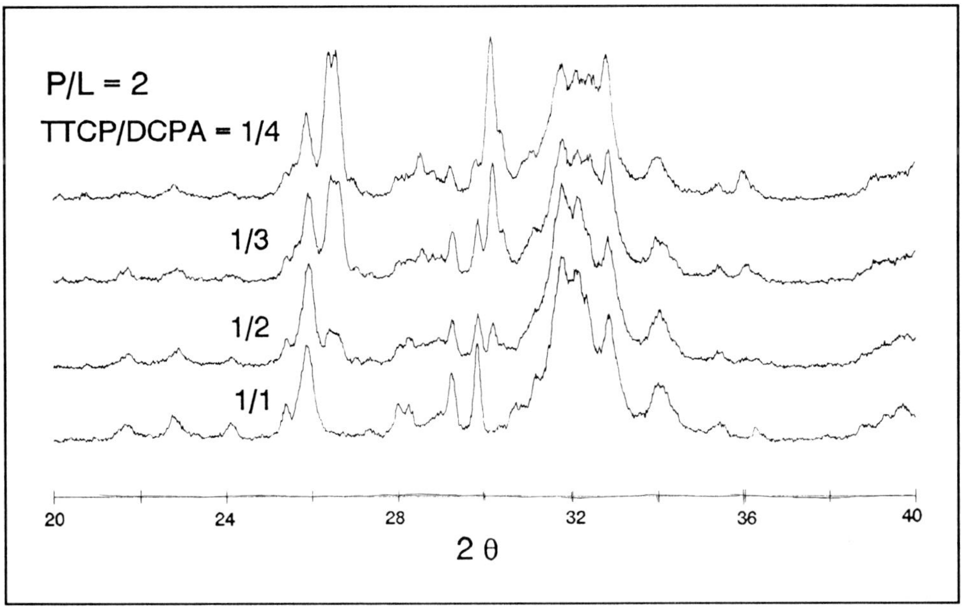

Figure 1. XRD patterns of 24-h CPC specimens with different TTCP/DCPA ratios and a P/L ratio of 2.

Calcium deficient OHAp can be considered as an inter-layering composite of OHAp and OCP.[27] Following this model the Ca/P ratio of calcium-deficient OHAp in the three component system, $Ca(OH)_2$-H_3PO_4-H_2O, can have a value ranging from the Ca/P ratio of OHAp (1.67) to that of OCP (1.33). In the present study, we examined the reactions of TTCP and DCPA in the form of cements (P/L = 2, 3, and 4) with a TTCP/DCPA ratio ranging from 1/1 to 1/4, leading to a Ca/P ratio from 1.67 to 1.33. The results show that in cements that contained a greater amount of water initially, i.e., with P/L of 2, only small DCPA or TTCP peaks appeared in the XRD patterns in the cements with TTCP/DCPA ratios of 1/1 and 1/2, suggesting near complete conversion to OHAp. In contrast, significant amounts of residual DCPA appear to be present in cements with TTCP/DCPA ratios of 1/3 and 1/4, as indicated by the pronounced DCPA peaks in the XRD patterns. At the higher P/L ratio of 4, the DCPA peaks were quite pronounced for all cements except the one with TTCP/DCPA ratio of 1/1 (Fig. 2). Residual TTCP (29.2 and 29.8° 2θ) peaks were also present in these samples, indicating that the reaction was incomplete in cements that contained very small amounts of water initially. It is interesting to note that after the cement was set, the residual TTCP and DCPA did not react even when the samples were immersed in water for approximately 24 h prior to the XRD analysis.

The presence of large amounts of residual DCPA in samples with a TTCP/DCPA ratio of 1/3 or 1/4, regardless of the P/L ratio used, indicates that the Ca/P of the calcium-deficient apatite formed is not predominantly determined by the amounts of TTCP and DCPA available for reaction. In fact, one would expect that the Ca/P ratio of the mineral formed is determined by the solution composition at the time the crystal lattice is formed. Thus, the results suggest that the formation of apatite with a Ca/P ratio below 1.5 was not favored by the solution compositions present in the cements studied. The two cements with a TTCP/DCPA ratio of 1/1 or 1/2, while having different Ca/P ratios, each formed a phase pure OHAp, suggesting that solution composition in the TTCP/DCPA cements favor the formation of apatites with Ca/P ratio only in the range of 1.67 and 1.5, as suggested by Brown and Fulmer.[17]

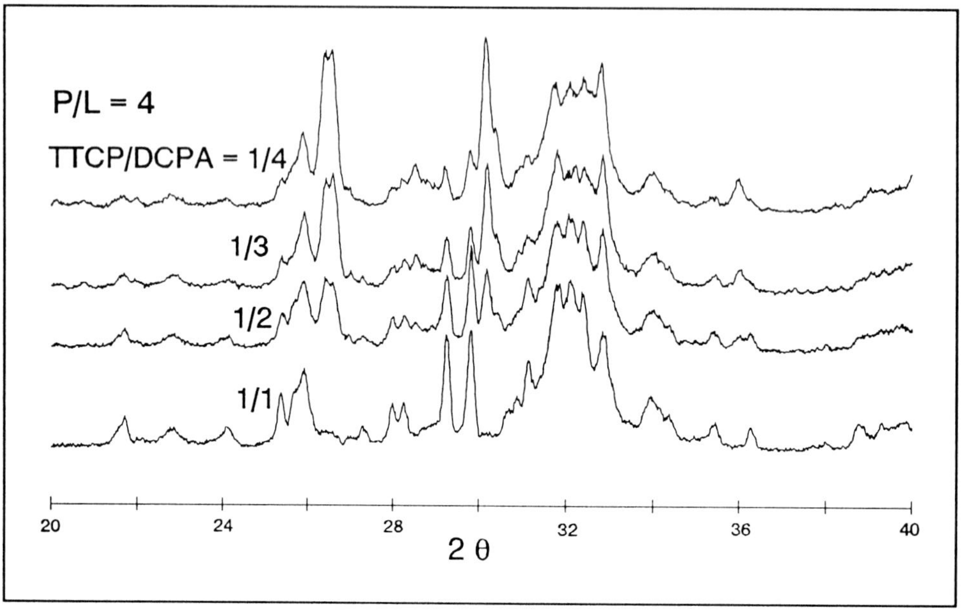

Figure 2. XRD patterns of 24-h CPC specimens with different TTCP/DCPA ratios and a P/L ratio of 4.

SEM examinations show the presence of crystals with plate-like morphology in all samples, suggesting that OCP may have been formed as a reaction intermediate. However, the main OCP peak at 4.8° 2θ was not detected in XRD patterns of any of the samples, indicating the absence of phase-pure OCP in the product.

DTS measurements show that, at a P/L ratio of 3, the DTS values (mean ± s.d., n = 5) were 12.9 ± 0.7, 8.1 ± 0.6, 6.5 ± 0.4, and 4.3 ± 0.7 MPa for cements with TTCP/DCPA ratios of 1/1, 1/2, 1/3, and 1/4, respectively. These results clearly indicate that the cement that formed stoichiometric OHAp had the highest mechanical strength.

B. EFFECTS OF THE PHOSPHATE CONCENTRATION OF THE CEMENT LIQUID

Ishikawa and Eanes[28] reported that the rate of OHAp formation in the hydrolysis of DCPA was significantly increased by phosphate. Since in the three component system the phosphate concentrations in solutions with neutral or alkaline pH's are extremely low,[29] the addition of phosphates in the liquid phase of the cement could also increase the rate of the cement setting reaction. It is important to note that the addition of phosphoric acid does not raise the phosphate concentration significantly, e.g., to 0.1 mol/L, until the pH is significantly lowered, e.g., to about 4 or below, which may interfere with the cement setting reaction. On the other hand, the phosphate concentration would increase in direct proportion to the amount a phosphate salt, e.g., Na_2HPO_4, added. This is because the Na^+ ions in the solution require an equivalent amount of anions to balance the electrical charges, and phosphate ions are the only anions that are present at a significant level. This concept of electroneutrality unbalance was thoroughly described by Lehr et al.[30]

In the present study, the effect of phosphate concentration on OHAp formation in the TTCP + DCPA cement was investigated. The rate of OHAp formation, expressed as the percent of starting materials converted to OHAp (eqn. 1) as a function of time, was found to be greatly enhanced by phosphate concentration of 0.25 mol/L and above (Fig. 3). In the presence of added phosphate, 40 to 60% of the CPC powder had converted to OHAp by 0.5 h, in contrast to about 5 to 10% conversion in the absence of phosphate. These results are consistent with the findings of Fulmer and Brown[21] that addition of 0.1 mol/L of Na_2HPO_4 accelerated the OHAp formation in TTCP + DCPA slurries. The rapid OHAp formation in these cements caused a much more rapid hardening of the cements (5 min) compared to the conventional CPC (25 min).

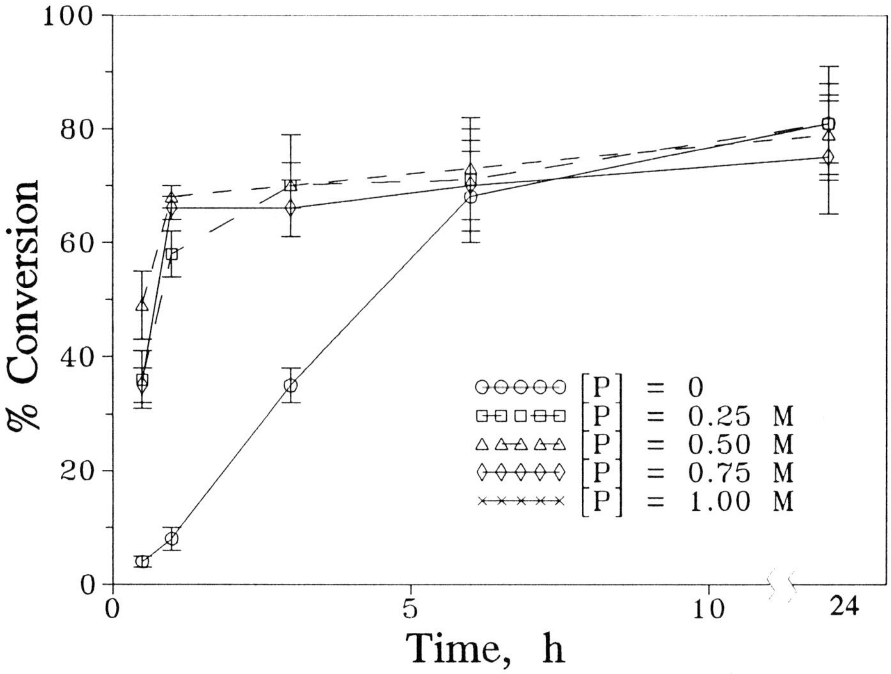

Figure 3. Percent conversion of TTCP and DCPA to OHAp as a function of time: effect of phosphate concentration.

IV. FORMATION OF OHAp IN THE TTCP + MCPM SYSTEM

Fulmer et al.[20] reported that reactions of TTCP and MCPM in a slurry system (P/L of 0.01) formed calcium deficient OHAp as the only product. In the present study, the reaction of TTCP and MCPM in the form of a cement, i.e. P/L of 3, was studied. Following the reaction stoichiometry represented by eqn. (5), a cement mixture with a TTCP/MCPM molar ratio of 7/2 was prepared, and the OHAp formation was followed by XRD as before.

$$7\,Ca_4(PO_4)_2O + 2\,Ca(H_2PO_4)_2 \cdot H_2O \rightarrow 6\,Ca_5(PO_4)_3OH + 3\,H_2O \qquad (5)$$

XRD patterns (Fig. 4) show that most of the MCPM in the cement has converted to DCPD in 2 min (the shortest time that the sample could be frozen to stop the reaction); the DCPD subsequently reacted with TTCP to form OHAp. The reactions in the cement system appear to be the same as the reactions that occurred in the slurry system reported by Fulmer et al.[20] The formation of DCPD as a reaction intermediate is very much expected because of the high solubility of MCPM, which quickly leads to the formation of DCPD, especially in a small amount of water.[31] The above results indicate that the cement-forming reaction that occurs in the TTCP + MCPM system is essentially the same as that in the TTCP + DCPD system with the exception that the former system includes an initial reaction of dissolution of MCPM and subsequent formation of DCPD.

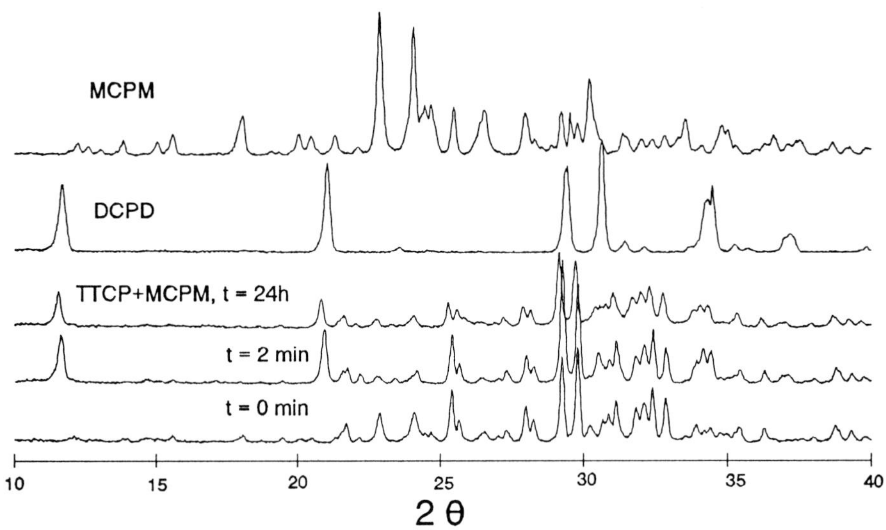

Figure 4. XRD patterns of a cement consisting of TTCP and MCPM at 0 min, 2 min, and 24h showing that DCPD was formed as an intermediate. Also shown are patterns of DCPD and MCPM.

V. FORMATION OF OHAp IN THE TTCP + α-TCP, TTCP + ACP AND TTCP + OCP SYSTEMS.

As described above, cement setting occurs readily in systems that contain TTCP and DCPA, DCPD, or MCPM as the cement powders and water as the liquid. Despite the fact that slurries that contain TTCP and one or more calcium phosphates from the group, α-TCP, β-TCP, OCP, and ACP, also produce solution compositions that are supersaturated with respect to OHAp,[16] it has not been shown that these systems form cements or significant amounts of OHAp. This is probably because the solubilities of these latter salts are too low to support rapid OHAp formation. Since the addition of phosphate significantly accelerated OHAp formation in the TTCP + DCPA system as described above, we investigated the formation of OHAp from reactions of TTCP and these less soluble calcium phosphates in the presence of a high phosphate concentration in the solution. Mixtures of TTCP with α-TCP, β-TCP, ACP, or OCP were prepared with molar ratios of the salts corresponding to the stoichiometry of the reactions described by eqns. (6) and (7), and cement samples were prepared with a 1 mol/L Na_2HPO_4 solution as the liquid.

$$Ca_4(PO_4)_2O + 2\ Ca_3(PO_4)_2 + H_2O \rightarrow 2\ Ca_5(PO_4)_3OH \qquad (6)$$

$$3\ Ca_4(PO_4)_2O + Ca_8H_2(PO_4)_6 \cdot 5H_2O \rightarrow 4\ Ca_5(PO_4)_3OH + 4\ H_2O \qquad (7)$$

XRD patterns of 24-h specimens show that near complete conversion of the starting materials to OHAp occurred in the systems, TTCP + α-TCP (Fig. 5), TTCP + ACP (Fig. 6), and TTCP + OCP (Fig. 7), but not in the TTCP + β-TCP system (Fig. 8). Based on the solubility phase diagrams of calcium phosphates,[29] β-TCP is less soluble than any other calcium phosphate except OHAp in the pH range of approximately 6 and above. This may be the reason for the lack of reaction even in the presence of a relatively high phosphate concentration.

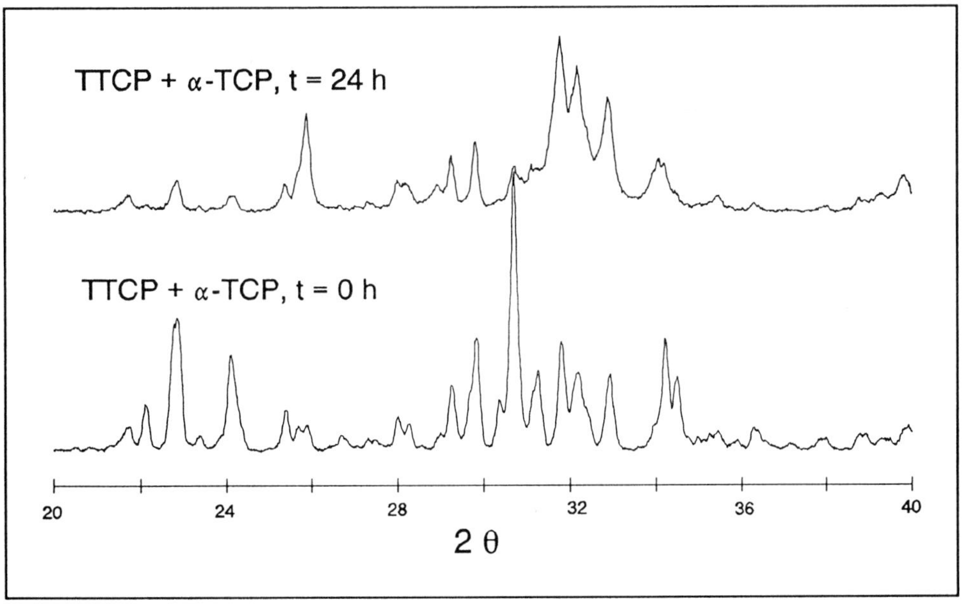

Figure 5. XRD patterns of a cement consisting of TTCP and α-TCP showing OHAp formation at 24 h.

Cementation occurred in the first three systems in which there was OHAp formation occurred readily and not in the TTCP + β-TCP system. These results indicate that OHAp formation is crucial for cement setting and that OHAp forming cements can be formulated in these systems provided that a phosphate-containing solution is used as the liquid phase.

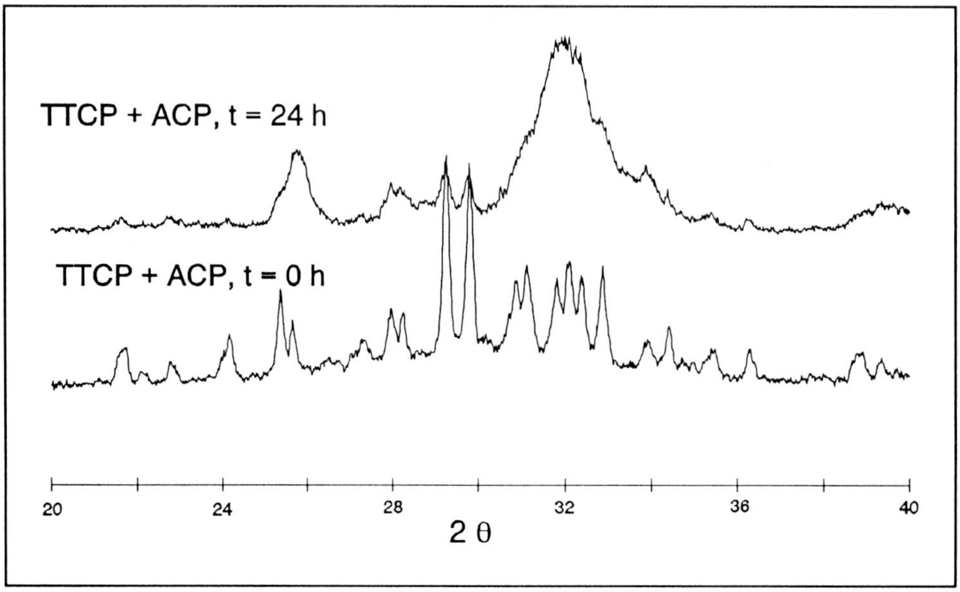

Figure 6. XRD patterns of a cement consisting of TTCP and ACP showing OHAp formation at 24 h.

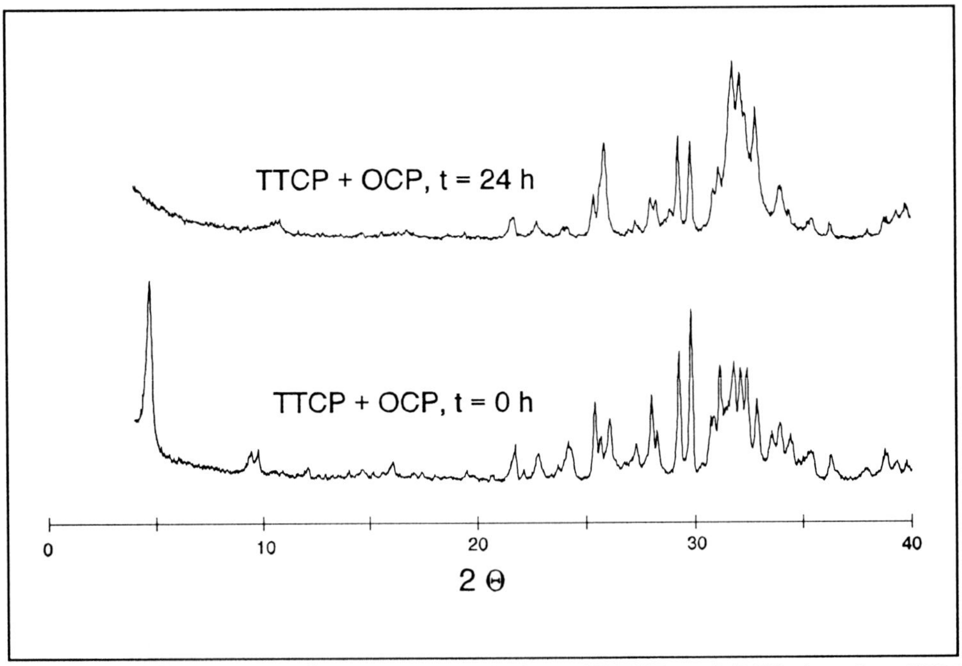

Figure 7. XRD patterns of a cement consisting of TTCP and OCP showing OHAp formation at 24 h.

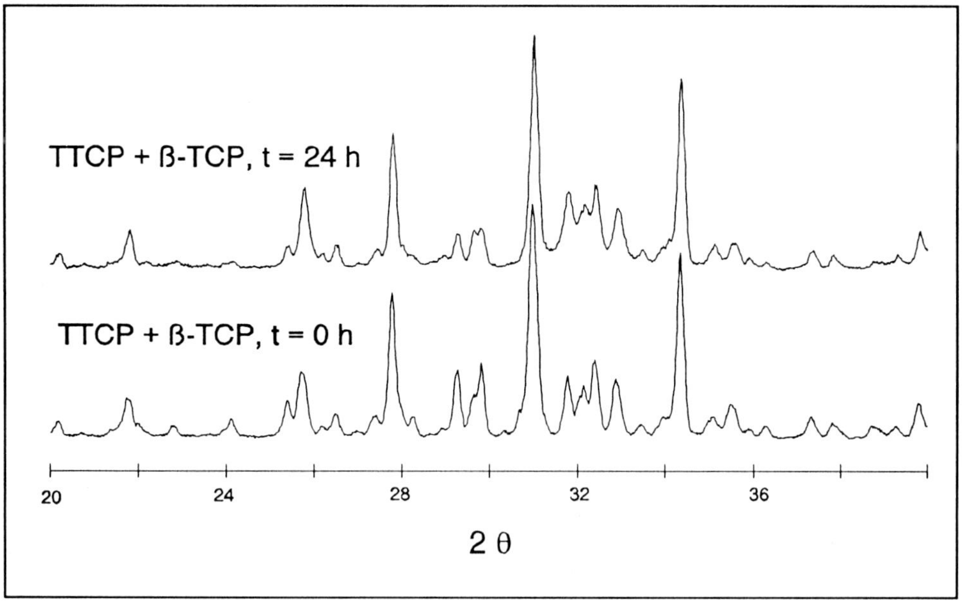

Figure 8. XRD patterns of a TTCP + β-TCP mixture showing lack of OHAp formation at 24 h.

ACKNOWLEDGEMENT

This study was supported in part by NIH grant DE05030.

REFERENCES

1. Chohayeb, A. A., Chow, L.C. and Tsaknis, P., Evaluation of Calcium Phosphate as a Root Canal Sealer-filler Material, *J. Endodon.*, 13, 384, 1987.
2. Sugawara, A., Chow, L. C., Takagi, S. and Chohayeb, H., In vitro Evaluation of the Sealing Ability of a Calcium Phosphate Cement When Used as a Root Canal Sealer-Filler, *J. Endodon.*, 16, 162, 1990.
3. Sugawara, A., Nishiyama, M., Chow, L. C. and Takagi, S., A New Biocompatible Material: Calcium Phosphate Cement - Biomedical Applications, *Tokyoto Shika Ishikai Zashi*, 38, 348, 1990.
4. Costantino, P. D., Friedman, C. D., Jones, K., Chow, L. C., Pelzer, H. J. and Sisson, Sr. G. A., Hydroxyapatite Cement. I. Basic Chemistry and Histologic Properties, *Arch. Otolaryngol Head Neck Surg.*, 117, 379, 1991.
5. Hong, Y. C., Wang, J. T., Hong, C. Y., Brown, W. E. and Chow, L. C., The Periapical Tissue Reaction to A Calcium Phosphate Cement in the Teeth of Monkeys, *J. Biomed. Mater. Res.*, 25, 485, 1991.
6. Friedman, C. D., Costantino, P. D., Jones, K., Chow, L. C., Pelzer, H. J. and Sisson, Sr. G. A., Hydroxyapatite Cement. II. Obliteration and Reconstruction of the Cat Frontal Sinus, *Arch. Otolaryngol Head Neck Surg.*, 117, 385, 1991.

7. Costantino, P. D., Friedman, C. D., Jones, R., Chow, L. C. and Sisson, Sr. G. A., Experimental Hydroxyapatite Cement Cranioplasty, *Plast. Reconstr. Sugr.*, 90, 174, 1992.
8. Sugawara, A., Nishiyama, M., Kusama, K., Moro, I., Nishiyama, S., Kudo, I., Chow, L. C. and Takagi, S., Histological Reactions of Calcium Phosphate Cement, *J. Japan Soc. Dent. Mater. Dev.*, 11, 11, 1992.
9. Yu, D., Wong, J., Matsuda, Y., Fox, J. L. and Higuchi, W. I., Self-Setting Hydroxyapatite Cement: A Novel Skeletal Drug-Delivery System for Antibiotics, *J. Am. Pharm. Sci.*, 81(6), 529, 1992.
10. Shindo, M. L., Costantino, P. D., Friedman, C. D. and Chow, L. C., Facial Skeletal Augmentation Using Hydroxyapatite Cement, *Arch. Otolaryngol Head Neck Surg.*, 119, 185, 1993.
11. Brown, W. E. and Chow, L. C., A New Calcium Phosphate, Water-setting Cement, in *Cement Research Progress 1986*, Brown, P. W., Ed., American Chemical Society, Ohio, 1987, pp.352.
12. Fukase, Y., Eanes, E. D., Takagi, S., Chow, L. C. and Brown, W. E., Setting Reactions and Compressive Strengths of Calcium Phosphate Cements, *J. Dent. Res.*, 69(12), 1852, 1990.
13. Doi, Y., Takezawa, Y., Shibata, S., Wakamatsu, N., Kamemizu, H., Goto, T., Iijima, M., Moriwaki, Y., Uno, K., Kubo, F., and Haeuchi, Y., Self-setting Apatite Cement, I. Physicochemical Properties, *J. Japan Soc. Dent. Mater. Dev.*, 6, 53, 1987.
14. Takezawa, Y., Doi, Y., Shibata, S., Wakamatsu, N., Kamemizu, H., Goto, T., Iijima, M., Moriwaki, Y., Uno, K., Kubo, F. and Haeuchi, Y., Self-setting Apatite Accelerator, II. Hydroxyapatite as Setting Accelerator, *J. Japan Soc. Dent. Mater. Dev.*, 6, 426, 1987.
15. Chow, L. C., Takagi, S., Costantino, P. D. and Friedman, C. D., Self-setting Calcium Phosphate Cements, *Mater. Res. Symp. Proc.*, 179, 3, 1991.
16. Chow, L. C., Development of Self-setting Calcium Phosphate Cements, *J. Ceram. Soc. Japan*, 99, 954, 1991.
17. Brown, P. W. and Fulmer, M. T., Kinetics of Hydroxyapatite Formation at Low Temperature, *J. Am. Ceram. Soc.*, 74(5), 934, 1991.
18. Brown, P. W., Hocker, N. and Hoyle, S., Variation in Solution Chemistry During the Low-Temperature Formation of Hydroxyapatite, *J. Am. Ceram. Soc.*, 74(8), 1848, 1991.
19. Brown, P. W., Phase Relationships in the Ternary System $CaO-P_2O_5-H_2O$ at 25°C, *J. Am. Ceram. Soc.*, 75(1), 17, 1992.
20. Fulmer, M. T., Martin, R. I. and Brown, P. W., Formation of calcium deficient hydroxyapatite at near-physiological temperature, *J. Mater. Sci. Mater. Med.*, 3, 299, 1992.
21. Fulmer, M. T. and Brown, P. W., Effects of Na_2HPO_4 and NaH_2PO_4 on hydroxyapatite formation, *J. Biomed. Mater. Res.*, 27, 1095, 1993.
22. Martin, R. I. and Brown, P. W., Hydration of tetracalcium phosphate, *Advance in Cement Res.*, 5(19), 119, 1993.
23. Graham, S. and Brown, P. W., The low temperature formation of octacalcium phosphate, *J. Crystal Growth*, 132, 215, 1993.
24. Brown, W. E. and Epstein, E. F., Crystallography of Tetracalcium Phosphate, *J. Res. Nat. Bur. Stand.*, 69A, 547, 1965.

25. Tung, M. S., Eidelman, N., Sieck, B. and Brown, W. E., Octacalcium Phosphate Solubility Product from 4 to 37°C, *J. Res. Nat. Bur. Stand.*, 93(5), 613, 1988.
26. Eanes, E. D., Gillessen, I. H. and Posner, A. S., Intermediate States in the Precipitation of Hydroxyapatite, *Nature*, 208(5008), 365, 1965.
27. Brown, W. E., Mathew, M. and Tung, M. S., Crystal Chemistry of Octacalcium Phosphate, *Prog. Crystal Growth Charact.*, 4, 59, 1981.
28. Ishikawa, K. and Eanes, E. D., The Hydrolysis of Anhydrous Dicalcium Phosphate into Hydroxyapatite, *J. Dent. Res.*, 72(2), 474, 1993.
29. Brown, W. E., Solubilities of Phosphates and Other Sparingly Soluble Compounds, in *Environmental Phosphorous Handbook*, Griffith, E. J., Beeton, A., Spencer, J. M. and Mitchell, D. T., Eds., John Wiley and Sons, New York, 1976, pp. 203.
30. Lehr, R. J., Brown, W.E., and Brown, W.H., Chemical Behavior of Monocalcium Phosphate Monohydrate in Soils, *Soil Science Soc. Am.*, 23(1), 3, 1959.
31. Brown W. E., Behavior of Slightly Soluble Calcium Phosphates as Revealed by Phase-equilibrium Calculations, *Soil Science*, 90(1), 51, 1960.

OCTACALCIUM PHOSPHATE CARBOXYLATES. 5. INCORPORATION OF EXCESS SUCCINATE AND AMMONIUM IONS IN THE OCTACALCIUM PHOSPHATE SUCCINATE STRUCTURE

Milenko Marković,[a] Bruce O. Fowler,[b] and Walter E. Brown[a,c]

SUMMARY

Octacalcium phosphate succinate, $Ca_8(HPO_4)_{1.07}(succ)_{0.93}(PO_4)_4{\cdot}6H_2O$ (OCP-SUCC), has an ~50% larger hydrated layer volume than that of its parent compound, octacalcium phosphate, $Ca_8(HPO_4)_2(PO_4)_4{\cdot}5H_2O$ (OCP). The incorporation of structurally excess ions in OCP-SUCC was established by chemical analyses, X-ray powder diffraction, and infrared spectroscopy. Both excess succinate and counter ammonium ions were found to incorporate in the hydrated layer of the OCP-SUCC structure; this incorporation caused a slight expansion in the *a*-axis of up to 3%. Removal of these excess ions resulted in contraction of the *a*-axis to near that of OCP-SUCC. OCP-SUCC and particularly other OCP-carboxylates (OCPCs) that have larger hydrated layer volumes have a potential to incorporate various molecules and ions; these OCPCs could serve as vehicles to facilitate slow release of these additives into aqueous solutions.

I. INTRODUCTION

Octacalcium bis(hydrogenphosphate) tetrakis(phosphate) pentahydrate, $Ca_8(HPO_4)_2(PO_4)_4{\cdot}5H_2O$, well known as octacalcium phosphate (OCP), has a layered structure composed of alternating hydrated and apatitic layers.[1-3] Monma prepared OCP derivatives in which aliphatic dicarboxylate ions replaced HPO_4^{2-} ions in the OCP structure.[4,5] Recently, it was shown that these HPO_4^{2-} ions can also be replaced by various physiologically relevant di- and tricarboxylate ions and some of their hydroxy and keto derivatives.[6,7] Compositional and structural details have been determined for some of these OCP-carboxylates (OCPCs) by comparing their vibrational spectra and X-ray diffraction patterns with those of OCP.[8,9] It was found that of the two crystallographically nonequivalent HPO_4^{2-} ions designated (5) and (6) in the OCP structure,[2] only the HPO_4(5) ions located at the Ca-HPO_4-Ca pillars in

---

[a] American Dental Association Health Foundation, Paffenbarger Research Center, National Institute of Standards and Technology, Gaithersburg, Maryland 20899.

[b] National Institute of Dental Research, NIH, Bone Research Branch Research Program, National Institute of Standards and Technology.

[c] Deceased.

0-8493-4750-5/94/$0.00 + $.50

the hydrated layer of OCP were replaced by carboxylate ions[8,9] which caused an expansion of the unit-cell *a*-axis.

Among these OCPCs, octacalcium phosphate succinate (OCP-SUCC), with composition of $Ca_8(HPO_4)_{1.07}(succ)_{0.93}(PO_4)_4 \cdot 6H_2O$, where succ = $OOCCH_2CH_2COO$, has been characterized in detail[7,8] and its solubility and kinetics of formation have been investigated.[10] OCP-SUCC has an expanded unit-cell *a*-axis (d_{100} = 2.13 nm) and an ~50% larger hydrated layer volume than that of its parent compound OCP (d_{100} = 1.868 nm); incorporation of additional ions in this expanded layer is probable. In the present paper the incorporation of additional excess succinate and ammonium ions in the OCP-SUCC structure was investigated.

II. EXPERIMENTAL[d]

The α-tricalcium phosphate, α-$Ca_3(PO_4)_2$ (α-TCP), was prepared by heating a 1:1 molar homogenized pressed mixture of $Ca_2P_2O_7$ and $CaCO_3$ at 1200°C for 4 h and then allowing it to cool rapidly in air to room temperature. The $Ca_2P_2O_7$ was prepared by igniting reagent grade $CaHPO_4.2H_2O$ at 900°C for 12 h. Succinic acid stock solution (0.3 mol/L) was prepared from reagent grade chemical dissolved in triply distilled water.

The α-TCP (particle size less than 10 μm) was hydrolyzed in 0.25 mol/L succinate solution prepared from stock solution adjusted with ammonium hydroxide to the desired initial pH ($5.7 < pH_{init} < 6.7$).[7] The initial solid/solution ratio was 10 mg/mL. The experiments were performed in a double-wall, water-thermostated cell at 37°C under a nitrogen atmosphere; suspensions were stirred using glass-covered magnetic stirrers. After completion of α-TCP conversion into OCP-SUCC (8 to 24 h),[7] suspensions were centrifuged and then filtered through 0.22 μm Millipore filters. Precipitates collected after 8 h were slightly washed with one 20 mL portion of water whereas those collected after 24 h were thoroughly washed with three 50 mL portions of water; the samples were dried at reduced pressure (30 kPa) at 22°C for 16 h.

The collected precipitates were chemically analyzed for calcium, phosphate, carbon, hydrogen, and nitrogen. Calcium was determined by atomic absorption spectroscopy with a Perkin-Elmer Model 603 spectrophotometer. Phosphate was determined as the phosphovanadomolybdate complex with a Cary Model 219 spectrophotometer. The precisions of calcium and phosphate determinations were ±0.4 and ±0.2%, respectively.[8] The contents of carbon, hydrogen and nitrogen in solid phases were determined by chemical microanalysis (Galbraith Laboratories, Knoxville, TN) with precisions of ±4.6, ±7.1 and ±4.8%, respectively.

The solid phases were characterized by X-ray powder diffraction (XRD) and infrared spectroscopy (IR). XRD patterns were recorded in the 3 to 66° 2θ range with a Rigaku X-ray diffractometer using CuKα radiation and sodium

[d] Certain commercial materials and equipment are identified in this paper to specify the experimental procedure. In no instance does such identification imply recommendation or endorsement by the National Institute of Standards and Technology, the National Institutes of Health, or the ADA Health Foundation or that the material or equipment identified is necessarily the best available for the purpose.

chloride as an internal standard. In the range from 3 to 6° the 2θ values were obtained from averages of triplicate expanded-scale recordings with an uncertainty of ±0.01°. IR spectra (4000 to 300 cm^{-1}) of samples in KBr pellets were recorded with a Perkin-Elmer Model 621 spectrophotometer purged with dry CO_2-free air.

III. RESULTS AND DISCUSSION

Compositional analyses were performed on 8 h (slightly washed) and on 24 h (thoroughly washed) OCP-SUCC samples. The 8 h samples contained significantly higher contents of carbon and nitrogen. In Figure 1 the content of ammonium ions, Ca/P molar ratio, $2\theta_{100}$ and d_{100} values are given as functions of the content of succinate ions. In 24 h samples of OCP-SUCC (Figure 1, unfilled circles) the content of succinate was 10.8±0.8%, corresponding to 0.93±0.07 succinate ion per formula unit (structural succinate), and the content of ammonium ions was negligible. In 8 h precipitates (Figure 1, filled circles) the total contents of succinate and ammonium varied from 13 to 20% and from 0.7 to 2.2%, respectively. The molar ratio of excess succinate (total succinate less 10.8% of structural succinate) to ammonium was ~1:2 which is in accord with the electroneutrality balance. The empirical formula of these derivatives of OCP-SUCC with excess succinate and ammonium is $Ca_8(HPO_4)_{1.07}(succ)_{0.93}(PO_4)_4 \cdot 6H_2O \cdot z(2NH_4^+ + succ^{2-})$, where $z<0.8$. This excess in the 8 h samples could result from kinetic factors during early stages of precipitation. The XRD patterns of these compounds were overall almost identical to that of OCP-SUCC except for the position of the $2\theta_{100}$ diffraction line which was shifted to lower values showing expansion of the unit-cell *a*-axis. From Figure 1 it is evident that an increase of succinates (a) was paralleled by an increase in ammonium ions, (b) did not significantly change the Ca/P molar ratio, and (c) caused a decrease of $2\theta_{100}$ and increase of corresponding d_{100} values.

TABLE 1
Chemical Composition and $2\theta_{100}$ Values of OCP-SUCC Samples with an Excess of Succinate and Ammonium Ions (1 and 2) and of these Samples After 24 h Equilibration in Water (1′ and 2′).

Sample No.	Ca/P (molar ratio)	C (mass %)	N (mass %)	$2\theta_{100}$ (degree)
1	1.57	8.12	1.66	4.02
1′	1.55	4.28	0.20	4.12
2	1.54	5.47	0.77	4.06
2′	1.54	3.83	0.12	4.16

This excess amount of succinate and ammonium ions associated with OCP-SUCC could derive from: (i) replacement of calcium by ammonium and hydrogenphosphate by succinate ions, (ii) coprecipitation of ammonium

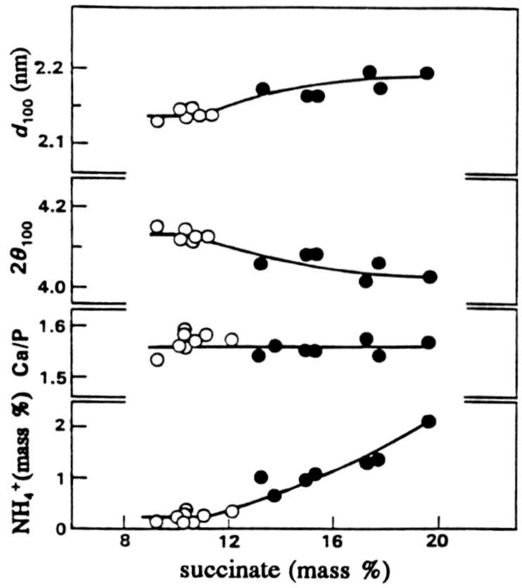

Figure 1. Contents of ammonium, Ca/P molar ratios, $2\theta_{100}$ and d_{100} values as functions of succinate contents for OCP-SUCC (unfilled circles) and for OCP-SUCC with an excess of succinate and ammonium ions (filled circles).

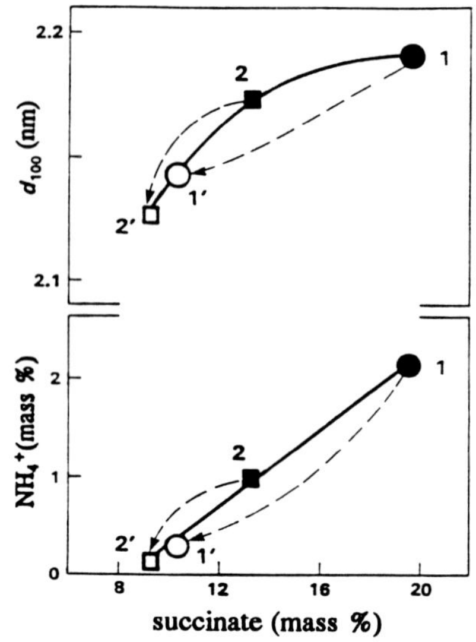

Figure 2. Contents of ammonium and d_{100} values as functions of succinate contents for OCP-SUCC samples with an excess of succinate and ammonium ions (filled symbols, denoted by 1 and 2) and for the same samples after 24 h equilibration in water (unfilled symbols, denoted by 1′ and 2′).

succinate salt, (iii) interlayering of ammonium succinate with OCP-SUCC, (iv) adsorption at the surface, and/or (v) incorporation in the hydrated layers (channels) of the OCP-SUCC structure. (i) The replacement of Ca^{2+} by NH_4^+ is not likely because of their ionic charge and size differences. This replacement, and especially hydrogenphosphate by succinate replacement, should cause considerable structural changes that were not observed in XRD patterns. (ii) The coprecipitation can be eliminated because XRD patterns of the precipitates with the highest contents of succinate and ammonium ions did not have diffraction lines of ammonium succinate salts, although the total mass % of these ions was ~10%. A physical mixture of crystalline ammonium succinate (9 mass %) and OCP-SUCC (91 mass %) showed XRD patterns for both compounds. (iii) The formation of a layered structure of OCP-SUCC and ammonium succinate is not very probable because of their structural dissimilarities. The additional layers could cause changes in XRD patterns that were not observed for these precipitates. (iv) If all these ions were adsorbed, no change in the d_{100} value would be observed. (v) The observed increase up to 3% in the d_{100} values (2.19 nm compared to 2.13 nm for OCP-SUCC) could arise from incorporation of excess succinate and ammonium counter ions in the hydrated layer of OCP-SUCC.

To further check if these barely significant d_{100} expansions were caused by structural incorporation of succinate and ammonium ions, additional experiments were performed. The 8 h precipitates of OCP-SUCC containing the larger amounts of succinate (higher carbon) and ammonium (higher nitrogen) were equilibrated in triply distilled water for 24 h at 37°C. In Table 1 chemical analyses and $2\theta_{100}$ values of the original (1 and 2) and the same samples after 24 h equilibration in water (1´ and 2´) are given. From these data, calculated ammonium ion contents and d_{100} values are shown as functions of succinate ion contents for these samples (Figure 2). In samples 1´ and 2´ the Ca/P molar ratios were nearly the same as in the original samples 1 and 2 (Table 1), but the contents of succinate (9.8±0.6%) were significantly lower and approached the value of structural succinate (10.8±0.8%), and correspondingly the content of ammonium dropped to the lower detection limits (Figure 2). The d_{100} values determined to a precision of ±0.2% showed that the *a*-axes in compounds 1´ and 2´ were contracted as compared to those in 1 and 2 (Figure 2). The decreases in ammonium and succinate contents, paralleled by a decrease in d_{100} values, indicate that these ions (or most of them) were incorporated in the hydrated layer of OCP-SUCC.

These results are supported by IR spectra shown in Figure 3 (the ammonium and carboxylate bands were normalized to the phosphate bands between about 700 to 500 cm^{-1}). The ammonium bands at 3140, ~3010, and 1400 cm^{-1} were only present in the original precipitate (Figure 3, spectrum 1), and the area of the carboxylate band near 1564 cm^{-1} was significantly smaller in the precipitate equilibrated in water (Figure 3, spectrum 1´; see reference 8 for a detailed spectrum of OCP-SUCC).

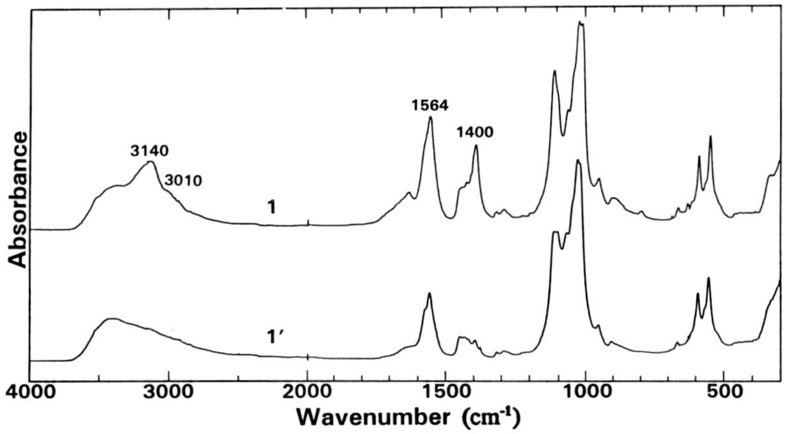

Figure 3. Infrared spectra of OCP-SUCC with an excess of succinate and ammonium ions (1) and of this sample after 24 h equilibration in water (1´). Band wavenumbers of ammonium (3140, ~3010 and 1400 cm^{-1}) and carboxylate (1564 cm^{-1}) ions are denoted. Sample designations correspond to those in Figure 2.

An *a*-axis contraction (decrease in the d_{100} value) concomitant with the removal of ions from the zeolitic hydrated layer of the OCP-SUCC structure has similarly been observed for progressively dehydrated OCP-adipate.[11] Moreover, the OCP-adipate structure was completely recovered by rehydration, showing the reversible change in the d_{100} value.[11]

Although excess succinate and ammonium counter ions were incorporated in OCP-SUCC which has an ~50% larger hydrated layer volume than that of OCP, some OCPCs, i.e. OCP-suberate, having an ~150% larger hydrated layer volume than that of OCP,[8] have higher potential for incorporation of excess ions. The OCPCs containing loosely-bound physiologically relevant ions and molecules in their large zeolitic hydrated layers could serve as vehicles for slow release of these additives into biological fluids. Investigation of these novel aspects of the OCPCs with emphasis on kinetics of incorporation and release of excess ions will be continued.

ACKNOWLEDGMENTS

This work was supported by the USA-Yugoslav Joint Fund for Scientific and Technological Cooperation in collaboration with the National Institute of Standards and Technology, Gaithersburg, MD (Grant PN 776), by the Ministry of Science, Technology and Informatics of Croatia and, in part, by USPHS Research Grant DE-05030 to the American Dental Association Health Foundation by the National Institutes of Health and is part of the dental research program conducted by NIST in cooperation with ADAHF. M. M. gratefully acknowledges financial support from the Fulbright Scholarship Exchange Program.

REFERENCES

1. Brown, W. E., Lehr, J. R., Smith, J. P., and Frazier, A. W., Crystallography of octacalcium phosphate, *J. Am. Chem. Soc.*, 79, 5318, 1957.
2. Brown, W. E., Crystal structure of octacalcium phosphate, *Nature*, 196, 1048, 1962.
3. Mathew, M., Brown, W. E., Schroeder, L. W., and Dickens, B., Crystal structure of octacalcium bis(hydrogenphosphate) tetrakis(phosphate)pentahydrate, $Ca_8(HPO_4)_2(PO_4)_4{\cdot}5H_2O$, *J. Crystal. Spectrosc. Res.*, 18(3), 235, 1988.
4. Monma, H. and Goto, M., Succinate-complexed octacalcium phosphate, *Bull. Chem. Soc. Jpn.*, 56, 3843, 1983.
5. Monma, H., The incorporation of dicarboxylates into octacalcium bis(hydrogenphosphate)tetrakis (phosphate) pentahydrate, *Bull. Chem. Soc. Jpn.*, 57, 599, 1984.
6. Marković, M., Fowler, B. O., and Brown, W. E., Incorporation of polycarboxylate ions in the octacalcium phosphate structure, *J. Dent. Res.*, 67(special issue), 270, 1988.
7. Marković, M., Fowler, B. O., and Brown, W. E., Octacalcium phosphate carboxylates. 1. Preparation and identification, *Chem. Mater.*, 1993, in press.
8. Marković, M., Fowler, B. O., and Brown, W. E., Octacalcium phosphate carboxylates. 2. Characteri- zation and structural considerations, *Chem. Mater.*, 1993, in press.
9. Fowler, B. O., Marković, M., and Brown, W. E., Octacalcium phosphate. 3. Infrared and Raman vibrational spectra, *Chem. Mater.*, 1993, in press.
10. Marković, M., Fowler, B. O., and Brown, W. E., Octacalcium phosphate carboxylates. 4. Kinetics of formation and solubility of octacalcium phosphate succinate, *J. Crystal Growth*, 1993, in press.
11. Monma, M. and Moriyoshi, Y., Zeolitic dehydration - rehydration of adipate-intercalated octacalcium phosphate, *J. Mater. Sci.: Mater. Med.*, 1, 21, 1990.

THE EFFECT OF ETHANOL ON THE SOLUBILITY OF HYDROXYAPATITE IN THE SYSTEM $Ca(OH)_2$-H_3PO_4-H_2O AT 25° AND 33°C

Ming S. Tung,[a] Changjian Lin,[b] Theresa H. Chow[c] and Pei Sung[d]

I. INTRODUCTION

Hydroxyapatite (HA), $Ca_5(PO_4)_3OH$, is the prototype of the inorganic constituent found in tooth and bone. Its physico-chemical properties have wide biological and industrial importance. Hence, its solubility in aqueous solutions has been extensively studied.[1-3] Although ethanol has been known to increase the association constants of ionic compounds and decrease their solubilities, the effect of ethanol on the solubility of HA has not been studied. Recently, ethanol has been reported to affect the precipitation of HA and other calcium phosphates.[4-5] This effect of ethanol may be due to the increase in precipitation rate or the effect on the solubility of HA or both. Therefore, the purpose of this study is to investigate the effect of ethanol on the solubility of HA.

II. EXPERIMENTAL METHODS AND MATERIALS

A. MATERIALS

Freshly boiled CO_2-free distilled water and reagent grade chemicals were used throughout the work. The HA was prepared by pumping phosphate and calcium solutions into a boiling ammonium acetate solution maintained at pH between 8.5 and 9.5 as described previously.[1] The HA was characterized by chemical, petrographic, infrared and x-ray methods, and scanning electron microscopy. The IR spectrum displayed the bands characteristic of well-crystallized HA. Weak bands in the regions of 1410 and 1640 cm^{-1} indicated slight contamination with carbonate and moisture. Hence, the HA was further heated at 850°C overnight before usage. The x-ray diffraction pattern was sharp and characteristic of well-crystallized pure HA with no extraneous peaks. The crystals appeared as irregularly shaped aggregates of needles smaller than 2 µm in the scanning electron microscope. The mean index of refraction (white radiation, 25°C) is 1.636 with a standard error of 0.002. This is lower than the indexes usually given for HA prepared hydrothermally, N_e=1.644 and N_w=1.651, and appears to be a characteristic of precipitated HA.[1]

---

[a] American Dental Association Health Foundation, Paffenbarger Research Center, National Institute of Standards and Technology, Gaithersburg, MD 20899.

[b] Xiamen University, Xiamen, Fujian, China, 361005.

[c] University of Maryland, College Park, MD, 20742.

[d] Food and Drug Administration, Rockville, MD, 20850.

0-8493-4750-5/94/$0.00 + $.50

B. ANALYTICAL METHODS

Various spectrophotometric methods were used to determine the concentrations of calcium and phosphate: calcium as the Ca-Arzenazo III complex,[6] and phosphate as the vanado-molybdate complex,[7] the molybdenum blue complex,[8] or the molybdate malachite green complex.[9] The estimated errors were 1.5% to 3% of the amounts analyzed. The pH was measured with a combination glass-calomel reference electrode and was calibrated with aqueous standards.

C. EQUILIBRATION PROCEDURES

Equilibrations were carried out in glass stopped flasks, which contained 2 g of HA and 50 ml of either water or phosphoric acid solution, and 0, 7.86, 16.04, 24.53, and 33.38 weight% of ethanol. Previous studies showed that equilibrium was attained within 7 days.[1-2] Therefore, the solutions were stirred by a magnet bar at 100 rpm at a fixed temperature for 1 week under nitrogen atmosphere. The solutions were then filtered. The pH values of the solutions were measured before and after filtration and averaged. The concentrations of calcium and phosphate were then analyzed.

D. CALCULATIONS

The solubility product of HA, K_{sp}, is defined here as

$$K_{sp}=(Ca^{2+})^5(PO_4^{3-})^3(OH^-) \text{ and } pK_{sp}= -\log(Ca^{2+})^5(PO_4^{3-})^3(OH^-)$$

for solutions in equilibrium with the HA solid. Parentheses indicate ionic activities obtained from the calcium and phosphate concentrations and pH and ionic strengths. A computer program,[2] which took into account the ion pairs and dissociation of phosphoric acid and water,[2,10] was used to calculate the ion activity coefficients through the use of the extended Debye-Huckel equation. The dielectric constants[11] and the equilibrium constants[10,12] used in the calculation are shown in the Tables 1 and 2. Some of the equilibrium constants of ethanol solutions were not available, and the constants for aqueous solutions were used. The effect of ethanol on the activity coefficient, expressed as "mean ionic medium effect," $_m\gamma$, is calculated as follows:[13]

$$\log {_m\gamma} =(pK_{sp}(\text{ethanol})-pK_{sp}(\text{water}))/N \qquad (1)$$

where $_m\gamma = 1$ in aqueous solution, and N is the number of the ions in one molecule and equals 9.

III. RESULTS AND DISCUSSIONS

The compositions of saturated HA solutions and pK_{sp}(HA) at 25° and 33°C are shown in Tables 1 and 2 respectively, where different trials use different initial concentrations of phosphoric acid. The pK_{sp} of HA in aqueous solution obtained in this study are 57.39 at 25°C and 57.31 at 33°C as compared to the literature values[1-3] of 57.43 to 58.52 at 25°C. The solubility of the HA prepared under the same conditions as the HA used here was reported[1] to have pK_{sp} of 57.43 at 25°C. Our study agreed with the report of Verbeck[3] that the solubility

Table 1
Solubility Products of Hydroxyapatite at 25°C.

Series 1. Ethanol wt. %=0

Trial	pH	[Ca]	[P]	pKsp
1	5.87	7.42E-4	1.43E-3	57.20
2	5.71	8.69E-4	1.73E-3	57.75

ε=78.3, pK_1=2.15, pK_2=7.20, pK_3=12.34, pKw=14.00.

Series 2. Ethanol wt. %=7.86

Trial	pH	[Ca]	[P]	pKsp
1	5.45	5.93E-4	1.25E-3	60.76
2	5.20	7.36E-4	1.55E-3	61.81

ε=74.0, pK_1=2.31, pK_2=7.33, pK_3=12.44, pKw=14.17.

Series 3. Ethanol wt. %=16.04

Trial	pH	[Ca]	[P]	pKsp
1	5.13	5.78E-4	1.22E-3	64.06
2	4.88	6.97E-3	1.49E-3	65.16

ε=69.3, pK_1=2.47, pK_2=7.46, pK_3=12.59, pKw=14.31.

Series 4. Ethanol wt. %=24.53

Trial	pH	[Ca]	[P]	pKsp
1	4.66	6.42E-4	1.35E-3	68.14

ε=64.3, pK_1=2.70, pK_2=7.61, pK_3=12.76, pKw=14.42.

Series 5. Ethanol wt. %=33.38

Trial	pH	[Ca]	[P]	pKsp
1	4.49	5.67E-4	1.22E-3	70.40
2	4.23	5.78E-4	1.26E-3	71.96

ε=59.0, pK_1=2.97, pK_2=7.80, pK_3=12.91, pKw=14.54.

Table 2
Solubility Products of Hydroxyapatite at 33°C.

Series 1. Ethanol wt. %=0

Trial	pH	[Ca]	[P]	pKsp
1	5.85	5.29E-4	1.02E-3	57.10
2	5.65	7.43E-4	1.55E-3	57.31

ε=75.5, pK_1=2.19, pK_2=7.19, pK_3=12.22, pKw=13.69.

Series 2. Ethanol wt. %=7.86

Trial	pH	[Ca]	[P]	pKsp
1	7.45	1.03E-5	1.95E-5	61.23
2	5.85	2.54E-4	5.30E-4	60.13
3	5.41	5.34E-4	1.14E-3	60.73

ε=71.2, pK_1=2.35, pK_2=7.32, pK_3=12.32, pKw=13.88.

Series 3. Ethanol wt. %=16.04

Trial	pH	[Ca]	[P]	pKsp
1	5.62	2.57E-4	5.76E-4	62.83
2	5.08	5.53E-4	1.17E-3	64.17

ε=66.6, pK_1=2.51, pK_2=7.45, pK_3=12.32, pKw=14.01.

Series 4. Ethanol wt. %=24.53

Trial	pH	[Ca]	[P]	pKsp
1	7.36	5.50E-6	9.10E-6	65.72
2	5.44	2.39E-4	5.49E-4	65.40
3	4.77	5.31E-4	1.15E-3	67.58

ε=61.8, pK_1=2.74, pK_2=7.60, pK_3=12.64, pKw=14.13

Series 5. Ethanol wt. %=33.38

Trial	pH	[Ca]	[P]	pKsp
1	4.83	2.82E-4	6.20E-4	70.39
2	4.46	5.04E-4	1.15E-3	71.11

ε=56.9, pK_1=3.01, pK_2=7.79, pK_3=12.79, pKw=14.25

of HA depends on the method of HA preparation. Ethanol decreased the solubility of hydroxyapatite, expressed as the apparent solubility product, from $pK_{sp} = 57.39$ in 0% ethanol to $pK_{sp} = 71.18$ in 33.38% ethanol at 25°C and from $pK_{sp} = 57.31$ in 0% ethanol to $pK_{sp} = 66.8$ at 33°C.

The Born equation[13] considers the electrostatic interactions in solvents with different dielectric constants and indicates that the decrease in the dielectric constant results in the decrease in solubility. The relation is expressed as

$$pK_{sp} - pK_{sp}^{w} = a\left(\frac{1}{\varepsilon} - \frac{1}{\varepsilon_w}\right)$$

where pK_{sp} and pK_{sp}^{w} are the negative logarithms of the solubility products in a mixed solvent with dielectric constant, ε, and water with dielectric constant, ε_w respectively. The fit of the Born equation with the data shown in Tables 1 and 2 is

$$pK_{sp} - 57.39 = 3629\left(\frac{1}{\varepsilon} - 0.0128\right) \text{ at } 25\text{°C and}$$

$$pK_{sp} - 57.31 = 3295\left(\frac{1}{\varepsilon} - 0.0133\right) \text{ at } 33\text{°C.}$$

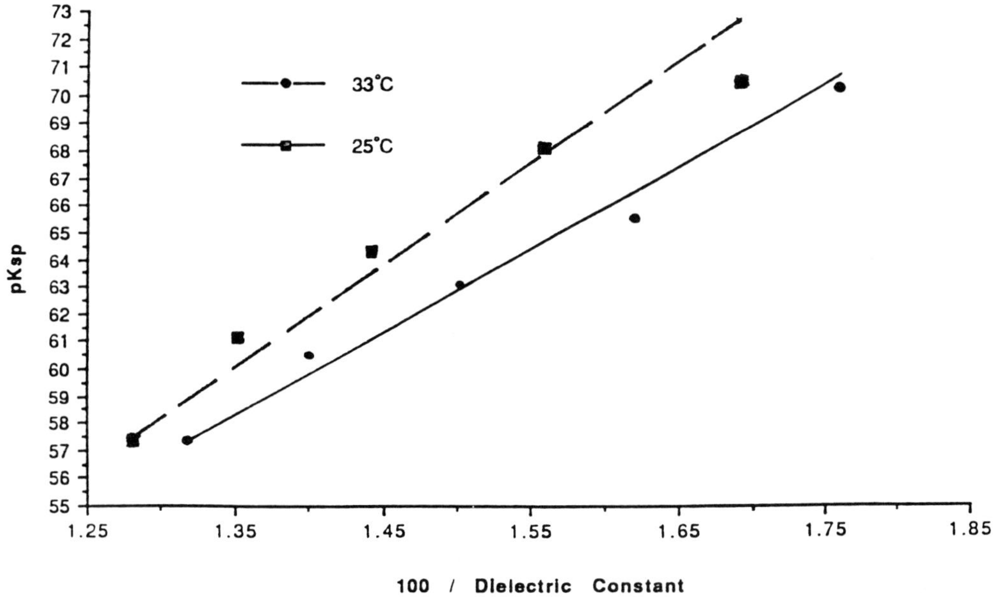

Figure 1. Negative logarithm of the solubility product vs. the reciprocal of the dielectric constant of the solvent. The fit of the Born equation: broken line, 25°C and solid line, 33°C.

The effects of ethanol and temperature on pK_{sp} are shown in Figure 1, where the values of pK_{sp} are plotted vs. the reciprocal of the dielectric constant of the solvent, together with the straight lines fitted to the Born equation. It is evident that the straight lines do not fit to the data as would be expected from the Born equation. There are many reasons for the deviations from the linear representation of the Born equation.[13] Perhaps, the most serious is that it oversimplifies the nature of ion-solvent interaction energies (solvation energies) in different media. The local effects of the ethanol on the ion-solvent interactions, at molecular level, are not taken into consideration. For example, ions dissolved in water form columbic hydration spheres. In the case of calcium ions in an aqueous HA system, there are six water molecules in the Ca hydration sphere. It is believed that ethanol weakens the hydration sphere and therefore decreases the solvation energy. The Born equation is incapable of taking the hydration sphere into account. Yet another source of the nonlinear relationship may be due to the problems in the measurement of the pH, i.e. the use of aqueous pH standard for the ethanol-water mixtures.

In the calculation of the ethanol effect, the aqueous standard state is retained for the ethanol-containing aqueous solution. Therefore, the decrease in solubility, i.e., the increase in pK_{sp}, is reflected by the increase in the activity coefficient due to the medium effect. The ethanol increases the activity coefficient of the chemical species, expressed as "mean ionic medium effect," $_m\gamma$, and shown in Table 3. Table 3 also lists the averaged solubility products of HA as pK_{sp}, obtained from average values of K_{sp}. The increase of the activity coefficient reflects changes in both interionic attractions and ion-solvent interactions. The ethanol decreases the dielectric constant and therefore increases the effective interionic forces. Ethanol also is believed to affect the ion-solvent interactions in such ways that it increases the activity coefficient.

Table 3

Averaged solubility product, K_{sp}, and Mean Ionic Medium Effect, $_m\gamma$

Temperature		**Ethanol wt. %**				
		0	**7.86**	**16.04**	**24.53**	**33.38**
25°C	pK_{sp}	57.39	61.02	64.33	68.14	70.69
	$_m\gamma$	1	2.53	5.90	15.65	30.05
33°C	pK_{sp}	57.31	60.48	63.11	65.71	70.62
	$_m\gamma$	1	2.25	4.41	8.58	30.12

IV. CONCLUSIONS

Solubility values of HA were determined in 0, 7.86, 16.04, 24.53, and 33.38% (by weight) ethanol-water mixtures at 25 and 33°C. The solubility of HA, expressed as solubility product (K_{sp}), decreased from pK_{sp} = 57.39 and 57.31 in 0% ethanol to 71.18 and 66.8 in 33.38% ethanol, respectively, at 25° and 33°C. This decrease is attributed to the decreases in the dielectric constant and the effects of ethanol on the ion-solvent interactions. The apparent solubility products of HA were not significantly different at these two temperatures in the absence of ethanol and increased at higher temperature in the presence of ethanol. The simple Born equation was used to fit the results.

ACKNOWLEDGMENT

W. E. Brown introduced one of the authors (M.S.T) to the science of calcium phosphates and inspired him during this study. This investigation was supported, in part, by USPHS Research Grant DE08916 and is part of the dental and medical research program conducted by the National Institute of Standards and Technology in cooperation with the American Dental Association Health Foundation.

[Certain commercial materials and equipment are identified in this paper to specify the experimental procedure. In no instance does such identification imply recommendation or endorsement by the National Institute of Standards and Technology or the ADA Health Foundation or that the material or equipment identified is necessarily the best available for the purpose.]

REFERENCES

1. Moreno, E. C., Gregory, T. M. and Brown, W. E., Preparation and solubility of hydroxyapatite, J. Res. Nat. Bur. of Stand., 72A(6), 773, 1968.
2. McDowell, H., Gregory, T. M. and Brown, W. E., Solubility of $Ca_5(PO_4)_3OH$ in the system $Ca(OH)_2$-H_3PO_4-H_2O at 5°, 15°, 25°, and 37°C, J. Res. Nat. Bur. of Stand., 81A(2), 273, 1977.
3. Verbeek, R. M. H., Steyaer, H., Thun, H. P. and Verbeek, F., Solubility of synthetic calcium hydroxyapatites, J.C.S. Faraday I, 76, 209, 1980.
4. Joost Larsen, M., Thorsen, A. and Jensen, S. J., Ethanol-induced formation of solid calcium phosphates, Calcif. Tissue Int. 37, 189, 1985.
5. Lerner, E., Azoury, R. and Sarig, S., Rapid precipitation of apatite from ethanol-water solution, J. of Crystal Growth 97, 725, 1989.
6. Mchaylouva, V. and Ilkova, P., Photometric determination of microamounts of calcium with Arsenazo 3, Anal. Chem. Acta. 53, 194, 1971.
7. Gee, A. and Deitz, V. R., Determination of phosphate by differential spectrophotometry, Anal. Chem., 25(1), 320, 1953.
8. Murphy, J. and Riley, J. P., A modified single solution method for the determination of phosphate in natural waters, Anal. Chem. Acta 27, 31, 1962.
9. Hess, H. H. and Derr, J. E., Assay of inorganic and organic phosphate in the 0.1-5 nanomole range, Analyt. Biochem., 63, 607, 1975.
10. Tung, M. S., Eidelman, N., Sieck, B. and Brown, W. E., Octacalcium phosphate solubility product from 4 to 37°C, J. Res. Nat. Bur. of Stand., 93, 613, 1988.
11. Woolley, E. M., Hurkot, D. G. and Hepler, L. G., Ionization constants for water in aqueous organic mixtures, J. Phys. Chem., 74, 3908, 1970.
12. Tossidis, I., Ueber die dissoziation von phosphor- und arsensaeure in wessrig-organischen loesungsmitteln, Inorg. Nucl. Chem. Letters, 12, 609, 1976.
13. Bates, R. G., Determination of pH, Chapter 8, Wiley, New York, 1973.

Section II.

Contributed Papers

CONSTANT-COMPOSITION STUDY OF THE PRECIPITATION BEHAVIOUR OF CALCIUM PHOSPHATE IN THE PRESENCE OF NON-COLLAGENOUS BIO-CHEMICALS

A.T.-C. Wong and J.T. Czernuszka
Department of Materials
University of Oxford
Parks Road, Oxford, OX1 3PH, U.K.

ABSTRACT

Whether a phosphorylated amino acid facilitates the precipitation of calcium phosphate and the transformation of precursor phases to hydroxyapatite depends firstly on the carbon chain to which the phosphoryl end group is attached and secondly on its concentration in the calcifying solution relative to the total calcium content. A highly electronegative phosphoryl group and a sterically flexible carbon chain favour the approach of free Ca^{2+} ions in the solution for the formation of essential intermediates in the precipitation process. However, the concentration of these organic additions needs to be carefully chosen in order to ensure a significant amount of uncomplexed Ca^{2+} ions available for the subsequent growth of calcium phosphate nuclei.

I. INTRODUCTION

A sound understanding of the precipitation behaviour of calcium phosphate is essential as it is directly related to hard tissue mineralisation. Throughout the years, there has been extensive research in the experimental crystallisation of calcium phosphate in purely ionic systems. Although these systems are relatively easy to control, they differ significantly from the physiological condition. Apart from calcium and phosphate ions, the body fluid contains a whole collection of organic and inorganic bio-chemicals, some of which have been found to play significant rôles in the calcification process. They can alter the nucleation and growth rates; induce the formation of precursor phases and their subsequent transformation to hydroxyapatite; and affect the morphology, the stoichiometry and the microscopic lattice structure of the resulting crystals.[1,2] It is therefore necessary to incorporate these compounds in the calcifying medium during precipitation experiments so that their effects can be examined.

Among the numerous bio-chemicals present in the body fluid, special attention has been drawn to bone-specific proteins. One common characteristic of most bone-specific proteins is that they all contain a high proportion of phosphorylated amino acid residues. These phosphoryl end groups are specifically involved in the mineralisation process due to their

0-8493-4750-5/94/$0.00+$.50

electronegativity and consequently their potential to bond to positive calcium ions. However, separate studies on individual phosphoamino acids suggested that not all phosphoryl end groups behave in the same manner.[1] Phosphoserine is found to promote secondary nucleation of tiny plate-like crystals whereas, for the same weight fraction, phosphatidylserine has an overall inhibitory effect on calcium phosphate precipitation. This implies a possible link between the side-chain and the calcium binding affinity of the phosphoryl end of the amino acids (Figure 1). Also, as calcium ions are likely to form complexes with these phospho-organics, the overall precipitation rate should be influenced by the concentration of these additives. This present work intends to verify these hypotheses.

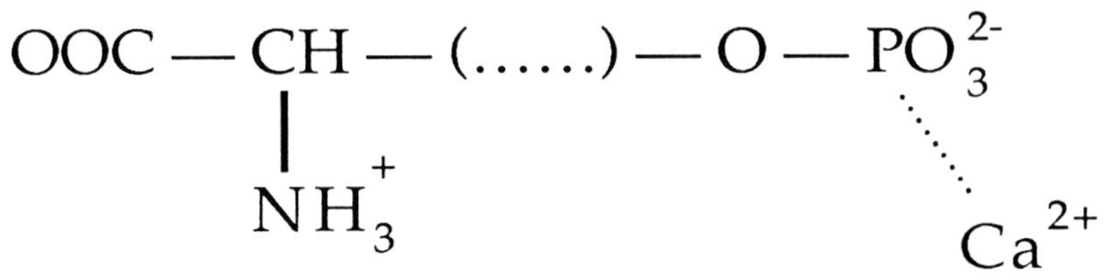

Figure 1. Possible link between the main carbon chain and the affinity of the electronegative phosphoryl end group for calcium ions in a phosphorylated amino acid.

Table 1. List of phosphorylated amino acids used in this study.

Chemical	Symbol	Formula
O-phospho-L-serine	SerP	$^{-}OOC-CH(NH_3^+)-CH_2-O-PO_3^{2-}$
O-phospho-L-threonine	ThrP	$^{-}OOC-CH(NH_3^+)-CH(CH_3)-O-PO_3^{2-}$
O-phospho-L-tyrosine	TyrP	$^{-}OOC-CH(NH_3^+)-CH_2-C_6H_4-O-PO_3^{2-}$
Phospho-L-arginine	ArgP	$^{-}OOC-CH(NH_3^+)-(CH_2)_3-NH-C(=NH)-NH-PO_3^{2-}$

II. MATERIALS AND METHODS

A. Stock solution

A supersaturated calcium phosphate solution with total calcium and phosphate contents of respectively 2 mM and 1.2 mM was prepared by dissolving synthetic hydroxyapatite powder (Aldrich Chemicals) in distilled water acidified with 0.1 M hydrochloric acid. The *p*H of this metastable solution was adjusted to 7.4 by the addition of 0.5 M potassium hydroxide. Potassium chloride was dissolved to give an ionic strength of 0.1 M.

B. Phosphorylated amino acids

The phosphoamino acids in Table 1 (Sigma) were chosen for this set of experiments. Amongst these compounds, SerP is the smallest and most flexible molecule. The bulkiness increases either due to the presence of bigger side groups (ThrP), or as a result of stiffened (TyrP) or lengthened (ArgP) main carbon chain.

Table 2. Compositions of calcifying solutions.

Expt. no.	Total Ca content (mM)	Total P content (mM)	Organic addition: Compound	Organic addition: (mM)	Ionic strength (M)	Temp. (°C)
Series 1						
1-1			—	(control)		
1-2			SerP			
1-3	2.00	1.20	ThrP	0.20	0.10	37.0
1-4			TyrP	(10% molar)		
1-5			ArgP			
Series 2						
2-1			—	(control: 0%)		
2-2				0.02 (1%)		
2-3				0.10 (5%)		
2-4	2.00	1.20	SerP	0.20 (10%)	0.10	37.0
2-5				0.50 (25%)		
2-6				1.00 (50%)		
2-7				2.00 (100%)		

C. Constant-composition experiments

The dual constant-composition technique as developed by Ebrahimpour *et al.* was adopted in this study.[3,4] Working solutions of compositions as given in Table 2 were prepared. Hydroxyapatite substrates were prepared in a similar manner as previously explained[1,5] and introduced to the solution at the inception of the experiments. In each experiment, the solution was stirred by a magnetic stirrer and the reaction chamber placed in a water bath. Nitrogen gas was bubbled through the solution to eliminate any dissolved carbon dioxide gas. The composition of the solution was monitored by a combined *p*H electrode and a Ca^{2+} ion electrode coupled with a calomel reference electrode. *p*H and $p[Ca^{2+}]$ values from a precision *p*H meter and an ion analyser were constantly monitored by a computer, and the addition of titrants through autoburettes was triggered by any deviation of the *p*H or $p[Ca^{2+}]$ value in excess of 0.003. The compositions of the titrants were calculated as described elsewhere.[3]

D. Characterisation of precipitate

Solid samples were removed from the reaction chamber at regular intervals and were then characterised by means of scanning electron microscopy, X-ray powder diffractometry and wavelength dispersion analysis.

III. RESULTS AND DISCUSSION

A. Effects of the side-chains of phosphorylated amino acids

In the first series of experiments, equal quantities (mol/mol) of organics were present in different batches of the stock solution in order to evaluate the relationship between the side-chains and the overall effect of the phosphorylated amino acids on calcium phosphate precipitation. Figure 2 shows the total calcium uptake rates as functions of time. It is obvious that, compared to the results from the control experiment, the whole precipitation rate was most significantly accelerated by SerP, the smallest and most flexible amongst the organic compounds. This promotional effect tailed off with increasing bulkiness of the additive and, indeed, in the presence of TyrP and ArgP, the overall crystallisation rate was slowed down.

Figure 3 displays the ratio of uptake rates of calcium against phosphate for the different experiments. It can be seen that, in every case, the initial Ca/P ratio was close to 1.3 which corresponds to the stoichiometry of octacalcium phosphate (OCP, Ca/P ratio 1.33). Thus, although the systems were under the influence of different bio-chemicals, the precursor phase to hydroxyapatite formation was still predominantly determined by the ionic product of total calcium and total phosphate. However, these organics did affect the subsequent phase transformation to thermodynamically stable hydroxyapatite (HAP, Ca/P ratio 1.67). Again, SerP induced the earliest transformation; and with increasing bulkiness of the individual amino acids, the transformation rate was accordingly retarded. Scanning electron micrographs of solid specimens removed after 48-54 hours (Figure 4) clearly depicted the growth of a secondary phase over a primary crystal coverage only in the case of SerP addition. These primary and secondary phases were confirmed to be respectively octacalcium phosphate and hydroxyapatite by X-ray diffraction spectra and wavelength dispersion analyses. Indeed, comparable degrees of transformation were achieved only after considerably longer periods (around 90 hours) in the control experiment and in the case of ThrP. After 144-160 hours, transformation to hydroxyapatite was complete in the control as well as with SerP and ThrP. However, no visible transformation was observed in the case of ArgP, while for TyrP, the nucleation rate was so slow that only large plates of OCP were obtained (Figure 5).

The differences in precipitation and transformation rates imply a direct dependence on the nature of the organic additives. As phosphoamino acids are involved in these processes by complexing with Ca^{2+} ions which subsequently bind to free phosphate ions, their effectson the crystallisation rate reflect the ease with which the appropriate free ions approach the phosphoryl end group.

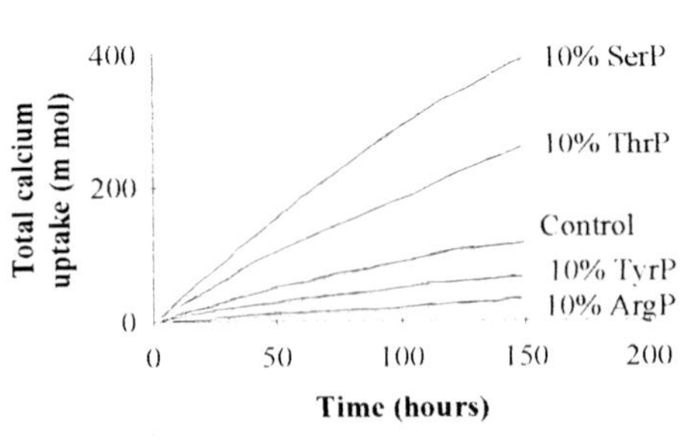

Figure 2. Total calcium uptake rates under the influence of 10% (mol/mol) of various additives.

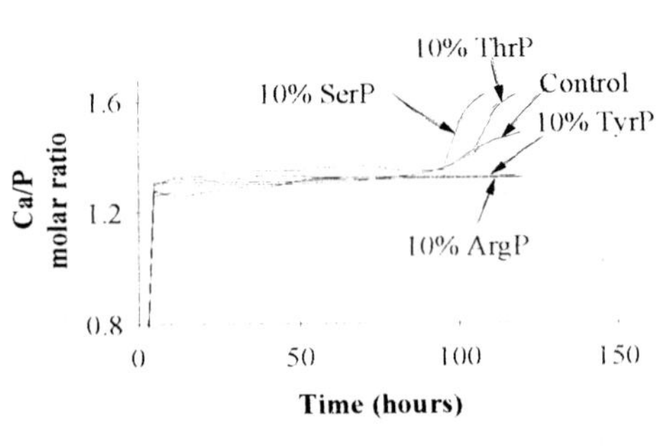

Figure 3. Molar ratios of calcium and phosphate uptake rates for Series 1 experiments.

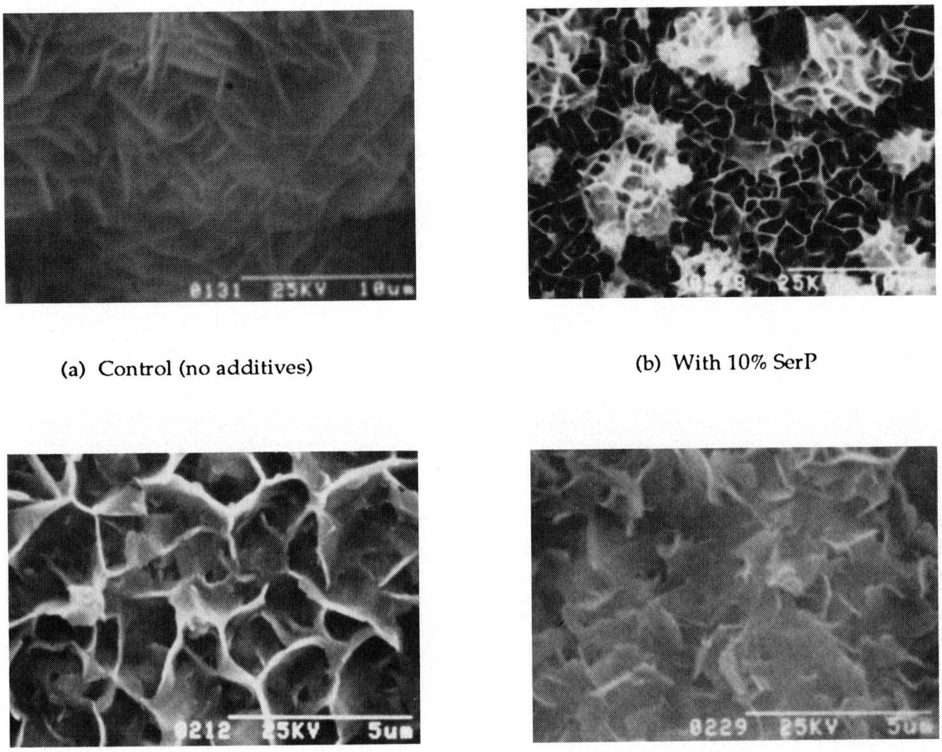

(a) Control (no additives)

(b) With 10% SerP

(c) With 10% ThrP

(d) With 10% ArgP

Figure 4. Scanning electron micrographs of solid samples removed from the reaction chambers after 48 to 54 hours.

Firstly, it is physically more feasible for ions in solution to access less bulky and sterically more flexible organic molecules in the correct orientation. Also, the electrostatic attraction between the amino acids and the calcium ions depends on the electronegativity of the phosphoryl group, which in turn is influenced by the nature of the side-chains. In this set of experiments, the observed trends of precipitation and transfromation rates not only agree with the physical consideration, but are also consistent with the relative reactivity in terms of electrostatics.

B. Effects of percentage concentration of additives

In addition to their chemical compositions, there is also a possible link between the relative concentration of organic additives and their effects on the precipitation phenomenon. To verify this, a second series of constant-composition precipitation experiments were performed, this time with varying amounts of SerP as in Table 2.

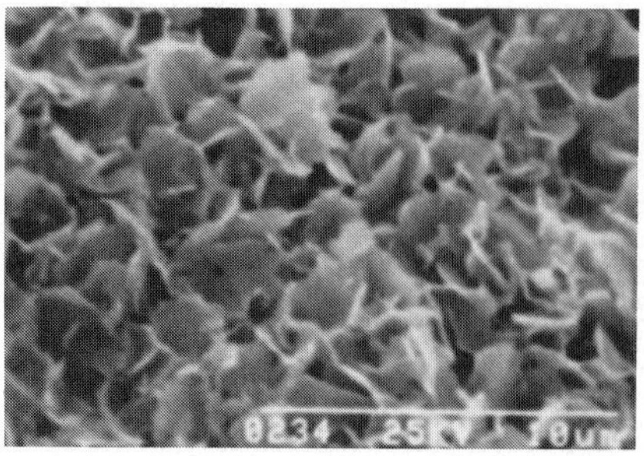

(a) Control (no additives)

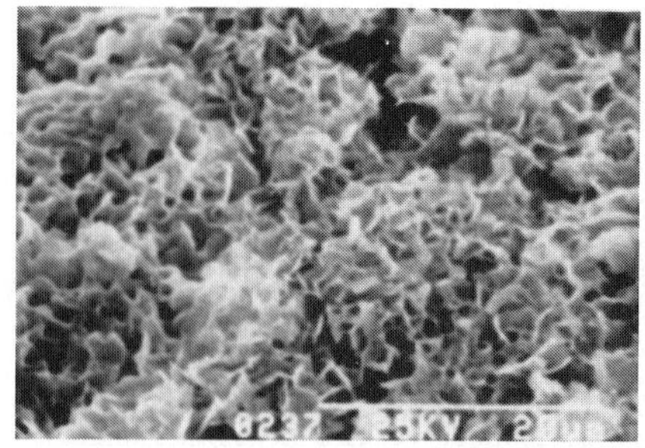

(b) With 10% SerP

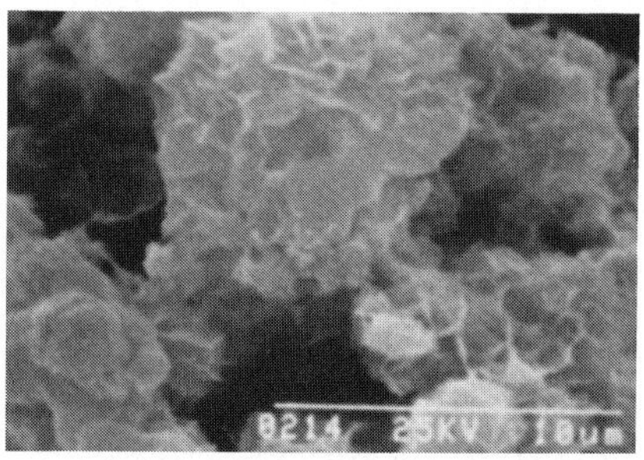

(a) With 10% ThrP

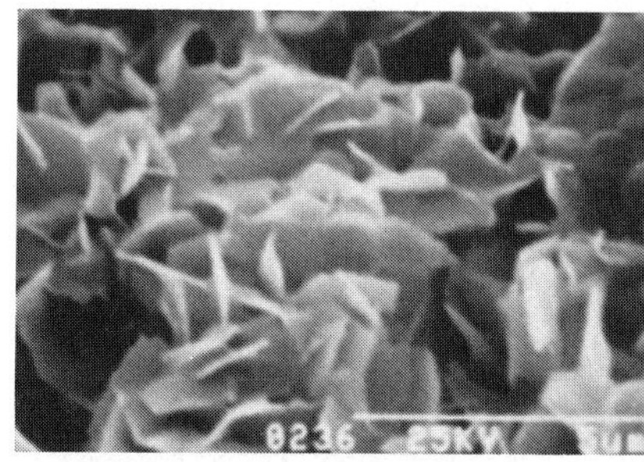

(b) With 10% ArgP

Figure 5. Scanning electron micrographs of solid samples removed from the reation chambers after 144 to 160 hours.

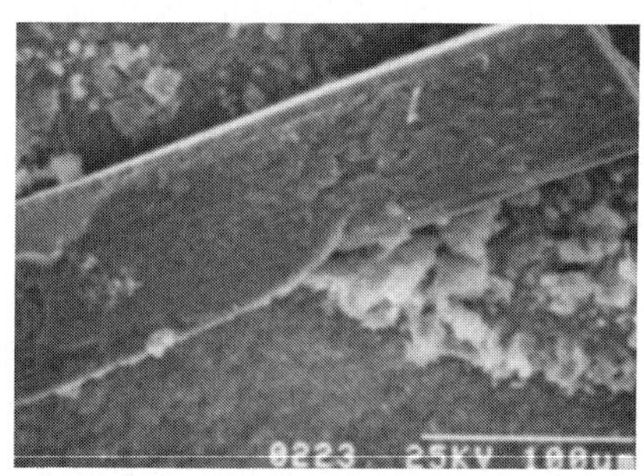

(e) With 10% TyrP

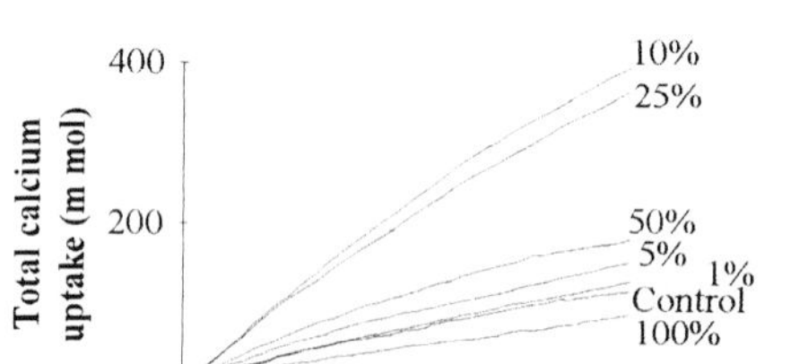

Figure 6. Total calcium uptake rates under the influence of different concentrations of SerP.

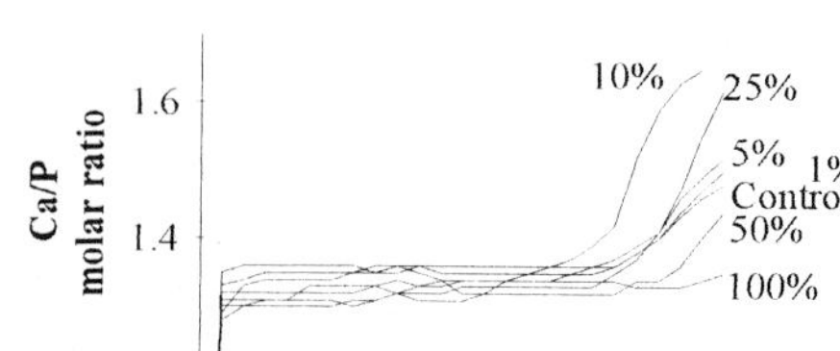

Figure 7. Molar ratios of calcium and phosphate uptake rates for Series 2 experiments.

The total calcium uptake rates are shown in Figure 6. With small amounts of addition (<10%), the overall precipitation rate increased with increasing concentration of SerP. Between 10% and 25% SerP, there appeared to be an optimum concentration beyond which additional SerP only imparted a decelerating effect. A parallel trend was observed for the transformation rates (Figure 7). The promotional effect on the transformation rate from OCP (precursor phase again unaffected by inclusion of SerP) to HAP again reached a peak between a concentration of 10% and 25%.

Although SerP has a high tendency to complex with Ca^{2+} ions to form intermediates crucial for accelerating the precipitation process, at the same time it essentially diminishes the supply of free Ca^{2+} available for the growth of nuclei. Thus, the apparent optimum SerP concentration reflects the condition at which these two conflicting factors were best compromised. As the same complexing mechanism should apply to other phosphoamino acids, it will not be surprising if similar trends are exhibited.

IV. CONCLUSIONS

The effects of a phosphorylated amino acid on calcium phosphate precipitation depend on the structure of the main carbon chain. Precipitation and phase transformation are both facilitated by phosphoamino acids with sterically flexible carbon chains and phosphoryl groups of enhanced electronegativity. However, as the complexing between Ca^{2+} and phosphoamino acid molecules essentially lowers the availability of free Ca^{2+} ions for crystal growth, there is, for each amino acid, an optimum concentration with respect to the total calcium content in the solution at which maximum promotional (or minimum inhibitory) effects are exhibited.

ACKNOWLEDGEMENTS

Financial support to this project from the Rhodes Trust and the Royal Society is greatly appreciated.

REFERENCES

1. Wong, A.T.-C., Czernuszka, J.T., *Mat. Res. Soc. Symp. Proc.*, 252, 49, 1992.
2. Clarke, K.I., Graves, S.E.,Wong, A.T.-C., Francis, M.J.O., Triffitt, J.T., Czernuszka, J.T., *J. Mat. Sci.: Mat. in Med.*, 1993 (in print).
3. Ebrahimpour, A., Zhang, J., Nancollas, G.H., *J. Crystal Growth*, 113, 83, 1991.
4. Zhang, J., Ebrahimpour, A., Nancollas, G.H., *J. Colloid & Interf. Sci.*, 152, 132, 1992.
5. Clarke, K.I., Wong, A.T.-C., Czernuszka, J.T., Dowling, B., Triffitt, J.T., *Bioceramics*, 4, 107, 1991.

DUAL CONSTANT COMPOSITION KINETICS STUDIES OF CERAMIC HYDROXYAPATITE AND HYDROXYAPATITE PLASMA COATED IMPLANTS

E.P. Paschalis, B.E. Tucker, S. Mukhopadhyay, K. Wikiel, N.B. Beals,* J.A. Bearcroft,* M. Spector,† and G.H. Nancollas
State University of New York at Buffalo, Buffalo NY;
*Smith & Nephew Richards Inc., Memphis, Tennessee;
†Brigham and Women's Hospital, Boston, Massachusetts.

INTRODUCTION

The CC method has found wide application in kinetics studies of the nucleation, growth and dissolution of calcium phosphate phases.[1-3] The extension of this technique to the simultaneous control of two ionic species has enabled dual constant composition (DCC) studies to be made of concurrent dissolution and growth processes, the simultaneous growth or dissolution of mixed calcium phosphate phases and crystalline phase transformation reactions,[4-6] Since it is now well established that a number of calcium phosphate phases such as octacalcium phosphate (OCP), tricalcium phosphate (TCP), as well as hydroxyapatite (HAP), are involved during many biomineralization processes,[7-9] such reactions may include the formation of calcium phosphate metastable intermediates which subsequently transform into thermodynamically more stable phases as the reactions proceed.

In addition to these synthetic calcium phosphates, other materials such as ceramic hydroxyapatite (CHAP) and hydroxyapatite plasma coated titanium implants (HPCTI) are of considerable importance. There is little doubt that the surface composition of a prosthetic device will dictate the *in vivo* response to aqueous media such as serum, and will control the biological reactions that take place immediately following implantation. In the present work, the DCC method has been modified in order to study the dissolution kinetics of calcium phosphates such as CHAP, β-TCP, and HPCTI.

MATERIALS AND METHODS

Solutions were prepared in grade A volumetric glassware using Reagent grade chemicals and triply distilled carbon dioxide-free water which had been filtered twice (0.22μ Millipore) before use. Calcium chloride solutions were standardized by EDTA titration. Phosphate concentrations were determined spectrophotometrically as the phosphovanadomolybdate complex. Potassium hydroxide solutions were prepared from washed pellets in a nitrogen atmosphere and standardized against potassium hydrogen phthalate. The DCC method incorporated two potentiostats (Metrohm) in conjunction with two ion specific sensors to provide constant composition devices for the control of calcium and hydrogen ion activities. Calcium phosphate solutions, of the appropriately calculated relative undersaturation with respect to synthetic calcium

0-8493-4750-5/94/$0.00+$.50

phosphate phases, were prepared in double-walled thermostatically controlled Pyrex vessels by mixing calcium chloride, potassium dihydrogen phosphate, sodium chloride and either potassium hydroxide or hydrochloric acid, to achieve the required pH. The onset of dissolution of the calcium phosphate surfaces introduced into the undersaturated solutions was detected using glass (Orion) and calcium (Orion) ion selective electrodes. By means of potentiostats, these changes in activities of the lattice ions were compensated for by the automated addition of titrant solutions.

During the dissolution reactions, aliquots of the working solutions were periodically withdrawn, filtered (0.22μ Millipore) and analyzed for calcium and phosphate. Any changes in these concentrations were used to compute the stoichiometry of the dissolving phases and to redesign DCC experimental conditions in order to achieve constant undersaturation.

In those cases, such as HPCTI, where the dissolution reactions involved an immediate release, into the working solution, of significant amounts of ionic species other than the principal phase, an initial surface preconditioning step (PC) was carried out in order to monitor the adjustment of the surfaces to the undersaturated conditions. The release of calcium-containing "impurities" such as calcium oxide, was monitored by following the pH and calcium ion activities of the preconditioning solutions as a function of time. When either equilibrium or the desired surface calcium to phosphate stoichiometry had been achieved, the surfaces were then subjected to DCC dissolution kinetics procedures.

Table 1
Typical experimental conditions

	T_{Ca} $/10^{-3}$ M	T_P $/10^{-3}$ M	IS /M	pH	HAP	TCP
CHAP	13.6	8.31	0.10	4.50	0.00337	-0.71
CHAP	13.6	8.14	0.10	4.50	-0.00329	-0.712
CHAP	8.00	4.80	0.10	4.50	-0.35	-0.825
CHAP	0.80	0.480	0.10	4.50	-0.913	-0.982
HPCTI	0.125	0.075	0.15	6.50	-0.50	-0.91
-TCP	0.604	0.040	0.15	6.50	1.03	-0.55

The relative undersaturation of the working solutions was calculated from the free ionic concentrations of the species computed by taking into account ion-pair and complex formation. These calculations were made using expressions for mass-balance, electroneutrality and the appropriate equilibrium constants, by successive approximations for the ionic strength. Relative undersaturations, σ_{HAP}, with respect to HAP were calculated from equation (1):

$$\sigma HAP = [(Ca)^5 (PO_4)^3 (OH) / K_{spHAP}]^{1/9} - 1 \qquad (1)$$

where the parenthesis enclose ionic activities and K_{spHAP} is the thermodynamic solubility product of HAP.

RESULTS AND DISCUSSION

Experimental conditions are summarized in Table 1. The marked dependence of the CHAP dissolution on the relative undersaturation is illustrated in Fig. 1, in which the rate of dissolution, expressed as equivalent moles of HAP, is plotted as a function of time. In another experiment, the solution was maintained at near saturation ($\sigma_{HAP} \approx 0$) with respect to HAP. It can be seen in (Fig. 2), in which the rate of dissolution (expressed as equivalent moles of HAP) is plotted as a function of time, that the CHAP surfaces

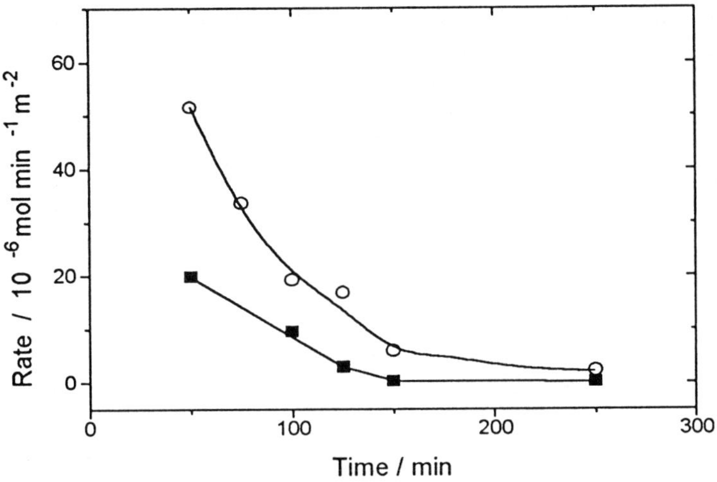

Figure 1. Rate of DCC dissolution of CHAP at different relative undersaturations as a function of time; (O) σ_{HAP} = -0.35 , (■) σ_{HAP} = -1.56×10^{-4}.

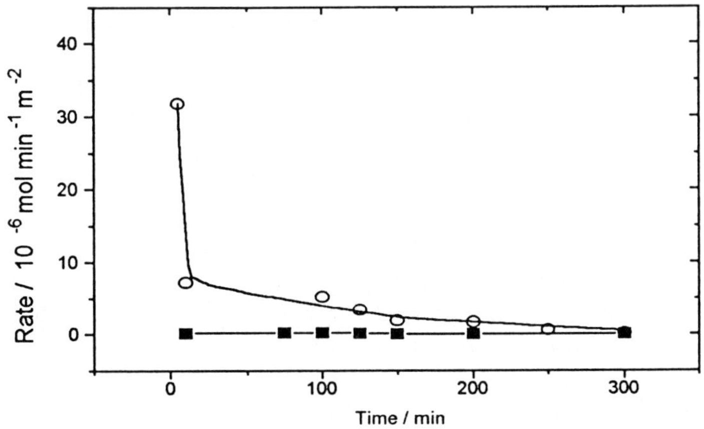

Figure 2. Comparison of DCC dissolution rates for (O) CHAP and (■) synthetic HAP at $\sigma_{HAP} \approx 0$.

underwent dissolution, conclusively showing the presence of calcium-containing phases other than the thermodynamically most stable hydroxyapatite. These "impurity" phases dissolved rapidly upon exposure to calcium phosphate solutions. Scanning electron micrographs of the seed material before and after dissolution suggest that the dissolution of CHAP occurs at specific sites as evidenced by the formation of "voids." These probably reflect the location of the "impurity" deposits within CHAP, which dissolve more rapidly than HAP.

Typical results of preconditioning (PC) experiments with HPCTI are summarized in Fig. 3, in which pH, Ca/P ratio, and relative supersaturation with respect to HAP of the solution are plotted as a function of time. It can be seen that the pH increased to values near 10, while the relative supersaturation reached values of almost 18. The latter observation is most significant since the system contains a calcium phosphate-coated implant surface which would be expected to initiate precipitation in the PC solution. It is likely that the relatively high Ca/P ionic ratio of the solution may markedly influence not only the rate of growth of the calcium phosphate phases but also their ability to nucleate at the implant surfaces.

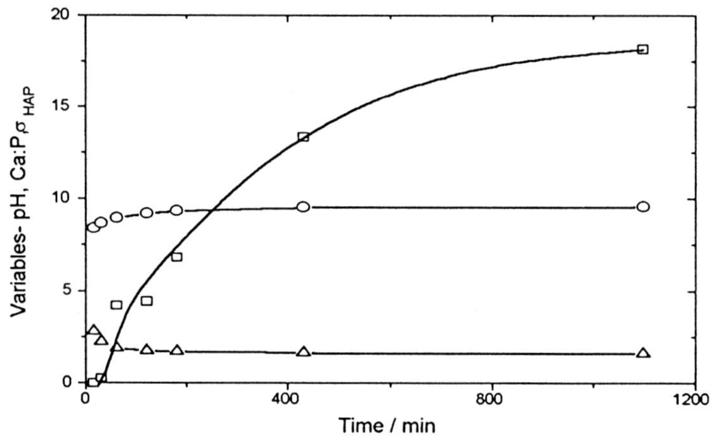

Figure 3. Profiles of (O) pH, (□) σ_{HAP} and (Δ) Calcium/Phosphate ionic ratio during the pre-conditioning procedure in 0.15 M NaCl.

The dissolution of HPCTI was studied as a function of pH and the results are shown in Fig. 4 as time plots of moles of acid titrant solution added in order to maintain the pH of the working solution constant. Three pH values were selected for study; 5.5 - a typical local pH of traumatized tissue; 7.4 - physiological; and 9.0 - close to the equilibrium value of a typical PC solution. It can be seen in Fig. 4 that experiments at pH 5.5 and 7.4 required the addition of acidic titrant solution (HCl) in order to maintain constant pH whereas at the pH 9.0 conditions involved a demand for base (KOH) as the titrant solution. This again points to the release of a more acidic phosphate species at the highest pH studied.

The variability of the dissolution characteristics of HPCTI obtained from different manufacturers was also examined and typical results are presented in Fig. 5 as plots of acid titrant added as a function of time for two typical samples that had been cleared for *in vivo* use by the FDA on the basis of their x-ray spectra. These data all indicated the presence of hydroxyapatite of various crystallinities. The titanium disks supporting the coatings were exposed to identical undersaturated calcium phosphate solutions (σ_{HAP} = -0.50) and it may be seen that they exhibited widely different dissolution kinetics behavior.

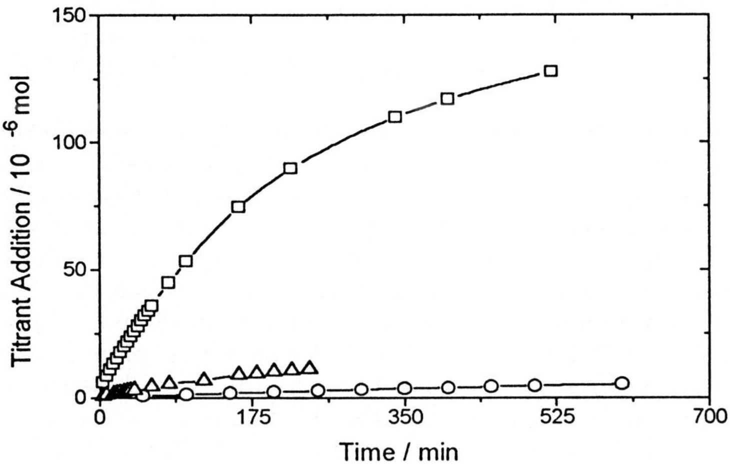

Figure 4. Comparison of titrant addition during DCC dissolution of HPCTI at pH (□) 5.5, (Δ) 9.0, and (O) 7.4. Titrant concentrations: (□, O)[HCl] = 3.0×10^{-3} M; (Δ) [KOH] = 3.0×10^{-3} M.

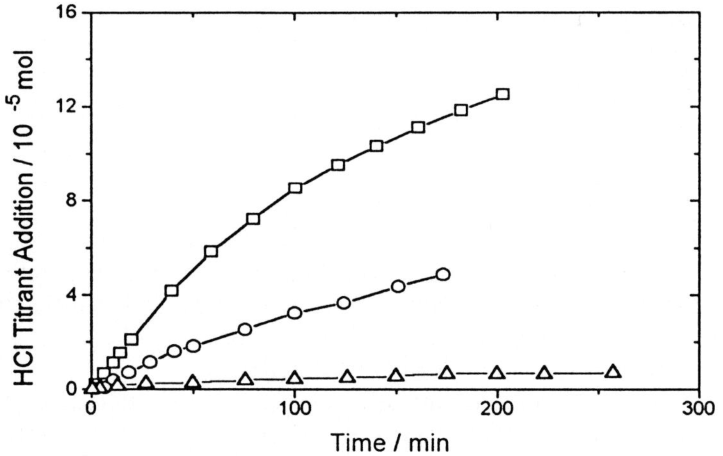

Figure 5. Comparison of HCl titrant addition during DCC dissolution at σ_{HAP} = -0.50 of (□) β-TCP, (O) Implant 1, (Δ) Implant 2.

The results of these studies clearly show that many ceramic hydroxyapatites, CHAP, cannot be represented by a single calcium phosphate phase. Surface layers may incorporate calcium-containing impurities, possibly calcium oxide and β-TCP, that are formed during their high temperature synthesis. The presence of such phases, that dissolve much more rapidly than the thermodynamically most stable hydroxyapatite, is best illustrated by the fact that CHAP may undergo dissolution in solutions that are saturated with respect to HAP. Furthermore, morphological studies, before and after dissolution kinetics studies, suggest a "patchy" pattern of dissolution resulting in the formation of voids. This may have important implications on the performance of these surfaces when used as implant material in stress-bearing devices.

HPCTI, in which the titanium is plasma coated with calcium phosphate, exhibited an even more reactive surface as evidenced by the results of the preconditioning experiments. In the early stages of the reaction, the pH rose dramatically to basic values and in many cases, calcium ions were released into the solution without accompanying phosphate species. Furthermore, the dissolution behavior during the PC and DCC experiments was clearly dependent on the manufacturing source despite the general description of the implants as "hydroxyapatite" coated. After the PC procedures, the solutions were appreciably supersaturated with respect to HAP but were apparently incapable of nucleating calcium phosphate phases on the plasma mineral surfaces. A recent study has shown that thermodynamic driving force for crystal growth and dissolution may not be the only consideration in determining the rate of reaction. Lattice ionic ratios in the working solutions and electrical potentials at the surface may also be important factors.[10] In the present case, changes in the Ca/P ionic ratios may also be important in determining the ability of the implant surfaces to nucleate calcium phosphate phases. In order to investigate these processes, the present work shows that the DCC method is uniquely suited for quantifying both the dissolution of surfaces such as CHAP and HPCTI and the calcium-containing impurity phases that may participate during the initial responses of the implant surfaces to *in vivo* conditions.

ACKNOWLEDGEMENTS

We thank the NIH (AR40427) and Smith & Nephew Richards Inc. for grants in support of this work.

REFERENCES

1. Ebrahimpour, A., Zhang, Z., Nancollas, G. H. Dual Constant Composition Method and its Application to Studies of Phase Transformation and Crystallization of Mixed Phases, *J. Crystal Growth*, 113, 83-91, 1991.
2. Tomson, M.B., Nancollas, G.H., Mineralization kinetics: A constant composition study, *Science*, 200, 1059-1060, 1978.
3. Ebrahimpour, A., Perez, L., Nancollas, G. H., The Induced Crystal Growth of Calcium Oxalate Monohydrate at Hydroxyapatite Surfaces. The Influence of Human Serum Albumin, Citrate, and Magnesium, *Langmuir*, 7, 577-583, 1991.
4. Zhang, J., Ebrahimpour, A., Nancollas, G. H., Dual Constant Composition Studies of Phase Transformation of Dicalcium Phosphate Dihydrate at Constant Supersaturation, *J. Coll. Interface Sci.*, 152, 132-140, 1992.
5. Ebrahimpour, A., Paschalis ,E. P., Zhang, J., Nancollas, G. H., Physical Chemical Studies of Mineralization and Demineralization of Apatites, in *Mechanisms and Phylogeny of Mineralization in Biological Systems*, Suga, S., Nakahara, H., Eds., Springer-Verlag Tokyo, 1991, pp. 273-280.
6. Johnsson, M. S-A., Paschalis, E. P., and Nancollas, G. H., Kinetics of Mineralization, Demineralization and Transformation of Calcium

Phosphates at Mineral and Protein Surfaces, in *The Bone-Biomaterial Interface,* Davies J., Ed., the University of Toronto Press, 1991, pp. 68-75.
7. Ellies, L., Carter, L., Natiella, J., Featherstone, J., Nelson, D., Quantitative Analysis of early *in vivo* Tissue Response to Synthetic Apatite Implants, *J. of Biomedical Mater. Res.,* 22, 137-148, 1988.
8. McCarty, D., Lehr, J., Halverson, P., Crystal Populations in Human Synovial Fluid, *Arthritis and Rheum.,* 26, 1220-1224, 1983.
9. Radin, S., Ducheyne, P., The Effect of Varying the Calcium Phosphate Composition and Structure on Dissolution and Precipitation Reactions in Simulated Interstitial Fluid, in *17th Annual Meeting of The Society for Biomaterials,* Scottsdale, AZ, 1991.
10. Zhang, J., Nancollas, G.H., Influence of calcium/sulfate ratio on the growth rate of calcium sulfate dihydrate at constant supersaturation, *J. Crystal.Growth,* 118, 287-294, 1992.

COMPARATIVE UTILITY OF MINERALIZED COLLAGEN AS AN OSTEOINDUCTIVE MATERIAL

Subramanian Gunasekaran, Ian C. Bathurst[†] Brent Constantz, James Quiaoit, John Ross,[††] Philip J. Barr,[†] and Denis Gospodarowicz[†]
Norian Corporation, 1025 Terra Bella Ave., Mountain View, CA 94043
[†] Chiron Corporation, 4560 Horton Street, Emeryville, CA-94608
[††] Department of Chemistry, Stanford University, Stanford, CA - 94305

INTRODUCTION

In prior work we have studied the mineralization of collagen, in the absence of other non-collagenous proteins, by nucleation and precipitation of calcium phosphates.[1] In this article we describe the results of an *in vivo* experiment with this mineralized collagen. The experiment is designed to test the material as a potential substitute for autograft bone and for delivering bone growth factors like BMPs (bone morphogenic proteins) to foster bone formation. Collagenous matrix[2] and demineralized bone[3-5] are being used for delivering such bone inducing growth factors. Other bio-active matrices being considered are polylactide-glycolide co-polymers,[6] fibrin,[7] porous hydroxyapatite,[8] tricalcium phosphate[9] and other calcium-rich minerals.[10,11] The overall objective of this study is the evaluation of mineralized collagen, nanophase composite of collagen and hydroxyapatite, for its osteoconductivity and its ability to express the incorporated bone morphogenic protein-2 (BMP-2) *in vivo.* Further these properties of mineralized collagen are compared with other bio-active matrices: [a] type-I collagen, [b] polylactide glycolide (1:1) co-polymer, and [c] fibrin glue. The results of the study demonstrate that mineralized collagen may serve as a substitute for autograft bone and for the delivery of BMP-2.

MATERIALS AND METHODS

The mineralization process of collagen has been described by Constantz and Gunasekaran.[12] Commercially available collagen (type I) from bovine Achilles tendon was pre-sterilized with ethylene oxide and used as the main ingredient for mineralized collagen. All other chemicals used were ACS grade and the mineralization process was done under aseptic conditions.

0-8493-4750-5/94/$0.00 + $.50

ANIMAL EXPERIMENTS

A total of thirty one adult New Zealand White rabbits weighing 3.0 to 4.5 kg were used for the study. All surgical procedures were performed with animals under general anesthesia using aseptic surgical techniques. An approximately 2-3 inch long mid-line skin incision was made and the parietal bone of the skull was exposed. Nine mm diameter circular portions of the bone were removed on either side using a slow speed dental burr. During this process, excessive heat was avoided by frequent interruption of drilling as well as by irrigating the surgical site with sterile saline solution.

The skull defect was filled with one of the following matrix materials: [1] Mineralized Collagen Disk, [2] Collagen (Type I) Disk, [3] Fibrin Glue (Beriplast®) Disk, [4] Polylactide/glycolide copolymer (PLG-CP), [5] Autologous Bone Disk (removed from the contra-lateral side of the rabbit's skull), and [6] Un-implanted control (empty hole negative control). To each experimental matrix material, a growth factor (Bone Morphogenic Protein-2, BMP2) was added prior to implantation (as outlined in Table 1).

Table 1
Experimental Design: The table lists the number of implantation sites referred as "n" for each type of matrix with the stated amount of BMP-2 incorporated prior to implantation.

MATRIX	**BMP-2 (μg/implant)**				
	0	**5**	**10**	**25**	**50**
Mineralized Collagen	n = 6	n = 1	n = 1	n = 1	n = 1
Collagen	n = 2	n = 1	n = 1	n = 0	n = 0
Fibrin	n = 3	n = 1	n = 1	n = 1	n = 0
PLG-CP	n = 3	n = 1	n = 1	n = 1	n = 1

Mineralized Collagen (Ultrafibre®)

UltraFibre is a nanophasic composite material consisting of type I collagen and apatitic mineral crystals well adhered to collagen.[1] Mineral/Collagen weight ratios were determined by ashing methods. X-ray diffraction, Fourier-transform infrared and transmission electron microscopy scans identified Ultrafibre as a composite of collagen and poorly crystalline hydroxyapatite.

Collagen- (Type-I)

Type-I collagen was purified from bovine Achilles tendon and characterized by ash weight, heavy metal content, shrink temperature, and amino acid analysis.

Fibrin Glue (Beriplast®)

Sterile fibrin glue material (Behring Werke) was obtained as a kit. The kit consists of fibrinogen and thrombin components which form a fibrin clot upon setting. These kits were used to make 9 mm diameter sterile discs to fill in the skull defects.

Polylactide/glycolide copolymer (PLG-CP)

Gamma sterilized microspheres (100-225 μm size) of polylactide/glycolide copolymer (PLGA, DL 100 - Lot No. SR 103B-89) were obtained from Medisorb-Dupont, Wilmington, Delaware. A mixture of 100 +/- 2 mg PLGA copolymer and 100 μl of blood drawn from the subject animal with sterile technique were mixed in a mold to form a 9 mm diameter disc implant.

Autologous Bone

Native or autologous bone removed from the contralateral side of the rabbit's skull was used to implant the defect region in the same animal. It was implanted as one intact piece without any grinding or mixing with blood. Autologous bone functioned as a positive control in the experiment.

Un-implanted Control Defect

A circular defect region was filled with no implant or growth factor. This empty hole was used to gauge bony ingrowth and repair without the benefit of a matrix material. It functioned as a negative control in the experiment.

Bone Morphogenic Factor-2 Added to the Various Implants

The growth factor, BMP-2, was incorporated in the implants at differing dosage levels (0, 5, 10, 25, and 50 micrograms). BMP-2 was prepared from an SF-9 insect cell line infected with recombinant baculovirus containing full length BMP-2. Purified BMP-2 as judged by SDS-PAGE migrated at 32-35 kD non-reduced and 15 kD when reduced. It was stored at neutral pH in 40% acetonitrile at -20°C. Protein concentration was measured using the Pierce BCA assay (**13**) and confirmed by amino acid analysis. The protein was isolated, purified, and characterized by Chiron Inc., Emeryville, CA, and filtered to yield a sterile preparation. In BMP-2 treated animals, appropriate amounts of the sterile growth factor as listed in Table-1 were added prior to implantation.

Animals after implantation were maintained in separate cages and received food and water *ad lib.* Three animals died of anesthesia, and six died of diarrhea. Pathological examination showed that the cause of death was not related to local infection or rejection of the implant. These animals were eliminated from consideration in the study. Due to such accidents the experimental design resulted as shown in Table 1. All rabbits were euthanized twenty-eight days post-op. The skull region containing both defects was harvested, fixed in neutral, buffered formalin and radiographed.

The harvested bone with the enclosed implant (dotted square in Figure-1) was cut along the fronto-parietal axis into two equal halves. One-half of each implant was subjected to undecalcified histologic analysis. These samples were dehydrated, embedded in LR White resin and polished following thin sectioning (0.6-1.0 mm) on a Buehler isomet saw.

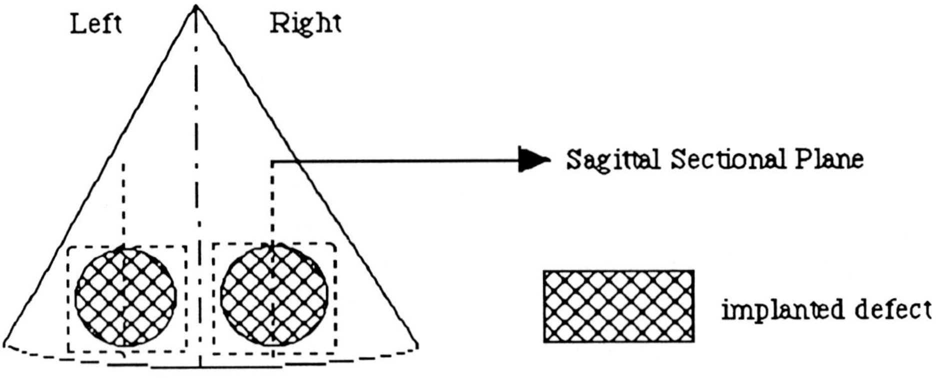

Figure 1. Diagramatic representation of skull defect analysis.

The sectioned sample was gold coated on a sputtering device, and mounted for electron microscopic evaluation in the back scattered mode (BSE). Hitachi S-570 SEM and Robinson backscatter detector (RBH-570RL) were used. Micrographs were taken with Polaroid 54 film and a montage of the entire defect was pieced together. The amounts of new bone, soft tissue, marrow and remaining implant in the surgical defect area were quantified by overlaying the montage with a grid transparency and point counting. The results were expressed as a percentage of the total defect area. Statistical analysis of histologic response between groups was performed by students t-test.

RESULTS

We list the experimental results in the order of description of different implant materilas in the "Materials and Methods" section. For each implant group we show back-scattered SEM montages of the mid-sectional image of the implant after 28 days of implantation.

Mineralized Collagen, Figure 2: The image shows that the new bone in the implant region , located between the two arrows, forms from the endosteal region to the periosteal region. The gray areas towards the periosteal region show remaining mineralized collagen, whereas the new bone closest to the endosteal region has replaced the implant entirely. It is calculated that the mineralized collagen alone without any BMP-2 yields good osteoconduction with $48.5 \pm 6.8\%$ new bone in the defect.

Type-I Collagen, Figure 3: Very little, if any, new bone has been formed in the defect region. Instead of bone, that region is mostly filled in with a fibrous tissue (the streaming lines indicated by arrows marked as FT) connecting the defect edges.

Fibrin Glue (Beriplast®) Figure 4: There is no new bone growth in the defect region within 4 weeks post implantation. As in the collagen sample there is a fibrous connective tissue formation (indicated by arrows marked as FT) replacing the implanted material.

Polylactide/glycolide copolymer (PLG-CP), Figure 5: There is no new bone nor a dense fibrous tissue ingrowth in the defect region.

Autologous Bone, Figure 6: The autologous bone implant has integrated well with the neighbouring old bone.

Un-implanted Control Defect, Figure 7: New bone growth occurs from the edges of the defect (indicatedby two arrows) towards the center. There is only partial bone ingrowth (24.8± 5.3 %) after 28 days post surgery and the image shows it as a non-healing model at this time interval.

Bone Morphogenic Factor-2 (BMP-2), Figures-8 20: The images in Figures 8-11 correspond to 5, 10, 25 and 50 micro gram quantities of BMP-2 respectively in the mineralized collagen implants. Incorporation of a minimum of 5μg of BMP-2 (Fig.-8) into the mineralized collagen resulted in full thickness new bone bridging the skull defect There is no remaining mineralized collagen seen within the new bone formed. Some remaining mineralized collagen is seen on either side of the newly formed bone in the endosteal and periosteal regions. The image in Fig. 9, shows new bone growth in nearly the entire defect. In some areas, the thickness of the new bone exceeds the normal thickness of the skull. Some mineralized collagen is not yet resorbed. In Figs. 10 and 11, the larger quantities of BMP-2 lead to new bone growth wherever the mineralized collagen with the added BMP-2 was implanted. Bone growth in excess of normal skull thickness is noticed in both the images. The new bone growth shown in these images (Figs. 10 and 11) has thinner bone-trabeculae than that of the new bone growth in the images of Figs. 7 and 8).

The images in Figures 12-20 respectively correspond to 5 and 10 micro gram quantities of BMP-2 in the collagen implants; 5, 10 and 25 micro gram quantities of BMP-2 in the Fibrin (Beriplast®) implants; 5, 10, 25 and 50 micro gram quantities of BMP-2 in the Polylactide/glycolide copolymer (PLG-CP) implants. The images demonstrate that the BMP-2 incorporation in collagen, Fibrin or PLG-CP does not significantly improve bone formation.

Percent new bone formed and the remaining implant in the defect are represented by the bar charts shown in Figs. 21 and 22.

DISCUSSION

The autologous or native bone attracts appropriate osteogenic cells for proper healing within a 4 week time interval. The mineralized collagen, to some extent without growth factor but fully with growth factor, leads to osseous healing response in the defect site similar to that of the autologous bone graft. Further the mineralized collagen appears to be a very effective matrix for BMP-2 compared to the other matrices studied in this screening model. Neither the the type-I collagen (or) fibrin glue nor PLG-CP alone was found to form more new bone than the empty controls. Fibrin glue and the collagen disk were possibly inhibiting bony ingrowth by promoting more soft tissue in the defect region.

In conclusion, the mineralized collagen, a nanophasic composite of collagen and hydroxyapatite, seems to possess chemical and structural resemblance with native bone and therefore may potentially serve as an osteoconductive material and may also be a more effective carrier to facilitate the osteoinductive properties of BMP-2 *in vivo*.

2

3

4

5

6

7

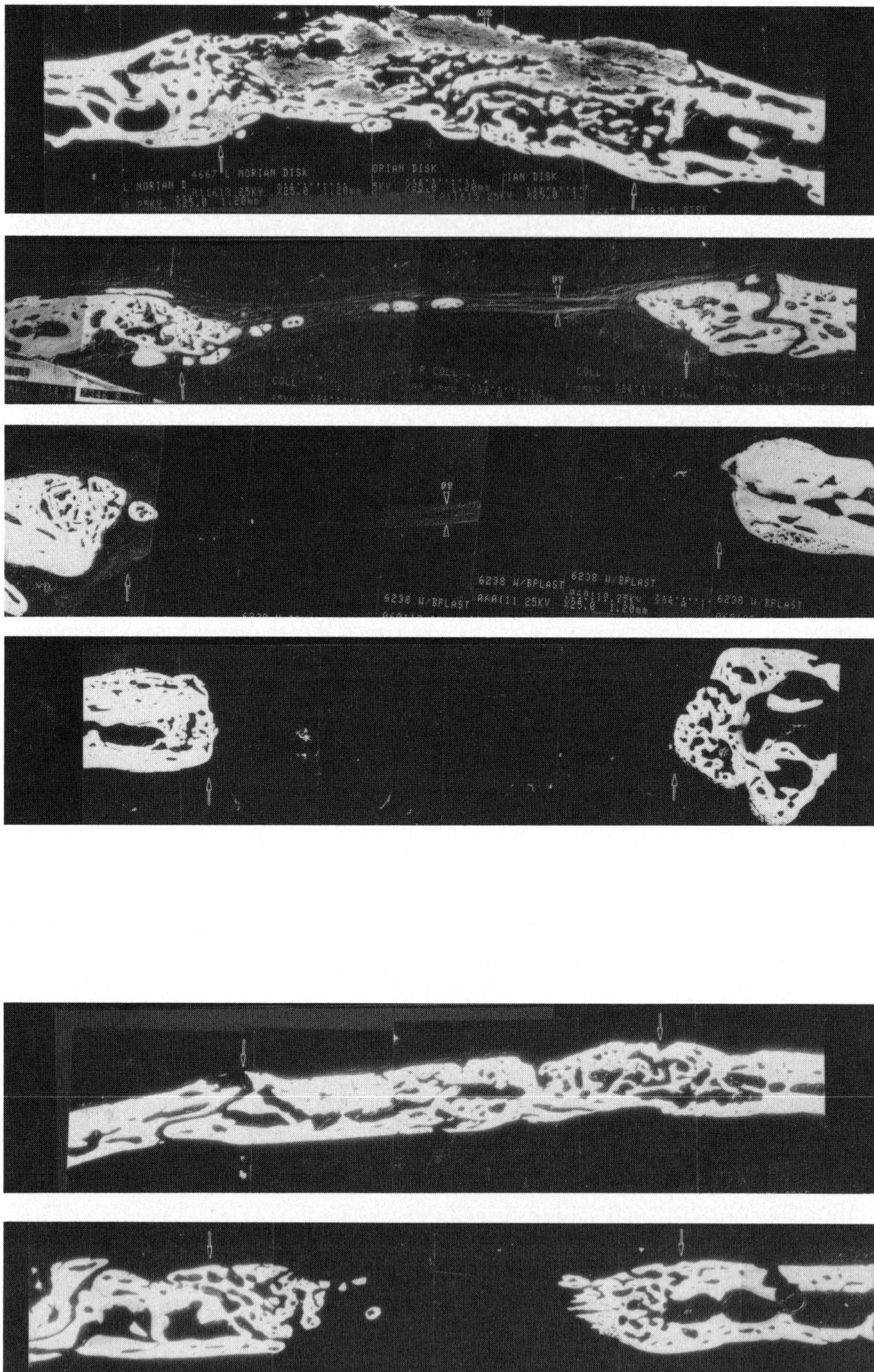

SEM back scatter image montages of implants (sagittal sections) at 28 days post surgery. The two arrows mark the defect boundary. Fig. 2. Mineralized Collagen; Fig. 3. Type-I Collagen; Fig. 4. Fibrin Glue (Beriplast®); Fig. 5:. Polylactide/glycolide copolymer (PLG-CP); Fig. 6. Autologous Bone; Fig. 7. Un-implanted control. MC= remaining mineralized collagen; FT= fibrous tissue formed in the defect.

8

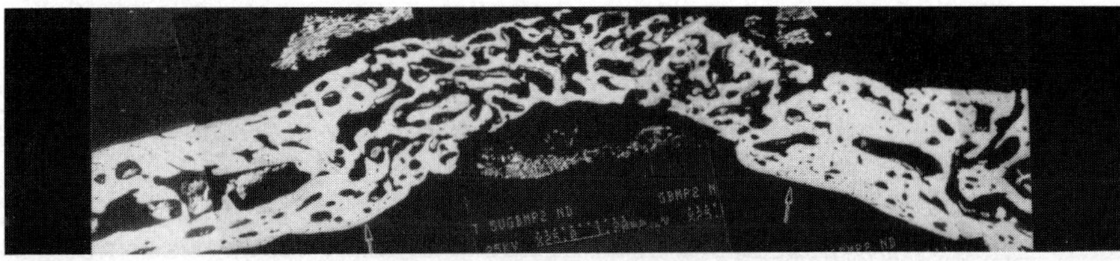

9

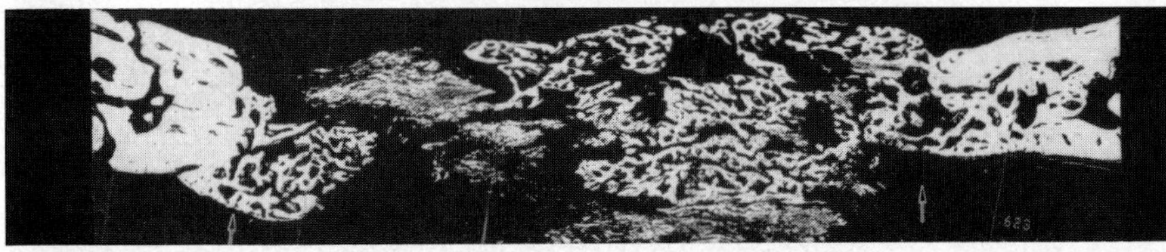

10

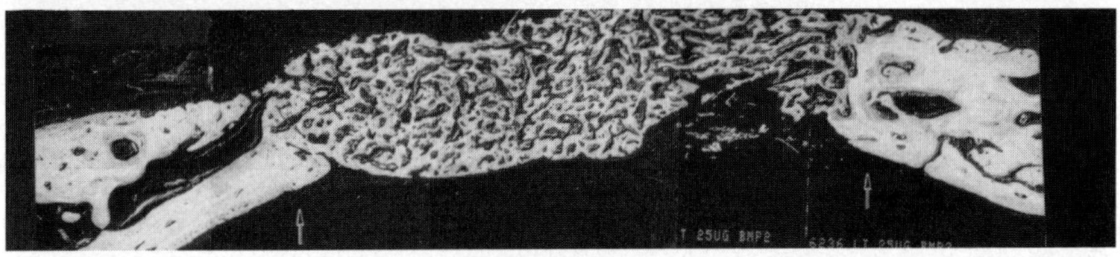

11

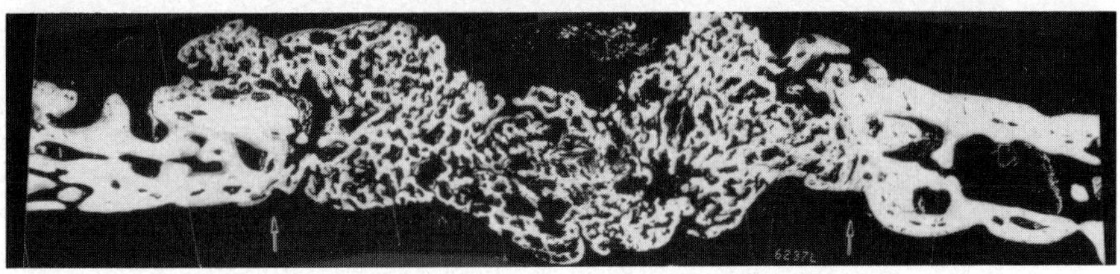

12

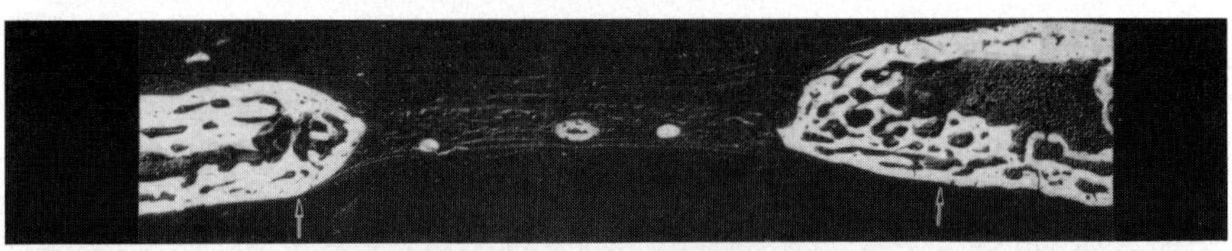

13

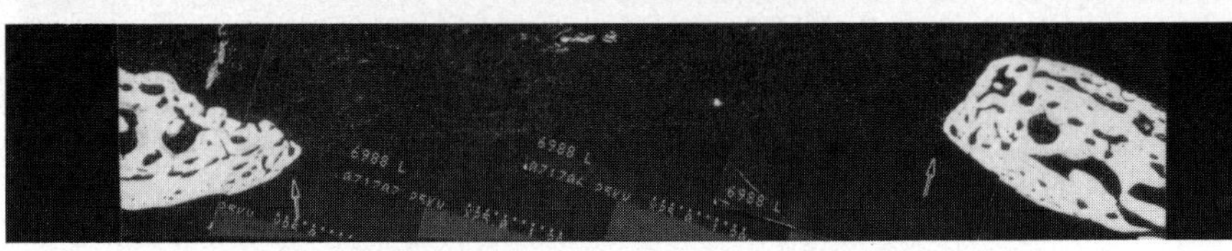

SEM back scatter image montages of implants (sagittal sections) at 28 days post surgery. The defect perimetry is indicated by two arrows. Fig. 8. Mineralized Collagen + 5 ug of BMP-2; Fig. 9. Mineralized Collagen + 10 ug of BMP-2; Fig. 10. Mineralized Collagen + 25 ug of BMP-2; Fig. 11. Mineralized Collagen + 50 ug of BMP-2. Mineralized collagen, even with the lowest dosage of 5 ug of BMP-2, resulted in full thickness bone bridging with some remaining implant seen on either sides of the new bone. The specimens with 25 and 50 ug BMP-2 resulted in bone with narrower trabecular struts. Fig. 12. Type-I Collagen + 5 ug of BMP-2; Fig. 13. Type-I Collagen + 10 ug of BMP-2. Collagen implants with BMP-2 do not result in considerable osteo-induction.

14

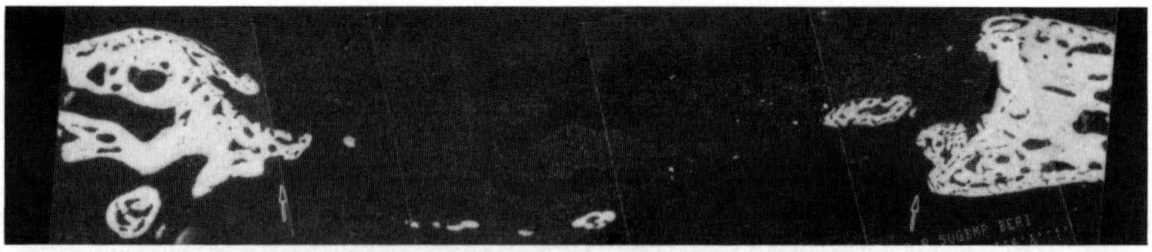

15

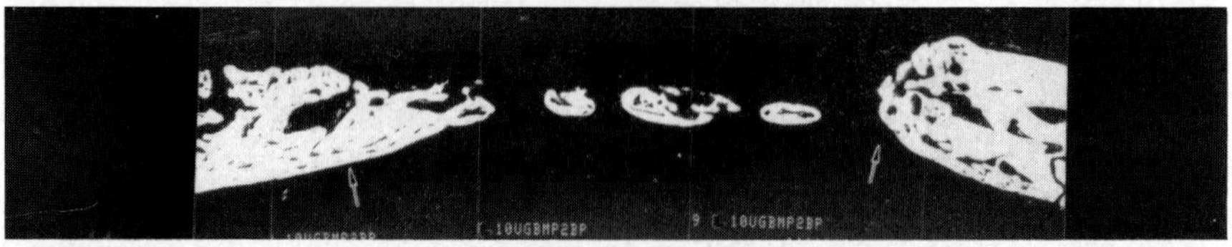

16

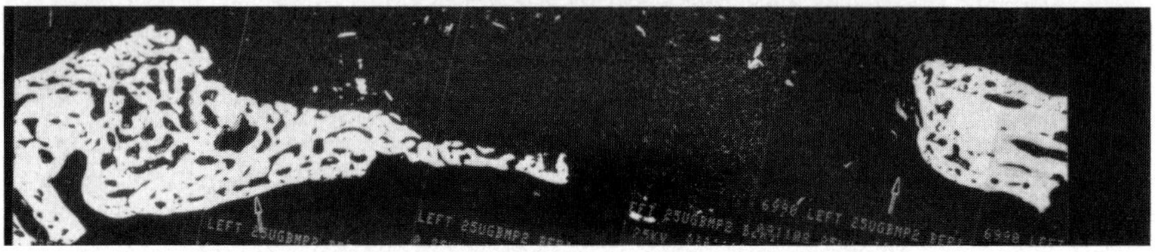

17

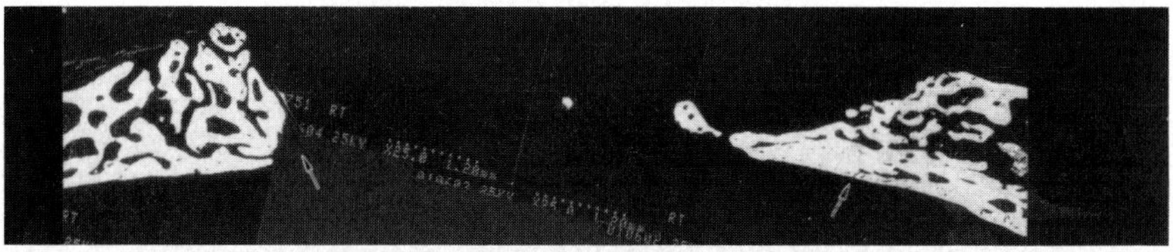

18

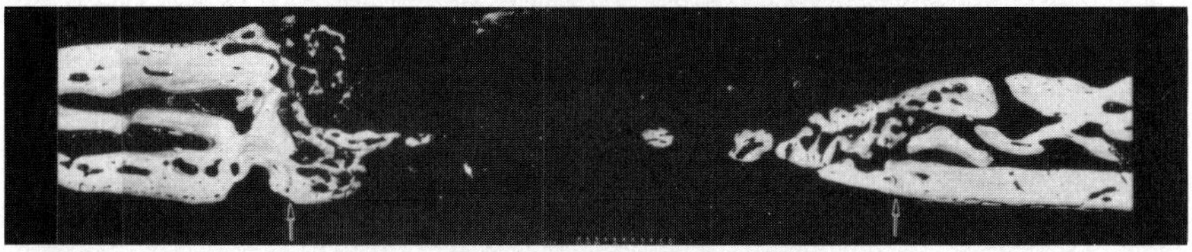

19

20

SEM back scatter image montages of implants (sagittal sections) at 28 days post surgery. The defect perimetry is indicated by two arrows. Fig. 14 . Fibrin Glue + 5 ug of BMP-2; Fig. 15. Fibrin Glue + 10 ug of BMP-2; Fig. 16. Fibrin Glue + 25 ug of BMP-2; Fig. 17. PLG-CP + 5 ug of BMP-2; Fig. 18. PLG-CP + 10 ug of BMP-2; Fig. 19. PLG-CP + 25 ug of BMP-2; Fig. 20. PLG-CP + 50 ug of BMP-2. BMP-2 incorporation in fibrin or PLG-CP implants does not significantly improve the bone formation.

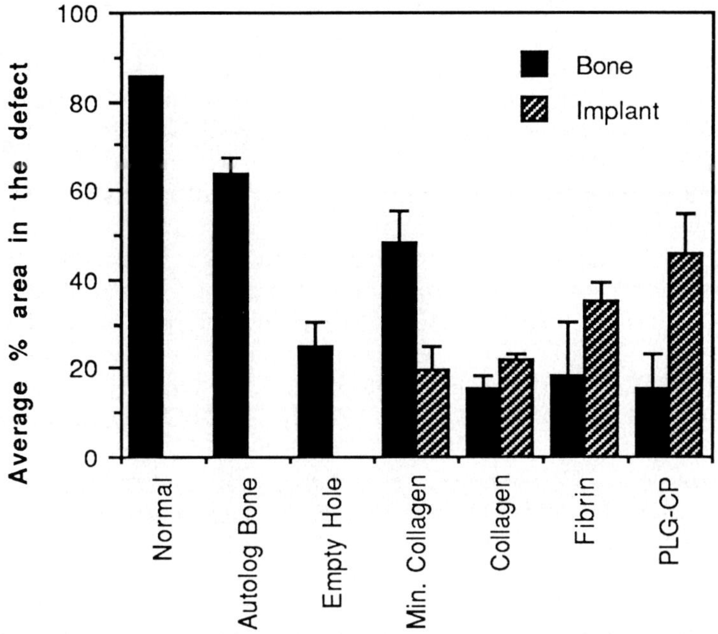

Figure 21. Comparison of the average percent of bone and implant in the defect (28 days after surgery). The new bone formed in the mineralized collagen sample (48.5 ± 6.8 %) is next best to that of the autologous bone implant (63.9 ± 3.1 %). The negative control (empty hole) and the other test materials formed significantly lesser amounts of new bone in the defect (below 18.6 %)

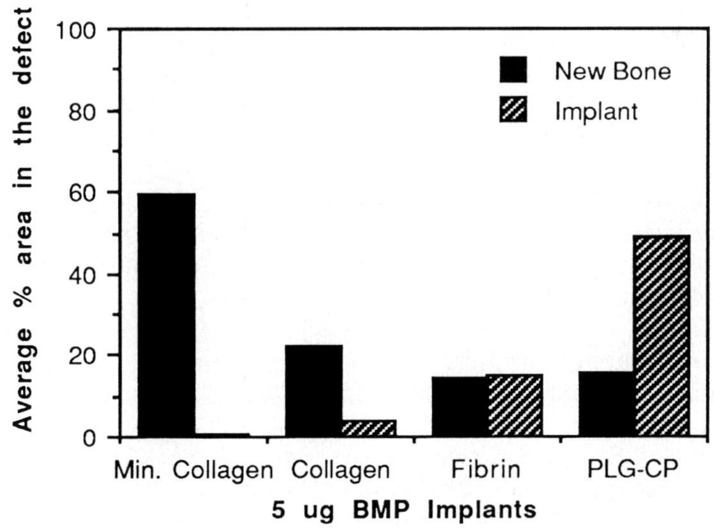

Figure 22. Comparison of the average percent of new bone formed and remaining implant (incorporated with 5 ug of BMP-2) in the defect for mineralized collagen, collagen, fibrin, and PLG-CP. Osteo-induction in collagen, fibrin and PLG-CP matrices with the bone morphogenic protein is only about one third of that in the mineralized collagen implant sample.

REFERENCES

1. Constantz, B.R., Gunasekaran, S., and Ross, J. Is there a need for a nucleating protein in collagen for bone mineral formation? *Proc. International Conference on Mineralized Tissues*, San Diego, CA, (4): 1992.
2. Katz, R.W., Felthousen, G.C., Reddi, A,H., Radiation sterilized insoluble collagenous bone matrix is a functional carrier of bone induction. Calcified Tissue International, 47:183-185 (1990).
3. Gebhart, M., Lane, J., A radiographical and biomechanical study of demineralized bone matrix implanted into a bone defect of rat femurs with and without bone marrow. Acta Orthopedica Belgica, 57 (2): 130-143, 1991.
4. Sampath, T.K., Maliakal, J.C., Hauschka, P.V., Jones, W.K., Sasak, H., Tucker, R.F., White, K.H., Coughlin, J.E., Tucker, M.M., Pang, R.H. Recombinant human osteogenic protein - 1 (hOP-1) induces new bone formation *in vivo* J. Biol. Chem., 267 (28):20352-62, 1992.
5. Gombatz, W.R., Pankey, S.C., Bouchard, L.S., *Controlled Release of TGF-B From a Biodegradable Matrix For Bone Regeneration,* Fourth World Biomaterials Congress April 24-28, p 179 1992.
6. Yasko, A.W., Fellinger, E.J., Waller, S., Tomin, A., Peteson, M., Wang, E.A., and Lane, J.M. Comparison of biological and synthetic carriers for rhBMP-2 induced bone formation. 38th Annual Meeting, Orthopedic Research Society, p. 71, 1992
7. Hotz, G., Alveolar ridge augmentation with hydroxyapatite using fibrin sealant for fixation. Part II: Clinical application. J. Oral Maxillofac. Surg., 20:208-213, 1991.
8. Holmes, R. and Hagler, H., Porous hydroxyapatite as a bone graft substitute in maxillary augmentation: An histometric study. J. Cranio-maxillofacial Surg., 16: 199-205, 1988.
9. Urist, M.R., Nilsson, O., Rasmussen, J., Hirota, W., Lovel, T., Schmalzreid, T,. and Finerman, G.A.M., Bone regernation under the influence of a Bone Morphogenic Protein (BMP) beta Tricalcium phosphate (TCP) composite in skull trephine defects in dogs. Clinical Orthopedics and Related Research. (214): 296-304, 1987.
10. Rosenblum, S.F., Frenkel, S., Ricci, J.L., Alexander, H., *The Effect of Fibroblast Growth Factor Released From A Calcium Sulfate Carrier on Bone Ingrowth Unsing A Canine Model,* Fourth World Boimaterials Congress April 24-28, p. 75, 1992.
11. Damien, C.J., Parsons, J.R., Benedict, J.J., and Weisman, D.S., Investigation of a hydroxyapatite and calcium sulfate composite supplemented with an osteoinductive factor. J. Biomedical Materials Research. 24 (6): 639-54, 1990.
12. Constantz, B.R., and Gunasekaran, S., Mineralized Collagen. US Patent # 5,231,169, Issue Date: July 27, 1993.
13. Davis, L.C., Radke, G.A., Measurement of protein using analysis with bicinchoninic acid (BCA). Anal. Biochem., 161: 152-156, 1987.

MATURATION OF POORLY CRYSTALLINE SYNTHETIC AND BIOLOGICAL APATITES.

C. Rey,* H-M. Kim, M.J. Glimcher
*Laboratoire des Matériaux - Physicochimie des Solides, Toulouse, France
Laboratory for the study of Skeletal disorders and Rehabilitation, Department of Orthopaedic Surgery, Harvard Medical School,
The Children's Hospital, Boston, MA

I. INTRODUCTION

The change of composition and short range order of poorly crystalline apatites after they have been precipitated (maturation) is one of the most important factors affecting their reactivity and interaction properties which are directly related to their biological functions. The aim of this report is to give a more precise description of the *in vitro* carbonate uptake and its exchanges during the maturation of carbonate apatites.

II. MATERIALS AND METHODS

A. SAMPLE PREPARATION

Poorly crystalline apatites were prepared by double decomposition of a solution of calcium nitrate ($Ca(NO_3)_2 \cdot 4H_2O$: 17.7 g in 250 ml H_2O) and a solution of ammonium phosphate containing sodium bicarbonate ($(NH_4)_2HPO_4$: 40 g; $NaHCO_3$ 20 g, concentrated ammonia solution 1 ml, in 500 ml H_2O). The calcium solution was rapidly poured into the phosphate solution. The large excess of phosphate and bicarbonate ions in the solution provided pH buffering. Maturation occurred in the mother solution, at room temperature, pH 7.4, without agitation. The maturation vials were stoppered to minimize the loss of CO_2 at this pH. After the maturation period the suspension was filtered on a large buchner funnel; the precipitate was rapidly washed with distilled water and lyophilized.

B. EXCHANGE EXPERIMENTS

The carbonate apatites equilibrated during maturation in a ^{12}C-carbonate solution for varying periods of time were centrifuged and resuspended in ^{13}C-carbonate solution of the same composition for 3 weeks.

C. CHARACTERIZATION

All samples were analyzed by X-ray diffractometry. All showed the typical reflections and characteristics of poorly crystalline apatite similar to bone mineral. Calcium concentration was determined by complexometry with EDTA, phosphate ions by spectrophotometry of phospho-vanado-molybdic acid and carbonate ions by coulometry.[1] The FTIR spectra were recorded on a Perkin

0-8493-4750-5/94/$0.00 + $.50

Elmer 1700 or an Analect FX 60/62 instrument. The intensity ratios and the resolution factors were determined as specified in a previous paper.[1] The relative amounts of $^{12}CO_3$ and $^{12}CO_3$ were determined by measurement of the area of the IR n_2 carbonate peaks with that of the n_4 phosphate peaks.

Table 1
Chemical composition of carbonateapatites after different maturation times.

Maturation time	Ca/P (atomic)	Ca/(P+C) (atomic)	Carbonate content (% weight)
0	1.44	1.41	0.90
1 hr	1.50	1.41	1.97
6 hrs	1.50	1.42	2.02
22 hrs	1.51	1.40	2.75
8 days	1.62	1.41	4.67
4 months	1.62	1.38	5.77

III. RESULTS

A. COMPOSITION CHANGES

The results of carbonate, calcium and phosphate analyses are shown in Table 1. An interesting feature is that apatites which were rapidly precipitated at room temperature in carbonate containing solutions at physiological pH contained only very small amounts of carbonate ions; most of the carbonate ions were incorporated during the maturation of the precipitate. As reported by a number of investigators, maturation of the crystals is associated with changes in the chemical composition resulting in an increase of the Ca/P ratio. However, as the carbonate is essentially substituted for phosphate ions the Ca/P ratio does not account for the variations in the stoichiometry of the crystals. This feature is best evaluated by the Ca/P+C ratio. This latter ratio remains essentially constant in our samples (approximately 1.40), indicating that the number of calcium vacancies in the lattice does not decrease significantly during maturation, and there is, therefore no evolution in the stoichiometry of the crystals toward a more perfect "pure" apatite under these *in vitro* conditions.

A similar evolution in composition has been observed in bone mineral of animals of different ages.[1,2]

B. FTIR STUDIES

The maturation of carbonate apatites induced small but significant structural changes observed in the carbonate bands in the n_2 domain (Figure 1).

Three bands can be detected in the spectra at 866, 871 and 878 cm^{-1} which have been respectively assigned to type A carbonate apatite (carbonate ions substituted for OH ions in the hydroxyapatite structure); type B carbonate (carbonate substituted for phosphate groups) and labile non-apatitic carbonate species, probably located at or close to the surfaces of the crystals.[3] The position of the A and B bands were constant in all samples and their resolution factors have previously been shown to be related to a crystallinity index of the solid phase.[1] The relative rate of evolution of the intensity ratios of the three carbonate bands and their resolution factors are shown in Table 2. Similar measurements of the apatite of the cortical bones of chickens of different ages have been reported[1]. In both the *in vitro* precipitated crystals and the crystals of chicken bone, the resolution factors (and thus the crystallinity of the solid phase) increased with time of maturation and the age of the animal. The intensity ratios of the *in vitro* precipitated carbonateapatite (A and B) were constant during maturation, as the carbonate concentration increased, demonstrating that both the A and B sites were being occupied at the same rate. In contrast, the relative amounts of labile, non-apatitic carbonate decreased with maturation time while the total carbonate content increased.

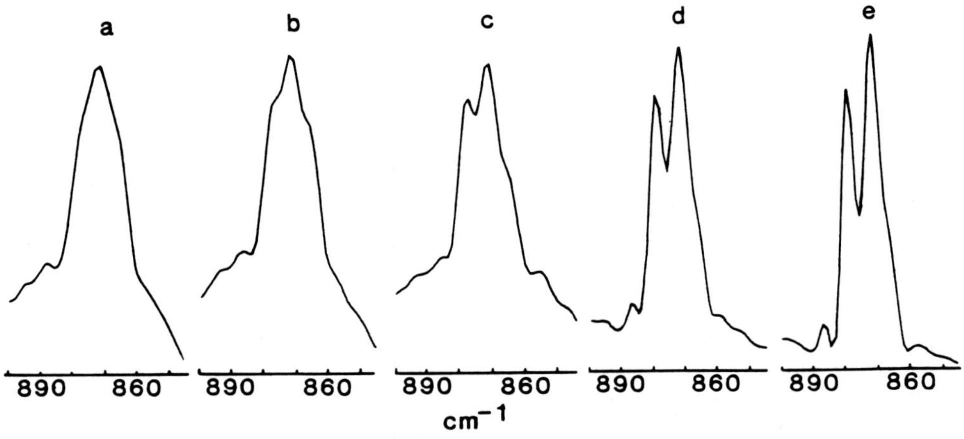

Figure 1. Resolution enhanced IR spectra of carbonate bands of apatites maturated in carbonate-containing solutions (Band width 8 cm^{-1}; Enhancement factor: 2.5; Triangular apodization).

Table 2
Main characteristics of IR carbonate bands of apatites maturated in carbonate-containing solutions.

Maturation time	Resolutio factor	A/B	Labile/B
0	0	0.76	0.77
4 hrs	0.05	0.79	0.69
33 hrs	0.20	0.81	0.50
3 days	0.39	0.83	0.42
9 days	0.41	0.82	0.40
2 months	0.54	0.81	0.39

In order to obtain more precise information on the carbonate mobility during maturation, the CO_3 exchange experiments described in Materials and Methods section were carried out.

C. ^{13}C - ^{12}C EXCHANGES

The relative amount of $^{12}CO_3$ and $^{13}CO_3$ taken up by the apatite crystals during *in vitro* maturation are shown in Figure 2 together with the initial $^{12}CO_3$ content of the samples.

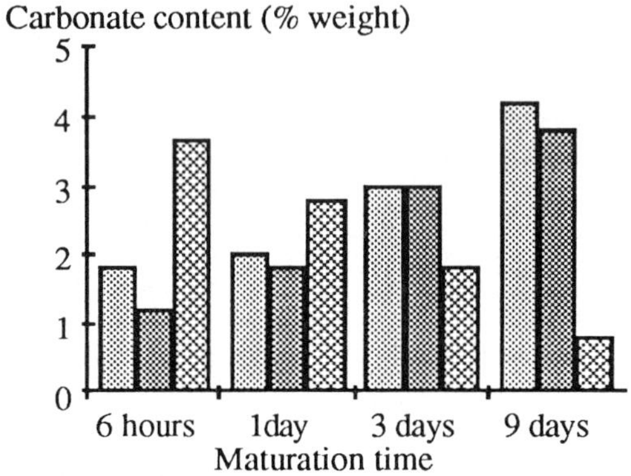

Figure 2.. Carbonate content of apatites maturated in ^{13}C carbonate solutions.

The most interesting observation is that the $^{12}CO_3$ initially incorporated by the crystals is not readily exchangeable during the first few weeks of equilibration with $^{13}CO_3$. Rather the increased carbonate content consists simply in a further uptake of $^{13}CO_3$ ions from the solution. The FTIR data obtained during this experiment is reproduced in Figure 3; the labile carbonate band appeared always more intense in the $^{13}CO_3$ peaks than in the $^{12}CO_3$, indicating that the last ions picked up by the precipitate occupied preferentially labile sites of the crystals.

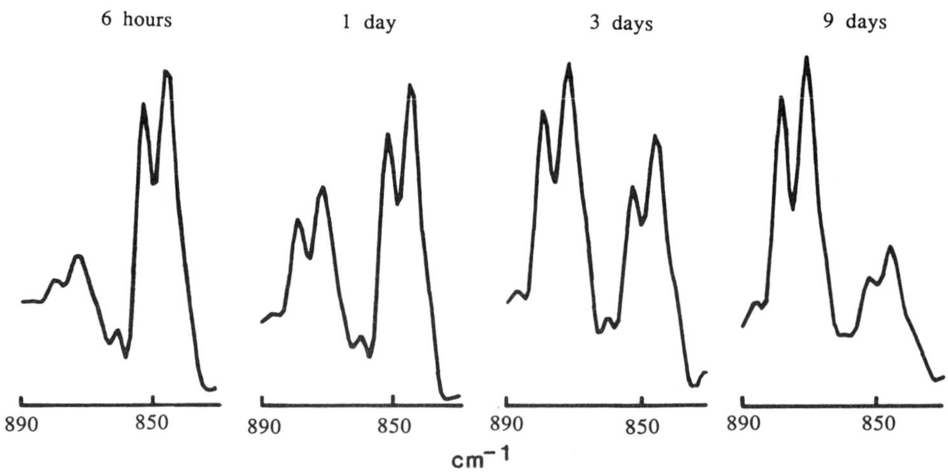

Figure 3. Resolution enhanced spectra of ^{12}C carbonateapatite maturated in ^{13}C carbonate-containing solution (same conditions as Figure 1).

IV. DISCUSSION

A. CARBONATE UPTAKE

The carbonate ions are not incorporated into the crystals in large numbers during the early rapid precipitation of the solid phase. Rather they enter the crystal lattice later during maturation. The same observation seems to be true for bone mineral, in which case the carbonate content increases as the turn over of the bone matrix crystals decreases. The stoichiometry does not vary much during maturation. The net result of these processes, with respect to the chemical composition of the crystals, corresponds to a replacement of HPO_4 ions initially present in the apatite by CO_3 ions, a suggestion proposed by Pellegrino and Blitz,[4] and later on by Legros et al.[2] The basis for this proposal is the analogy between the substitution scheme of the bivalent ions: their incorporation in the apatite lattice is associated with a cationic vacancy and a monovalent anionic vacancy.[5,6] The stability of the Ca/P+C ratio is more difficult to explain and may be related to the existence of the non-apatitic environments which will be discussed further in the paper.

B. CRYSTAL MODIFICATIONS

Although maturation of the crystals was associated with an increase in the crystallinity index, it did not appear to be related to an increase in the size of the crystals as determined by transmission electron microscopy and specific surface area determinations. Thus the processes are not simply due to dissolution of small crystals and the growth of larger crystals. The same observation relative to crystal size has been made for bone mineral crystals which showed only very small size variation as a function of age.[7] The increase of crystallinity deduced from carbonate bands resolution factors might be due to changes in the local short range environments of the sites where carbonate is located moving from disturbed atomic planes at the surface to the more regular atomic arrangements in the interior of the crystal. These conclusions are consistent with the resolution factors of the ^{13}C and ^{12}C carbonate bands in samples used for the exchange experiments which demonstrated that the $^{13}CO_3$ ions incorporated by the crystals in the late stages of the exchange generally had lower resolution factors than the $^{12}CO_3$ taken up at the beginning of maturation.

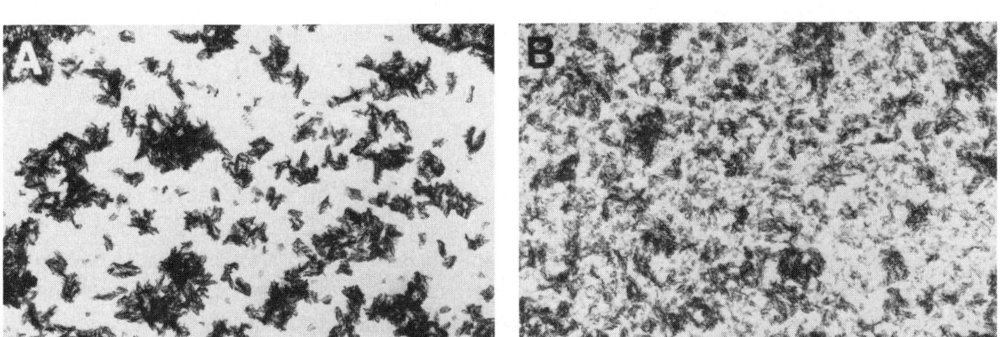

Figure 4. Electron micrography of apatite crystals (a) after precipitation (b) after 12 days maturation (magnification 26000).

The changes in carbonate environment during maturation and the stability of crystal habit shown by electron microscopy suggest a topotactic transformation, i.e. a transformation initiated in or on the crystals themselves. Such a transformation would begin on the surface of the crystals, by the fixation of carbonate ions in a labile environment. As the number of surface carbonate increased, it would induce a reorganization of the crystal structure corresponding to the development of a carbonate apatite out of the first formed HPO_4^{2-}-rich apatite. Such a proposal is consistent with the data obtained from bone and young enamel by Thermal Stimulated Currents (TSC) and IR analyses, respectively,[8,9] from which it was concluded that there were two types of apatite crystals in such tissues with respect to the internal atomic organization of the crystals.

C. DRIVING FORCE OF THE MATURATION

In addition to the modifications of the environments at the sites of the carbonate ions, maturation also involves a decrease of the labile environment of the non-apatitic phosphate ions which are found in highest concentration in the first formed crystals *in vitro*. Similar data has been observed as a function of the age of bone and enamel crystals.[10] These data suggest that the evolution of initially formed labile apatite crystals into more stable, carbonated apatite crystals *in vitro* and *in vivo*, is the driving force of the process. Once the carbonate apatite is formed it does not further evolve to a more stable phase at an observable rate despite the very large surface area of the crystals.

D. OUTLINE OF THE PRECIPITATION AND MATURATION OF APATITE CRYSTALS

The labile environments of some phosphate and carbonate ions in the poorly crystalline apatites are characterized by specific spectroscopic features corresponding to the processes of forming a more stable carbonate apatite. The precipitation of PO_4^{3-} ions from a neutral or slightly alkaline solution (pH 7.0-7.4), which contains for the most part protonated phosphate groups, induces a release of protons that locally decreases the pH during the very earliest phases of the formation of a solid phase. Thus, the crystals which form in an acidic environment, the extent of the acidity being proportional to the rate at which the solid phase is deposited, are not at this stage in equilibrium with the solution. These physical chemical conditions may lead to ionic environment within the newly formed crystals which resemble those existing in HPO_4^{2-}-rich phosphates such as brushite or octacalcium phosphate both of which have been proposed as precursors of the apatitic phase, both *in vitro* and *in vivo*.[11-12] Under these acidic conditions, the carbonate ions would be excluded from the solid phase during the first stages of its formation because they either cannot substitute for phosphate groups in the precursors or because of the shift in the acid-base equilibrium which favors the formation of HCO_3^- and CO_2 due to the local, acidic pH of the rapidly forming crystals. During maturation, however, the solid reached an equilibrium with the solution phase by virtue of its large surface area. The carbonate ions are thus able to be added to the newly formed apatite crystals and slowly develop to a more stable carbonate apatite while the number of labile apatite crystals rich in HPO_4^{2-} but containing only very few carbonate groups decrease accordingly.

CONCLUSION

The maturation of apatite crystals in carbonate containing solutions is not accompanied by the evolution of a Ca-P stoichiometry similar to pure hydroxyapatite, either *in vivo* or *in vivo*. Rather, the apparent non-stoichiometry (viz., the lower Ca/P ratio of the initial solid phase slowly changing with time to that of stoichiometric apatite during maturation) is the result of an increase in the CO_3 content replacing the hydrogenophosphate ions. Thus the Ca/P+C ratio is found to remain constant during the evolution of a stable carbonate apatite with time. The maturation is driven by an initially labile solid phase, rich in labile non-apatitic species, into a stable, more crystalline carbonate apatite possibly by a topotactic transformation while retaining the initial crystal habit and size.

REFERENCES

1. Rey, C., Renugopalakrishnan, V., Collins, B., Glimcher, M.J., Fourier Infrared spectroscopic study of the carbonate ions in bone mineral during aging, *Calcif. Tisue Int.* 49,251, 1991.
2. Legeros, R., Balmain, N., Bonel, G., Structure and composition of the mineral phase of periosteal bone, *J. Chem. Res.*, 1, 8, 1986.
3. Rey, C., Collins, B., Goehl, T., Dickson, I.R., Glimcher, M.J., The carbonate environment in bone mineral: a resolution enhanced fourier transform infrared spectroscopic study, *Calcif. Tisue Int.*,45, 157, 1989.
4. Pellegrino, E.D., Biltz, R.M., Mineralization in the chick embryo I. Monohydrogen phosphate and carbonate relationships during maturation of the bone crystal complex. *Calcif. Tisue Res.*, 10, 128, 1972.
5. Kuehl, G. Nebergall, H., Hydrogen phosphate- and carbonate apatite. *Z. Anorg. Allgem. Chem.* 324 (5-6), 313-20 (1963).
6. Labarthe, J.C., Bonel, G., Monter, G., Sur la structure et les propriétés des apatites carbonatées de type B phosphocalciques. *Ann. Chim.* 8, 127, 1972.
7. Bonar, L.C., Roufosse, A.H., Sabine, W.K., Grynpas, M.D., Glimcher, M.J., X-ray diffraction studies of the crystalliity of bone mineral in newly synthesized and density fractionated bone. *Calcif. Tisue Int.* 35, 202, 1983.
8. Rey C., Renugopalakrishnan, V., Shimizu, M., Collins, B., Glimcher, M.J., A resolution enhanced fourier transform infrared spectroscopic study if the environment of the CO_3^{2-} ion in the mineral phase of enamel during its formation and maturation, *Calcif. Tisue Int.* 49, 259, 1991.
9. Lamure A., Bennis, A., Moscane, F., Hitmi, N., Vignoles, M., Heughebaert M., Lacabanne C., Influence of defects on the physical structure of non-stoichiometric hydroxyapatite. *Fourth World Biomaterial Congres, Berlin*, 1992.
10. Rey, C., Shimizu, M., Collins, B., Glimcher, M.J., Resolution enhanced fourier transform infrared spectroscopic study of the environment of phosphate ions in the early deposits of the a solid phase of calcium phosphate in bone and enamel, and their evolution with age. I: Investigations in the n_4 PO_4 domain. *Calcif. Tisue Int.* 46, 384, 1990.
11. Francis, M.D., Webb, N.C., Hydroxyapatite formation from a hydrated calcium monohydrogen phosphate precursor. *Calcif. Tisue Res.*, 6, 335, 1971.
12. Brown, W.E., Crystal growth of bone mineral, *Clin. Ortho.*, 44, 205, 1966.

PREDICTION OF PRECIPITATION AND TRANSFORMATION BEHAVIOUR OF CALCIUM PHOSPHATE IN AQUEOUS MEDIA

A. T.-C. Wong and J. T. Czernuszka
Department of Materials
University of Oxford
Parks Road, Oxford, OX1 3PH, U.K.

ABSTRACT

Based on the Avrami-Johnson-Mehl expression, a model has been developed to describe the *ex vivo* crystallisation behaviour of calcium phosphate in supersaturated solutions. This model relates various thermodynamic and kinetic factors to the preferential formation of precursor phases and their subsequent stage-wise transformation to hydroxyapatite. The validity of the model is verified by a comparison with experimental data.

I. INTRODUCTION

Calcium phosphate, due to its existence in hard tissue mineral, has attracted vast interest in various fields of research. It is well-known that in spite of its thermodynamic stability, formation of hydroxyapatite [HAP, $Ca_5(PO_4)_3(OH)$] is very often preceded by precursor phases, such as dicalcium phosphate dihydrate [DCPD, $CaHPO_4{\cdot}2H_2O$] and octacalcium phosphate [OCP, $Ca_4H(PO_4)_3{\cdot}2.5H_2O$], during crystallisation in aqueous media.[1] This phenomenon is in accordance with Ostwald's rule of stages for the multi-phase precipitation of sparingly soluble inorganic salts, which states that the phase of highest solubility (and hence lowest supersaturation) is preferentially formed as a result of favourable kinetics; while thermodynamic driving forces subsequently impel the transformation to the more stable phase(s).[2]

Although the precipitation of calcium phosphate has been extensively studied, there are still no existing models which correlate the determining factors to the transformation process. This work aims to derive an expression to describe the overall precipitation behaviour by modifying the Avrami-Johnson-Mehl formula to adapt to aqueous ionic systems. The original Avrami expression made no assumptions regarding the type of reaction mechanism,[3-5] and should therefore be applicable to this particular system, which is likely to involve solvent-mediated redissolution and recrystallisation processes.

0-8493-4750-5/94/$0.00 + $.50

II. DEVELOPMENT OF PRECIPITATION MODEL

A. Avrami-Johnson-Mehl expression

Avrami *et al.* proposed that, for a three-dimensional nucleation and growth process involving randomly distributed nuclei, the fraction formation of a particular phase is given by:[3-5]

$$\phi = 1 - exp\left(-\frac{\pi}{3} N^{n/4} G^{3n/4} t^{n} \right) \tag{1}$$

where ϕ = fractional formation (by volume);
N = nucleation rate (number of nuclei $m^{-3}\ s^{-1}$);
Γ = growth rate or interface velocity ($m\ s^{-1}$);
t = time (s); and
n depends on the growth mechanism (see Table 1).[6]

Table 1
Values of n in: $f = 1 - exp\,(-k'\, t^n)$ under different conditions[6]

Interface-controlled growth		*Diffusion-controlled growth*	
Condition	n	Condition	n
Increasing nucleation rate	> 4	Growing from small dimensions	1.5 - 3
Constant nucleation rate	4	Needles and plates of long dimensions	1
Decreasing nucleation rate	3 - 4	Thickening of long cylinders (needles)	1
Zero nucleation rate	3	Thickening of very large plates	0.5

1. Nucleation rate, N

The classical equation for the homogeneous nucleation rate in supersaturated solution is:[7]

$$N^{homo} = K\ exp\left(-\frac{\Delta G_c^{homo}}{k\,T} \right) \tag{2}$$

where K = kinetic (frequency) factor (number $m^{-3}\ s^{-1}$);
k = Boltzmann constant = $1.3806 \times 10^{-23}\ J\ K^{-1}$;
T = absolute temperature (K); and
ΔG_c^{homo} = change in free energy due to homogeneous nucleation.

$DG_c^{homo}$is the summation of the reduction in Gibb's free energy of the system and the increase in surface energy at the solid-liquid interface. Numerically,[7]

$$\Delta G_c^{homo} = \frac{f\ v^2 \gamma_{SL}^3}{(kT)^2\ (ln\ \beta)^2} \tag{3}$$

where f = shape factor, $16\pi/3 \le f \le 32$;
v = volume per molecule in unit cell (m^3);
γ_{SL} = solid-liquid interfacial free energy of nucleus ($J\ m^{-2}$);
β = supersaturation = $\dfrac{\text{ionic product (IP)}}{\text{solubility product } (K_{sp})}$

The kinetic factor, K, in equation 2 is a function of the entropy of the system; and in the case of crystallisation in dilute solutions, it can be assumed to be proportional to the probability (P) that the appropriate constituent ions collide to form a nucleus. Hence,

$$K = K_1 \Pi \tag{4}$$

where K_1 is a constant (number $m^{-3}\ s^{-1}$) and P for each calcium phosphate phase is given previously to be:[7]

$$\Pi^{DCPD} = \frac{2!\,[Ca^{2+}]\,[HPO_4^{2-}]}{([Ca^{2+}] + [HPO_4^{2-}])^2}$$

$$\Pi^{OCP} = \frac{7!\,[Ca^{2+}]^4\,[HPO_4^{2-}]\,[PO_4^{3-}]^2}{4!\,2!\,([Ca^{2+}] + [HPO_4^{2-}] + [PO_4^{3-}])^7}$$

$$\Pi^{HAP} = \frac{9!\,[Ca^{2+}]^5\,[PO_4^{3-}]^3\,[OH^-]}{5!\,3!\,([Ca^{2+}] + [PO_4^{3-}] + [OH^-])^9} \tag{5}$$

However, since typical crystallisation processes involve heterogeneous nucleation on existing seeds rather than spontaneous homogeneous nucleation, certain modifications must be made in equation 2. The following expression relates homogeneous and heterogeneous nucleation rates:[6]

$$\frac{N^{hetero}}{N^{homo}} = \frac{\delta}{L}\, exp\left(\frac{\Delta G_c^{homo} - \Delta G_c^{hetero} - \Delta g^{strain}}{k\,T}\right) = \lambda \tag{6}$$

where δ = boundary layer thickness;
L = substrate crystal grain size; and
Δg^{strain} = strain energy due to lattice mismatch between precipitate and substrate.

Provided that precipitation takes place in a well-stirred working solution and that the substrate seeds are of uniform grain size, δ and L in equation 6 can be assumed constant. ΔG_c^{hetero} is a function of free energies of both the substrate and the precipitating phases as well as the solid-solid interfacial energy, γ_{xy}. The term Δg^{strain} comes into effect whenever the substrate is a different phase from the precipitate. Owing to the high similarity of their respective crystal structures along certain directions, Δg^{strain} is minimal at an OCP-HAP interface.[8,9] However, Δg^{strain} may be more prominent in the cases of DCPD-OCP and DCPD-HAP interfaces as a result of significant lattice distortions at the solid interface.[8-11] The dimensionless variable λ in equation 6, therefore, accounts for the combined effect of the heterogeneity of nucleation and the strain arising from lattice mismatch.

Combining equations 2 to 6, the rate of heterogeneous nucleation is in the form of:

$$N^{hetero} = K_2 \lambda \Pi \, exp\left[- \frac{f \; v^2 \; \gamma_{SL}^3}{(kT)^3 \, (ln \; \beta)^2} \right] \tag{7}$$

2. Growth rate, Γ

Growth of existing nuclei is controlled either by bulk diffusion or by interface reactions.[12] The value of n in equation 1 depends on the growth mechanism (Table 1). As there is little hindrance to diffusion in dilute aqueous solutions (i.e. the interfacial composition of the solution can be approximated to be the same as the bulk composition), crystal growth under these circumstances is very likely to be interface-controlled. Hence from Table 1, a value of n greater than 3 is expected.

The rate of crystal growth in a dilute solution is given by:[12]

$$\Gamma = K_3 \, k \, T \, ln \frac{IP^{1/v}}{K_{sp}^{1/v}} = \frac{K_4 \, T}{v} ln \; \beta \tag{8}$$

where v = number of ions or radicals per molecule.

3. Modified Avrami equation

Substituting equations 7 and 8 in equation 1, the original Avrami equation becomes:

$$\phi = 1 - exp\,[- (\kappa\lambda)^{n/4} \, \zeta^{n/4} \, t^n] \tag{9}$$

where $\kappa\lambda$ = transformation coefficient ($K^{-3} \, s^{-4}$); and

$$\zeta = \left(\frac{T \, ln \; \beta}{v}\right)^3 \Pi \, exp\left[- \frac{f \; v^2 \; \gamma_{SL}^3}{(kT)^3 \, (ln \; \beta)^2} \right] \tag{10}$$

Although ζ appears to be a rather complicated function, its value can in fact be determined for particular experimental conditions. Supersaturation (β) and collision probability (Π) are both functions of the respective concentrations of individual ions, which in turn can be calculated by considering the various complexing equilibria, the ionic strength and the *p*H of the calcifying solution, solubility constants and activity coefficients. Now, it is very difficult to precisely evaluate the shape factor (f) for new nuclei, but as long as their morphology remains uniform, it is reasonable to assume an intermediate value of 25. On the other hand, values of v and γ_{SL} can be obtained from existing literature. Thus the value of ζ should be calculable.

The only unknowns left in equation 9 are the transformation coefficient ($\kappa\lambda$) and n. In the transformation coefficient, κ is a constant term whereas λ, as previously explained, is the variable which accounts for the heterogeneous nature of the nucleation process. In order to use equations 9 and 10 for prediction, the values of these parameters need to be found out.

4. Evaluation of transformation parameters

It is possible to work out the values of the transformation parameters with the aid of experimental results.[13-16]

a. *Time exponent, n*

With reference to equation 9, by plotting $ln\{ln[1/(1-\phi)]\}$ against ln t, the value of n can be determined. This is shown in Figure 1, from which it is apparent that over quite a wide range of solution composition, the values of n, given by the slopes of the plots, are all within the limits of 3.36 ± 0.24, at a confidence level of 78% (χ^2 test). In comparison with Table 1, this corresponds to an interface-controlled growth mechanism with a decreasing nucleation rate.

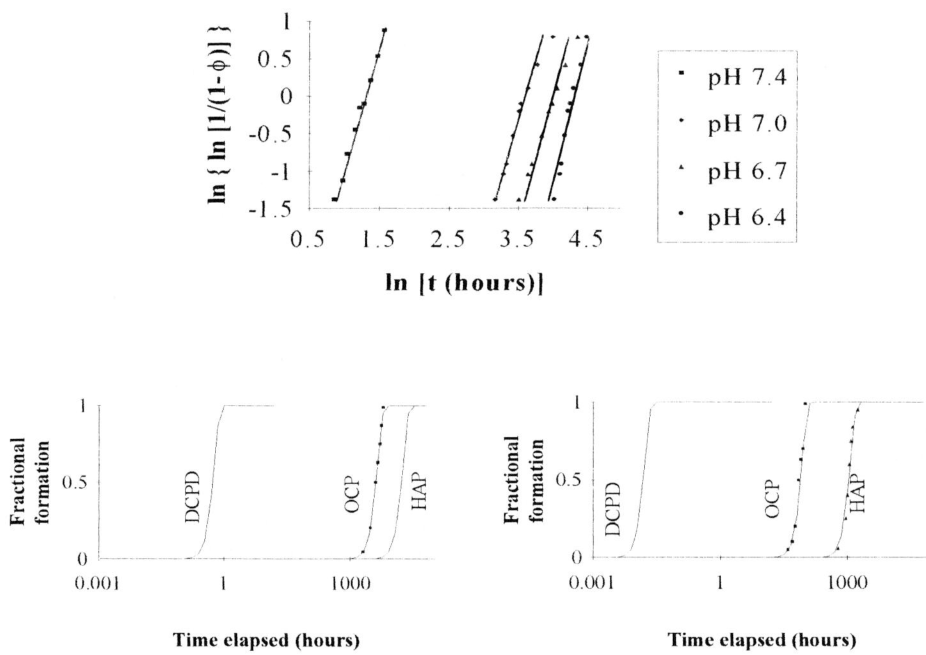

Figure 1. Plot of $ln\{ln\ [1/(1\text{-}f)]\}$ against ln t for calcium phosphate phase transformation. (DCPD-OCP data from references 13-16.)

b. *Transformation coefficient, $\kappa\lambda$*

Having found the value of n, it is then possible to estimate the transformation coefficient. As kl is a combination of various system parameters, this is achieved by iterating for values which, when substituted in equation 9, give the best fit to experimental data under different conditions. Figure 2 shows the relationship between time and the fractional formation of different phases in solution with a total calcium content of 2 mM at various *p*H values. It is obvious that the trend described by the modified Avrami expression is in close agreement with the actual event; and can be well-fitted to experimental results by adjusting the transformation coefficient alone. Surprisingly, although the λ

term is dependent on the physical conditions inside the reaction medium, the overall coefficient $\kappa\lambda$ varies only slightly within the limits of $10^{-10.63\pm0.35}$ K^{-3} s^{-4} (χ^2 confidence level 86.7%) over a *p*H range from 6.0 to 7.5. This relative constancy reflects the comparative insignificance of the variable term l with respect to the constant term κ, which implies that the heterogeneity of nucleation and the lattice strain energy have little effects on the overall activation energy. In fact, it is ζ in equation 10 which is most sensitive to changes in physical and chemical conditions, and is not uncommon to deviate in orders of magnitude up to 10 upon slight changes in system parameters.

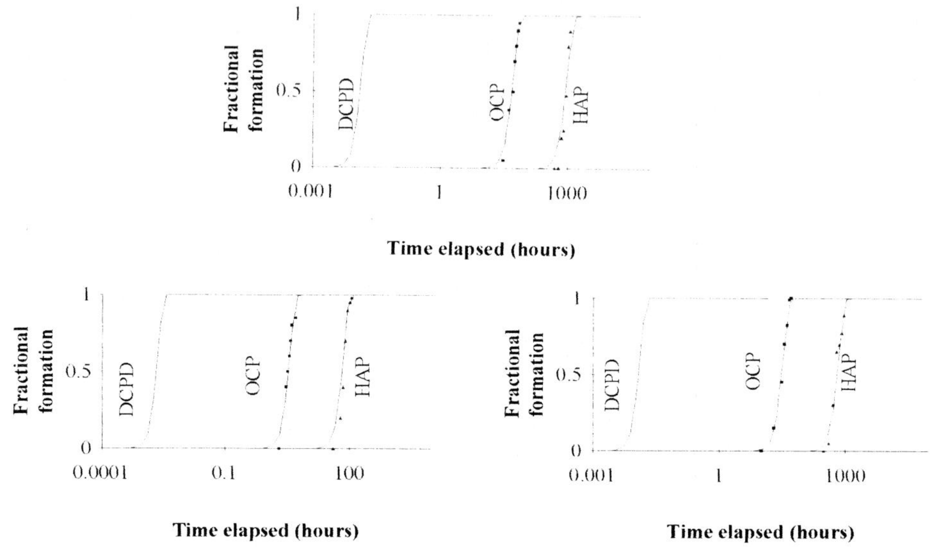

Figure 2. Formation of various calcium phosphate phases under different conditions as predicted by equations 9 and 10, compared to experimental results.[13-16] *Clockwise from top left:* (a) *p*H 6.0; (b) *p* 6.4; (c) *p*H 6.7; (d) *p*H 7.0; (e) *p*H 7.4. (All at 37°C, total calcium content 2 mM, ionic strength 0.1 M.) Experimental results: DCPD-OCP transformation (■); experimental OCP-HAP transformation (▲).

III. RELEVANCE OF PRECIPITATION MODEL TO BIOLOGICAL SYSTEMS

Although the modified Avrami expression has not been derived through an approach which is rigorously built on microscopic nucleation and growth mechanisms, it predicts the macroscopic *ex vivo* precipitation of calcium phosphate quite satisfactorily. However, additional factors need to be considered if this model is to be applied to biological systems. Physiological hard tissue calcification is different from experimental calcium phosphate precipitation in a good number of ways. Firstly, the physiological process involves a highly complex body fluid which contains, in addition to calcium and phosphate ions, a whole collection of biochemicals. Some of these compounds have been found to exert significant influence on the calcification process.[17,18] Furthermore, deposition of bone mineral occurs on a collagen substrate in the body instead of calcium phosphate seeds used in a typical precipitation experiment. On the one hand, collagen has a strong affinity for phosphate ions;[18] on the other hand, the collagen-mineral interface thus created exhibits very different physical properties. Consequently, the presence of collagen and biochemicals effectively alters various parameters in the present model: e.g. interfacial free energy (γ_{SL}), change in system free energy (ΔG_c^{hetero}), interfacial strain energy (Δg^{strain}), solution composition and supersaturation (β), transformation coefficient ($\kappa\lambda$) and ζ. Moreover, it has been widely reported of the presence of an amorphous calcium phosphate phase in natural hard tissues. Unfortunately as this is a metastable non-equilibrium phase, its presence is difficult to predict by the modified Avrami equation due to the lack of thermodynamic information. As a result, in order for the present equations to be applied to complex biological systems, there is still a necessity for a more detailed mechanistic approach to improve this preliminary model.

IV. CONCLUSIONS

Taking into account the nature of the reactions, the Avrami-Johnson-Mehl expression has been accordingly modified to predict the precipitation and transformation behaviour of calcium phosphate in dilute aqueous media. It relates the kinetic and thermodynamic factors, including termperature, solution composition and system free energies, to the formation of different phases during the multi-ionic precipitation process. The ensuing model is found to describe the *ex vivo* crystallisation phenomenon quite satisfactorily. However, improvement on this model is necessary before it can be applied to complex biological systems.

ACKNOWLEDGEMENTS

The authors would like to thank the Rhodes Trust and the Royal Society for their financial support to this research project.

REFERENCES

1. Wong, A. T.-C. and J. T. Czernuszka, Colloids & Surfaces, 1993 (in print).
2. Ostwald, W., Z. Phys. Chem., 22:289 (1897).
3. Avrami, M., J. Chem. Phys., 7:1103 (1939).
4. Avrami, M., ibid., 8:212 (1940).
5. Avrami, M., ibid., 9: 177 (1941).
6. Christian, J.W., in The Theory of Transformation in Metals and Alloys Part 1: Equilibrium and General Kinetic Theory, 2nd ed., Pergamon Press, Oxford (1975).
7. Boistelle, R. and I. Lopez-Valero, J. Crystal Growth, 102:609 (1990).
8. Brown, W.E., J. P. Smith, J. R. Lehr, A. W. Frazier, Nature, 196:1048 (1962).
9. Brown, W.E., M. Mathew, and M. S. Tung, Prog. Crystal Growth Charact., 4:59 (1981).
10. Clarke, K.I., A. T.-C. Wong, J. T. Czernuszka, B. Dowling, and J. T. Triffitt, Bioceramics, 4:107 (1991).
11. Kay, M.I. and R. A. Young, Nature, 204:1050, (1964).

12. Porter, D.A. and K. E. Easterling, in Phase Transformation in Metals and Alloys, Reinhold (1981).
13. Perez, L., L. J. Shyu, and G. H. Nancollas, Colloids & Surfaces, 38:295 (1989).
14. Ebrahimpour, A., J. Zhang, and G. H. Nancollas, J. Crystal Growth, 113:83 (1991).
15. Zhang, J., A. Ebrahimpour, and G. H. Nancollas, J. Colloids & Interf. Sci., 152:132 (1992).
16. Wong, A.T.-C., Czernuszka, J.T., in preparation.
17. Wong, A. T.-C., and J. T. Czernuszka, Mat. Res. Soc. Symp. Proc., 252:49 (1992).
18. Clarke, K.I., S. E. Graves, A. T.-C., Wong, M. J. O. Francis, J. T. Triffitt, and J. T. Czernuszka, J. Mat. Sci.: Mat. in Med., 1993 (in print).

THE ROLE OF INTERFACIAL CHEMISTRY IN SURFACE NUCLEATION AND GROWTH OF CALCIUM OXALATEMONOHYDRATE

Lin Song, Allison A. Campbell, and Bruce C. Bunker
Materials Sciences Department
Pacific Northwest Laboratory*
Richland, Washington 99352

ABSTRACT

The growth of calcium oxalate monohydrate (CaOx) on colloidal oxide particles has been studied to investigate the role of ion adsorption in heterogeneous nucleation and growth of crystalline phases from aqueous solutions. Electrosonic amplitude (ESA) titrations of colloidal suspensions of SiO_2, TiO_2 and Al_2O_3 were used to characterize native particle surface charges and to detect adsorption of Ca^{2+} and $Ox^{2-}(C_2O_4^{2-})$. For all three oxides, the results suggest that adsorption of divalent ions occurs on surfaces with opposite charges. The kinetics of CaOx nucleation on the colloidal oxides were determined using constant composition methods. Results indicate that induction times for CaOx nucleation are shortened by the presence of colloidal oxide particles. Analysis of the induction times as a function of solution supersaturation using classical nucleation theory suggests that at pH 6.5 SiO_2 and TiO_2 lower the surface energy barriers to nucleation while Al_2O_3 does not.

INTRODUCTION

Heterogeneous nucleation is of importance in controlling the deposition of ceramic films via biomimetic processing, for *in vivo* synthesis of biological materials such as teeth and kidney stones, and for undesired scale formation in industrial processes. There have been extensive studies on nucleation and crystal growth processes.[1] As described by classical nucleation theory,[2] the induction time for nucleation, number of nuclei formed, and size of critical nuclei are controlled by both solid liquid interfacial energy and solution supersaturation. The occurrence of nucleation and crystal growth must overcome the energy barrier caused by interfacial energy.

This work is aimed at investigating the effect of surface chemistry on the nucleation barrier. Three types of oxide colloids, SiO_2, TiO_2 and Al_2O_3, were selected for this purpose. These well studied and relatively simple model colloids have very different surface charge characteristics. At pH 6.5, Al_2O_3 has positive surface charge while SiO_2 surfaces are negatively charged and

---

* Operated for the U. S. Department of Energy by Battelle Memorial Institute under Contract 66DEAC0676RLO 1830.

0-8493-4750-5/94/$0.00 + $.50

TiO_2 surfaces are near neutral, which are ideal for systematic studies of surface charge effects.

A nucleation and crystal growth process occurs by a series of consecutive steps: bulk diffusion, surface adsorption, surface diffusion, and ion incorporation into the lattice.[3] By studying adsorption of Ca^{2+} and Ox^{2-} ions and CaOx formation on oxide surfaces, these studies address the basic mechanisms which control heterogeneous nucleation and crystal growth process. In addition, although solution pH greatly influences the surface charges of the selected particles, it does not influence the solubility of calcium oxalate over a wide range. Therefore, these studies will provide a unique approach towards understanding the relative importance of such parameters as pH effect, surface complex stability, and interfacial strain energy.

MATERIALS AND METHODS

The commercial products, α-Al_2O_3 (AKP30, Sumitomo), SiO_2 (PST3, Nissan) and TiO_2 (P25, Degussa) were used for electrosonic amplitude (ESA) and Constant Composition (CC) measurements. The powders had surface areas of 6.8 m^2/gm for Al_2O_3, 15.0 m^2/gm for SiO_2, and 56.9 m^2/gm for TiO_2 by BET methods. The colloidal suspensions were prepared by ultrasonic dispersion and adjusted to the desired pH by addition of hydrochloric acid or sodium hydroxide solutions. Oxide seed slurries were equilibrated in 0.01 M of NaCl at pH 6.5 and room temperature for at least three days prior to CC experiments.

Water was purified to 15 Megohms/cm or higher by reverse osmosis and carbon and ion exchange filtering using a Millipore system. Stock solutions of calcium chloride, potassium oxalate, and sodium chloride were prepared from reagent grade chemicals; (Fisher) using the deionized and CO_2 free water and were passed through 0.22μ Millipore filters before use.

A Matec ESA8000 system was employed for ESA measurements.[4] Kinetic studies of calcium oxalate formation on oxide colloidal surfaces were carried out using CC techniques.[5] The experiments were initiated by the addition of desired colloidal seed slurry with a total surface area of 2670 cm^2. The consumption of $CaCl_2$ titrant during the crystal growth process was recorded with time. All ESA and CC measurements were conducted in NaCl solutions at a constant ionic strength of 0.01 M and 25°C. Transmission electron microscopy (TEM) experiments were carried out on a Phillips 400 system at 120 keV.

RESULTS AND DISCUSSION

The surface charge properties of selected oxide particles were determined by acidbase potentiometric titration. The isoelectric points found for the particles were 1.9 for SiO_2, 6.5 for TiO_2 and 9.2 for Al_2O_3. This is in excellent agreement with previously reported results6. As illustrated in Figure 1, the presence of divalent Ca^{2+} in oxide suspensions at high pH resulted in a large increase in zeta potential, and changed the sign of surface charge from negative to positive. This suggested that specific Ca^{2+} adsorption was promoted on negatively charged surfaces. No Ca^{2+} surface association was observed on positively charged surfaces. On the other hand, the adsorption of oxalate anions Ox^{2-} was promoted on the positively charged surfaces and it reversed the surface charge from positive to negative. Solution analyses confirmed that at pH 6.5 there was extensive Ca2+ adsorption and negligible Ox^{2-} adsorption on negative SiO_2 colloidal surfaces, comparable but not so intense Ca^{2+} and Ox^{2-} adsorption on near neutral TiO_2 surfaces, and negligible Ca2+ adsorption and extensive Ox^{2-} adsorption on positive Al_2O_3 surfaces.

In Figure 2, the growth rates for CaOx were calculated from the steady state slopes of the calcium consumption vs. time, while induction times were calculated by extrapolating the steady state slopes back to zero calcium consumption. CC induction times for unseeded solutions and solutions containing SiO_2, TiO_2 and Al_2O_3 particles are shown as a function of supersaturation in Table I. The results show that all three colloids stimulate CaOx nucleation, leading to shorter induction times. At pH 6.5, the SiO_2 slurry exhibited the

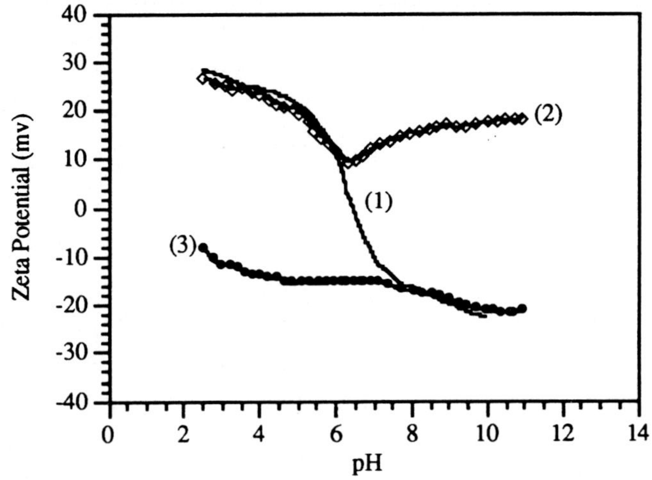

Figure 1. Zeta potentials as a function of pH for: (1) 0.5% (by volume) of TiO_2; (2) 0.5% of TiO_2 in 5.5 mM of $CaCl_2$; (3) 0.5% of TiO_2 in 5.5 mM of K_2Ox. Temperature = 23°C, ionic) strength = 0.01 M NaCl.

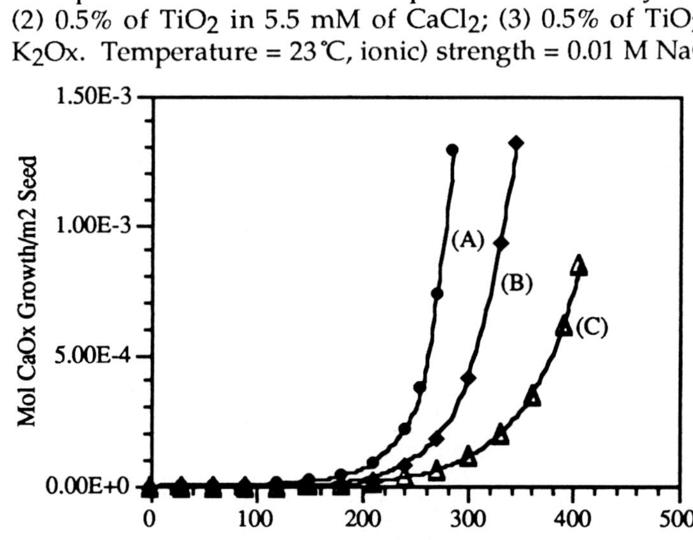

Figure 2. CaOx nucleation and growth on different colloidal surfaces as a function of time. (A) on SiO_2; (B) on TiO_2; (C) Al_2O_3. pH = 6.5, temperature = 25°C, Tca = Tox =2.00×10^{-4} M, ionic strength = 0.01 M NaCl.

shortest induction time (270 minutes), followed by TiO_2 (290 minutes), Al_2O_3 (360 minutes), and unseeded solutions (700 minutes).

The transmission electron micrograph of solids isolated 240 minutes after the start of the silica CC experiment shows that CaOx nucleation and growth occurs on the oxide surface as indicated by the arrows in Figure 3. Homogeneous nuclei were not observed. The measured thickness of the CaOx film on SiO_2 ranges from 818 nm, with the average thickness agreeing with the thickness calculated from the CC results (11 nm).

Table I. Nucleation and Growth of Calcium Oxalate at 25°C, pH 6.5, ionic strength = 0.01 M NaCl, and Different Supersaturation Ratios.

Seed	Tca=Tox/10^{-4}(M)	S	Induction Time (min)*
SiO_2	2.20	3.65	105
SiO_2	2.00	3.32	270
SiO_2	1.70	2.82	530
SiO_2	1.50	2.49	1540
TiO_2	2.00	3.32	290
TiO_2	1.80	2.99	370
TiO_2	1.70	2.82	980
TiO_2	1.50	2.49	1180
Al_2O_3	2.30	3.82	60
Al_2O_3	2.00	3.32	360
Al_2O_3	1.70	2.82	1500
unseeded	2.30	3.82	260
unseeded	2.00	3.32	700
unseeded	1.70	2.82	2500

* The measured induction times are reproducible within 12%. Total seed surface area = 2670cm^2 for each seeded experiment.

The data in Table I can be used to calculate the extent to which colloidal particles lower the barrier to CaOx nucleation using a modified Gibbs Thomson equation:[7]

$$\ln(1/\tau) = 1\text{nA} - \frac{\pi\sigma_{CL}{}^3 v^2}{3k^3T^3} \cdot \frac{1}{(1\text{nS})_2}$$

in which σ_{CL} is the interfacial energy for nucleation, τ is the induction time for calcium oxalate nucleation, S is the solution supersaturation ratio, A is a "pre-exponential factor," v is the molecular volume of CaOx, k is Boltzmann's constant, and T is the absolute temperature. Experimental data were analyzed by plotting $\ln(1/\tau)$ vs. $(\ln S)^{-2}$ (an example for SiO_2 is shown in Figure 4) and interfacial energies for different systems were calculated from the slopes of the regression lines (Table II).

As shown in Table II, the measured interfacial energies of SiO_2 and TiO_2 are significantly lower than those of homogeneous and spontaneous (or unseeded)

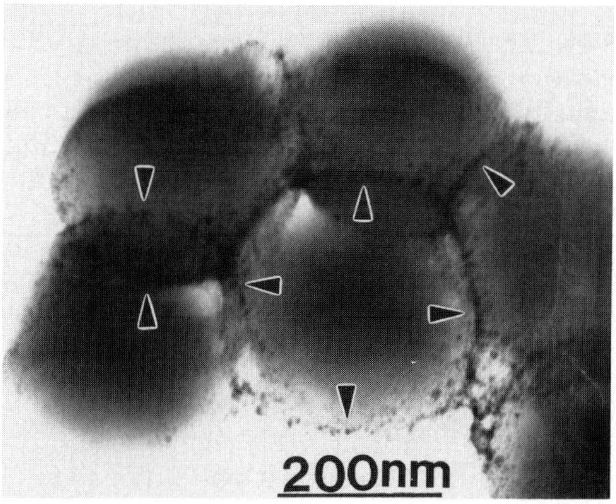

Figure 3. TEM of CaOx film formation on SiO_2 colloidal surfaces.

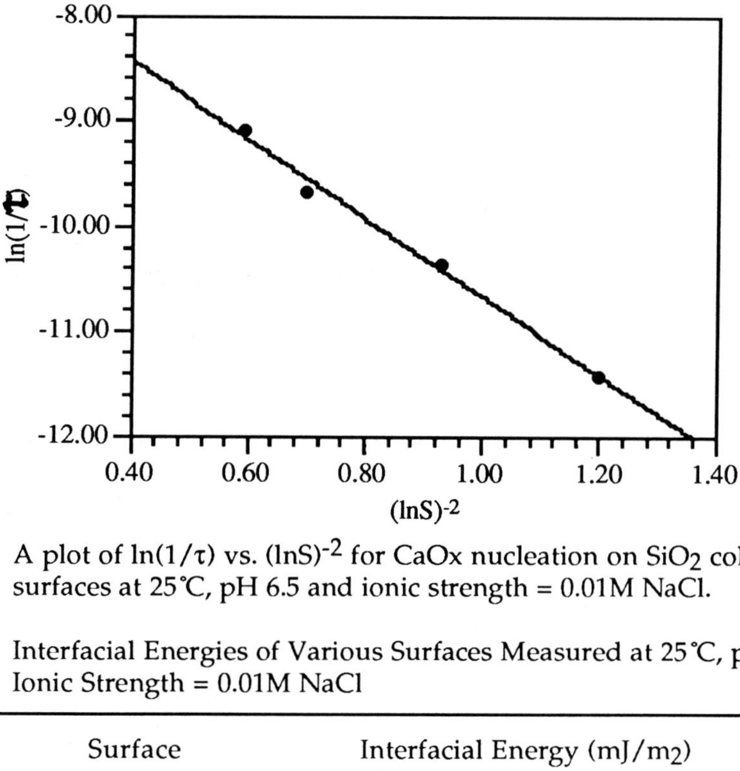

Figure 4. A plot of $\ln(1/\tau)$ vs. $(\ln S)^{-2}$ for CaOx nucleation on SiO_2 colloidal surfaces at 25°C, pH 6.5 and ionic strength = 0.01M NaCl.

Table II. Interfacial Energies of Various Surfaces Measured at 25°C, pH 6.5 and Ionic Strength = 0.01M NaCl

Surface	Interfacial Energy (mJ/m_2)
homogeneous	69*
spontaneous (unseeded)	32
Al_2O_3	35
TiO_2	26
SiO_2	27

*Reported in Refs. 7 and 8.

nucleation processes. The nucleation energy barrier on Al_2O_3 is comparable to spontaneous nucleation, which may explain the longest induction times observed. Our preliminary results seem to suggest that at pH 6.5 the negatively charged SiO_2 surface is the most effective at promoting heterogeneous nucleation. This observation is also consistent with the natural processes where proteins that stimulate biomineralization often carry negative charges. The lower interfacial energy for TiO_2 maybe resulted from the higher stability of titaniumoxalate surface complex, even though Ox2 species are more extensively adsorbed on positive Al_2O_3 surfaces and Ca^{2+} are adsorbed on a larger extent on negative SiO_2 surfaces at pH 6.5. However, as the interfacial energy is an average of many factors, the contributions of individual parameters need to be addressed in further experiments.

CONCLUSIONS

The preliminary results we obtained suggested all three selected oxide colloidal surfaces stimulate CaOx formation. The observation that SiO_2 and TiO_2 are more effective at inducing CaOx precipitation than Al_2O_3 can be explained by their significantly reduced interfacial energies or nucleation barriers. The results obtained to date suggest that negative surfaces capable of Ca^{2+} adsorption are more effective than positive surfaces which bind Ox^{2-} in promoting CaOx nucleation. However, further investigations will be required to establish the relative importance of parameters such as surface charge, surface complexation, and interfacial strain energy on surface nucleation processes.

Acknowledgements

This work was supported by the Office of Basic Energy Sciences, Department of Energy, under Grant ED3803000, and by Northwest College and University Association for Science (Washington State University) under Grant DEFG0689ER3375522 with the U. S. Department of Energy. We gratefully acknowledge Dr. Jun Liu for conducting TEM measurements.

REFERENCES

1. Nielsen, A. E., Electrolyte crystal growth mechanisms, J. Cryst. Growth, 67, 289, J1984.
2. Mohanty, R., Bhandarkar, S. and Estrin J., Kinetics of nucleation from aqueous solution, AIChE J., 36(10), 1536, 1990.
3. Chiang, P. and Donohue, M. D., Crystallization from ionic solution, AIC Symp. Series, 83(253), 8, 1987.
4. OBrien, R. W., The electroacoustic equations for a colloidal suspension, J. Fluid Mech., 212, 81, 1990.
5. Sheehan M. E. and Nancollas, G. H., Calcium oxalate crystal growth, a new constant composition method for modelling urinary stone formation, Invest. Urol., 17, 446, 1980.
6. Parks, G. A., The isoelectric points of solid oxides, solid hydroxides, and aqueous hydroxo complex systems, Chem. Rev., 65, 177, 1965.
7. Brown, C. M., Ackermann, D. K., Purich, D. L. and Finlayson, B., Nucleation of calcium oxalate monohydrate: use of turbidity measurements and computer assisted simulations in characterizing early events in crustal formation, J. Crystal. Growth, 108, 455, 1991.
8. Walton, A. G., in The Formation and Properties of Precipitates, p. 30, Kreiger, Huntington, New York, 1979.

EFFECT OF PARTICLE SIZE OF METASTABLE CALCIUM PHOSPHATES ON CRUSHING STRENGTH OF SELF-SETTING BIOACTIVE CALCIUM PHOSPHATE CEMENT

Makoto Otsuka, Yoshihisa Matsuda, Yoshiko Suwa,*
Jeffrey L. Fox,** and William I. Higuchi**
Kobe Women's College of Pharmacy, Kobe 658
*Kyoritsu Ceramic Materials Co., Nagoya 455 Japan
**Department of Pharmaceutics, University of Utah, Salt Lake City, UT

INTRODUCTION

Hydroxyapatite (HAP, $Ca_{10}(PO_4)_6(OH)_2$) is an important mineral component of hard tissues such as teeth and bone.[1] Therefore, when used in implanted artificial hard tissue, HAP has a high affinity for natural hard tissue in situ and can be molded to fill spaces created by physical damage to the bones and/or teeth. Some attempts[2] have been made to prepare bioactive materials for hard tissues using HAP. Yamamura et al.[3] applied HAP beads to bone filler with drug delivering ability, and reported the release of antibiotics from the beads, but it was not long enough for practical therapy since the drug was only absorbed on the surface.

On the other hand, Brown and Chow[4] reported that a bioactive self-setting calcium phosphate cement was formed *in situ* and molded to fill the space created by the absence of bone as reported that a bioactive self-setting calcium phosphate cement was formed *in situ* and molded to fill the space created by the absence of bone as an artificial hard tissue. Once formed and bonded with bone tissue, it is considered that controlled drug delivery may be achieved. From a pharmaceutical perspective, Otsuka et al.[5] investigated a system for delivering antibiotics using a patented self-setting calcium phosphate cement containing tetracalcium phosphate. We concluded that the drug release rate was controlled by a diffusion process in the pores in the cement, and the system continuously released drugs over a long term. However, in practical applications, the calcium phosphate cement does not have adequate mechanical strength after setting, which is the most serious problem of this system. Therefore, in this study, we investigated the effect of the particle size of metastable calcium phosphate as a raw material on the crushing strength of the cement in order to improve the mechanical strength of self-setting calcium phosphate cement used as a drug delivery system.

0-8493-4750-5/94/$0.00 + $.50

MATERIALS AND METHODS

MATERIALS

Tetracalcium phosphate (TECP, $Ca_4PO_4)_2O$) and dicalcium phosphate dihydrate (DCPD, $CaHPO_4\,2H_2O$) powders were obtained from Kyoritsu Ceramic Co., and Nakalai Co., Japan. HAP used as seed crystals was synthesized by precipitation[6] at 105℃. Powdered samples (10 g) of TECP and DCPD were ground for 0, 5, 15 and 30 min in a 350 ml agate centrifugal ball mill containing agate balls, respectively. The rotating speed of the mill was 225 rpm.

PRODUCTION OF THE SELF-SETTING CALCIUM PHOSPHATE CEMENT SYSTEM

The calcium phosphate cement powder[4] consisted of an equimolar mixture of various particle sizes of TECP and DCPD, and 40% HAP seed crystals. The cement formulations are summarized in Table 1. One gram of the cement powder was mixed and kneaded with various amounts of (0.50 ml) 25 mM H_3PO_4. The paste was poured into a mold 6 mm in diameter and 12 mm in thickness (Japan Industrial Scale), the mold was filled by the paste and stored at 37℃ and 100% RH for 24 h.

Table 1. Formulation of self-setting calcium phosphate cement.

	Specific surface area (m^2/g)		
	DCPD	TECP	HAP
		weight percent	
Sample	19.2w/w%	40.8w/w%	40.0w/w%
Cement A	0.760	0.140	21.9
Cement B	0.760	0.391	21.9
Cement C	0.760	0.632	21.9
Cement D	0.760	1.71	21.9
Cement E	1.41	0.140	21.9
Cement F	1.41	0.391	21.9
Cement G	1.41	0.632	21.9
Cement H	1.41	1.71	21.9
Cement I	3.02	0.140	21.9
Cement J	3.02	0.391	21.9
Cement K	3.02	0.632	21.9
Cement L	3.02	1.71	21.9
Cement M	4.93	0.140	21.9
Cement N	4.93	0.391	21.9
Cement O	4.93	0.632	21.9
Cement P	4.92	1.71	21.9

X-RAY DIFFRACTION MEASUREMENT

The x-ray powder diffraction profiles of the cement and drug-loaded cement samples were measured at room temperature with an x-ray diffractometer (Target, Cu; filter, Ni; voltage 35 kV, current, 15 mA; scanning speed 0.5° 2θ/min).

FOURIER TRANSFORMED INFRARED (FT-IR) SPECTROSCOPY

The sample powder was dispersed in a KBr powder (sample concentration 5%) and analyzed. FT-IR spectra were obtained by powder diffuse reflectance on an FT-infrared spectrophotometer and modified using the Kubelka-Munk equation.

MICROMETRIC CHARACTERIZATION

The true densities of the powders were determined using an air comparison pycnometer. The specific surface area (Sw) was measured with a gas adsorption apparatus using BET gas adsorption.

RESULTS AND DISCUSSION

CHARACTERIZATION OF SELF-SETTING CALCIUM PHOSPHATE CEMENT

After setting, all self-setting calcium phosphate cements showed typical x-ray diffraction patterns, except for cements A, B, E, I and M. The cements showed a small diffraction peak at 2θ=11.6° attributable to DCDP, indicating that the transformation from DCPD into HAP was incomplete. Since cements A, E, I and M contained the largest TECP particles (13.1 μm) and A and B contained the largest DCPD particles (3.33 μm), the dissolution rates of TECP and/or DCPD were controlled by the size of TECP and/or DCPD, indicating that the particle size of metastable calcium phosphate was an important factor in the transformation to HAP. Therefore, the other formulation cements could be transformed into HAP, because the raw materials were small enough to dissolve during kneading of the cement paste.

EFFECT OF METASTABLE CALCIUM PHOSPHATE PARTICLE SIZES ON THE CRUSHING STRENGTH OF SELF-SETTING CALCIUM PHOSPHATE CEMENT

The specific surface area (Sw) of TECP affected the crushing strength of fixed self-setting calcium phosphate cement. This was suggested by the following observation. The crushing strength of the cements containing smaller DCPD particles (Sw=4.93 m^2/g) was increased with increasing TECP Sw, but that of the cements containing larger DCPD particles (Sw=0.760 m^2/g) was not.

The Sw of DCPD affected the crushing strength of fixed self-setting calcium phosphate cement. This was suggested as follows: The crushing strengths of all cements increased with increasing of the Sw of DCPD, and that of the cements containing smallest TECP particles (Sw=1.71 m^2/g) was the highest.

Figure 1 shows the relationships between the diameter of the DCPD or TECP particles and the crushing strength of self-setting calcium phosphate cement, suggesting as follows: All cements containing the largest TECP particle powder had low mechanical strengths, the mechanical strength increased with a decrease in the sizes of TECP particles. However, the best mechanical strength was not the cement formulation (cement P) having the finest TECP and DCPD powders, but cement L (powder particle sizes of DCPD and TECP were 0.844 and 1.08 μm). In general, the nucleation and crystal growth processes during the cement setting were controlled by the degree of supersaturation, and the degree of supersaturation depended on the dissolution rate of the metastable calcium phosphates. At the initial stage of cement setting, the dissolution rate of the metastable substance is generally considered to be diffusion controlled, given by the Noyes-Whitney equation (eq. 1)[7] as follows:

$$dC/dt = k\,S/V\,(Cs - C) \qquad (1)$$

where k is the rate constant per unit area, S is the available surface area, V is the solvent volume, Cs is the solubility, and C is the solute concentration.

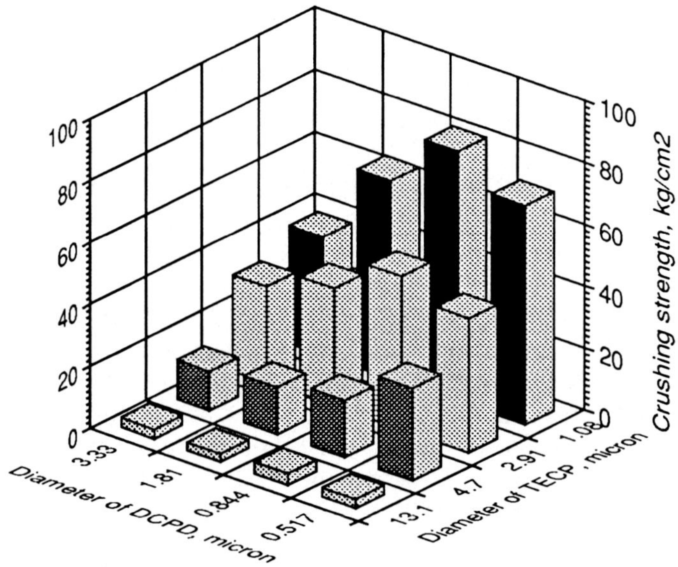

Figure 1. Effect of the particle size of DCPD and TECP on crushing strength of self-setting calcium phosphate cement.

The dissolution rates of the metastable calcium phosphates were controlled by the solubility and surface area of the solids. Therefore, after dissolution of the metastable form, the concentration reached supersaturation, after which the stable form of the crystal grew. Since the solubility of TECP was much higher than that of DCPD, the Sw of TECP affected the crushing strength more than that of DCPD.

RELATIONSHIP BETWEEN THE CRYSTAL STRUCTURE AND THE CRUSHING STRENGTH OF THE CEMENT AFTER SETTING

In general, the crystallite size was estimated by Scherrer equation[8] based on the x-ray powder diffraction profiles, as shown in Equation (2).

$$Dhkl = (K \lambda / \beta 1/2 \cos \theta) \tag{2}$$

where Dhkl is crystallite size, K is constant (0.9), λ is wave length of the x-ray (1.545Å), $\beta 1/2$ is half-width of the difference peak and θ is the diffraction angle.

The sizes of the HAP crystallites formed were estimated based on the diffraction peaks at 25.8 and 32.8° attributable to the 002 and 300 planes. The relationship between the crushing strength and the crystallite size of the cements after setting did not show significant relationship. However, it seems that the crushing strength depended slightly on the crystallite size attributable to the 300 and 002 planes. LeGeros et al.[9] reported the effect of the carbonate ion content on the crystal structure of HAP. The crystallinity and the a-axis length of the lattice parameter decreased with increasing the carbonate ion content, but the c-axis length increased. Scanning electron microphotographs showed that the size and shape of the crystallites changed from long needles to smaller rods to tiny spheroids. In this study, because HAP had a hexagonal crystal structure and grew along the C-axis, the crystallites in the stronger cement were smaller.

RELATIONSHIP BETWEEN THE CRYSTAL STRUCTURE AND THE SPECIFIC SURFACE AREA OF THE CEMENT AFTER SETTING

The relationship between the crystallite size and the specific surface area (Sw) of the cements after setting suggested the following: The crystallite size attributable to the 300 plane decreased with increasing Sw, but that attributable to the 002 plane showed no relationship.

Figure 2 shows the relationship between the crushing strength and the Sw of the cements after setting. The crushing strength of the cement increased with increasing Sw, and the relationship was linear. The results indicated that the Sw of the cement increased with the crystal growth along a- and/or b-axes, and became rod-type crystals as reported by LeGeros et al.[9] The stronger cement contained the fine particles, because the contact area between the particles was larger. Fine particles arise from a highly supersaturated mother liquid, because the driving force of the nucleation rate is the supersaturation. The supersaturation depended on the Sw of TECP or DCPD in this cement system as discussed in the previous section.

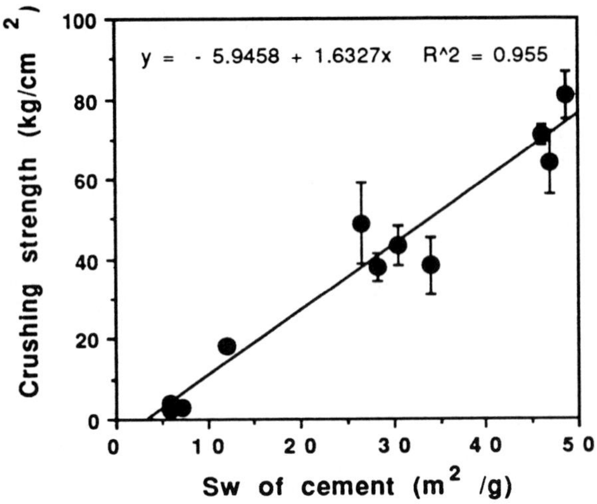

Figure 2. Relationship between the crushing strength and the specific surface area of hydroxyapatite in self-setting calcium phosphate cement.

REFERENCES

1. H. Aoki, "Science and medical applications of hydroxyapatite," pp. 137-163, Takayama Press, Tokyo (1991).
2. T. Tabata and M. Ogiso, "New concept of apatite ceramic implant," *J. Dent.*, 18:337 (1983).
3. K. Yamamura, G. Chou, and H. Iwata, "The development of antibiotics loaded hydroxyapatite beads," *Drug Delivery System*, 6:103 (1991).
4. W. E. Brown and L. C. Chow, U.S. Patent 4,612-053 (1986).
5. M. Otsuka, Y. Matsuda, D. Yu, J. Wong, J. L. Fox, and W. I. Higuchi, "Self-A novel skeletal drug-delivery system for antibacterial drugs using setting hydroxyapatite cement," *Chem. Pharm. Bull.*, 38:3500-3501 (1990).
6. Y. Doi, Y. Takezawa, S. Shibata, N. Wakamatsu, H. Kamemizu, T. Goto, M. Iijima, Y. Moriwaki, K. Uno, F. Kubo, and Y. Haeuchi, "Self-setting apatite cement I.: Physiocochemical properties," *J. Jpn. Dent. Mat. Dev.*, 6:53-58 (1987).
7. A. Noyes and W. I. Whitney, *J. Am. Chem. Soc.*, 19:930 (1897).
8. P. Scherrer, *Göttingen Nachr.*, 98 (1918).
9. R. Z. LeGeros, J. P. LeGeros, and W. P. Shirra, "Conversion of monetite, $CaHPO_4$ to apatite: Effect of carbonate on the crystallinity and the morphology of the apatite crystallites," *Adv. in X-ray Analysis*, 14:57-66 (1971).

AN HYDRAULIC CEMENT FOR BIOLOGICAL USES

E. Mejdoubi,* J. L. Lacout,* P. Michaud** and F. Rodriguez**
*Laboratoire des Matériaux - Physico-Chimie des Solides, ENSCT
INPT, URA 445 - 38, rue des 36 Ponts - 31400 Toulouse, France
**Laboratoire de Galénique, Faculté de Pharmacie, Université
Paul Sabatier, rue des Maraîchers - 31400 Toulouse - France.

ABSTRACT

A calcium-phosphate cement which hardens when added to water forming hydroxyapatite can be composed of a mixture of three phosphate compounds: monocalcium phosphate, tricalcium phosphate and tetracalcium phosphate. The relative proportions of the inital mixture modifies the setting time. A mechanism for the reaction is proposed.

A. INTRODUCTION

Self-setting calcium-phosphate cements have been the subject of considerable interest in recent years for orthopedic and dental applications. The cements harden at the site of application and forms solid calcium phosphate, which is well-known to be biocompatible, and especially hydroxyapatite which is said to be osteoconductive. Their applications are many. However calcium phosphate cements (i) do not generally have a suitable convenient setting time, (ii) do not have good mechanical properties, especially compressive and tensile strengths, (iii) do not generally retain their mechanical properties when disturbed during the setting period. Therefore, many fundamental and applied studies remain to improve their properties in their possible applications (1).

B. RESULTS AND DISCUSSION

The cements are prepared by addition of water to a mixture of acidic and basic calcium phosphate compounds. The main calcium phosphates are listed in Table 1 in order of increasing atomic calcium to phosphorus ratio (Ca/P) which corresponds to an increase in alkalinity.

Two main ways of preparing cements have been investigated by various authors according to the two reactions.

$$2Ca(HPO_4)\cdot 2H_2O + 2\ Ca_4(PO_4)_2 \rightarrow Ca_{10}(PO_4)_6(OH)_2$$

0-8493-4750-5/94/$0.00+$.50

$$Ca(H_2PO_4)_2{\cdot}H_2O + Ca_3(PO_4)_2 \rightarrow 4\ Ca(HPO_4){\cdot}2H_2O$$

The first reaction uses dicalcium phosphate and tetracalcium phosphate and induces the formation of hydroxyapatite (2,3). The setting time is quite long, more than four hours. The second one uses monocalcium phosphate and tricalcium phosphate and forms dicalcium phosphate. The setting time is very short, less than one minute (4).

Table 1. Main calcium phosphate compounds.

Ca/P	Compound	Formula
0.50	Monocalcium phosphate	$Ca(H2PO_4)_2{\cdot}H_2O$
0.50	Monocalcium phosphate anhydrous (MCPA)	$Ca(H_2PO_4)_2$
1.00	Dicalcium phosphate dihydrate (DCPD)	$Ca(HPO_4){\cdot}H_2O$
1.00	Dicalcium phosphate anhydrous (DCPA)	$Ca(HPO_4)$
1.33	Octacalcium phosphate (OCP)	$Ca_8H_2(PO_4)6.5H_20$
1.50	Tricalcium phosphate (β-TCP)	β -$Ca_3(P0_4)_2$
1.50	Tricalcium phosphate (α-TCP)	α-$Ca_3(P0_4)_2$
1.67	Hydroxyapatite (HAP)	$Ca_{10}(PO_4)_6(OH)2$
2.00	Tetracalcium phosphate (TTCP)	$Ca_4(PO_4)_2O$

In many applications, a suitable setting time must be in the range fifteen to sixty minutes. For our part, we examined a cement formed by a more complex mixture of monocalcium, tricalcium and tetracalcium phosphates, added to water. The quantities of the three solid phosphate compounds were calculated to obtain a final product with an apatitic composition, according to the overall reaction:

$$\alpha\ Ca_4(PO_4)_2O + bCa(H_2PO_4)_2{\cdot}H_2O + cCa_3(PO_4)_2 \rightarrow Ca_{10}(PO_4)_6(OH)_2$$

Of course, many factors influence the chemical result and the properties, the setting time, the mechanical strength, etc.

A first factor is the value of the coefficients a, b , c:. For the same final product with an apatitic composition they are dependent on each other but they can take different values. The ranges are: a between 0 and 0.67; b between 0 and 2.00; c between 1 and 2.33, with $b = 2 - 3a$ and $c = 1 + 2a$.

A good choice can greatly reduce the quantity of tetracalcium phosphate which is quite difficult to prepare, and modifies the mechanical properties and the setting time (5). Also the crystallographic form of the phosphate, dicalcium phosphate monohydrate or anhydrous, tricalcium phosphate or amorphous, plays a role on the setting time. Some others factors are also important such as the particle dimensions, the liquid-to-solid ratio, etc.

In this paper, only some results are presented. They were obtained with a cement with the composition a = 2; b = 2; c = 1 and the following starting materials: monocalcium phosphate mono hydrate, β-tricalcium phosphate, tetracalcium phosphate (6). The discussion will be focused on the different reactions which can occur during the setting period.

Figure 1 shows the X-ray patterns of this cement at three times during setting. The decreases of the lines due to tetracalcium phosphate can be observed alongside the formation of hydroxyapatite. After 3 days, the main compound is the apatite, but some tricalcium phosphate remains.

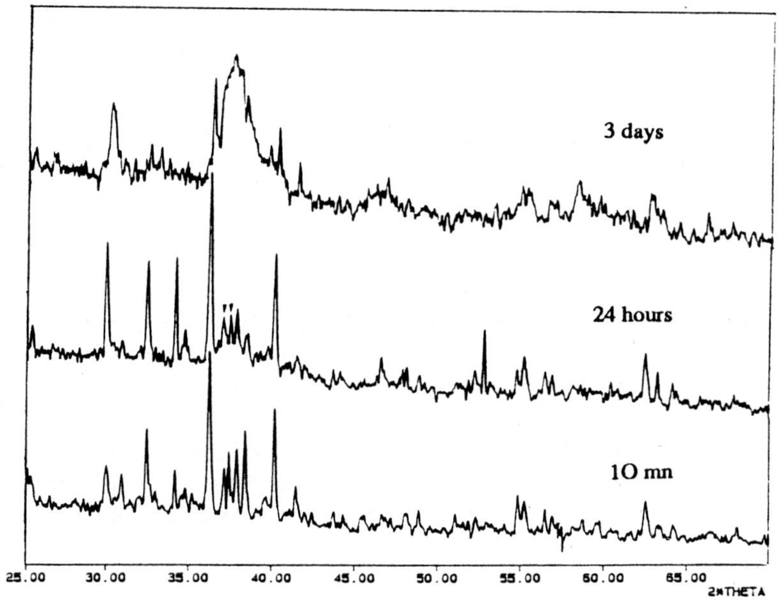

Figure 1. X-ray pattern of the cement at three times during setting.

Infrared spectra confirm these results infrared bands due to carbonate ions which substitute for PO_4 can be noticed (1300-1400 cm^{-1}) as can bands due to hydroxyl ions (3560 cm^{-1}).

The hardening of the cement was determined by the resistance to the penetration into the cement surface of a needle of 0.9 mm^2. The general shape is a two-stage curve which can be considered as the superimposition of two curves corresponding to two main reactions (Figure 2). The mixture of the four components (mono-, tri- and tetracalcium phosphate) reacts according to various mechanisms:

MCPM + TTCP → DCPD (fast)
MCPM + TCP → DCPD (fast)
DCPD + TTCP → HAP (slow)
TCP + TTCP → HAP (very slow)

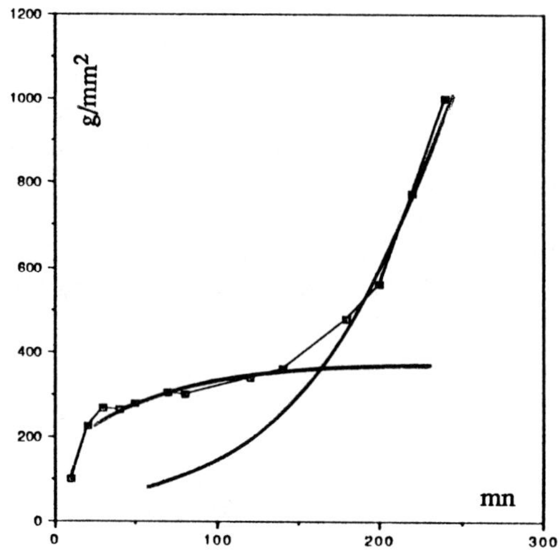

Figure 2.
General shape of the curve: setting of the cement vs. time.

At the beginning, when the liquid is added to the solid, the dissolution of monocalcium phosphate induces a strong decrease of the local pH and DCPD is formed via the two first reactions. The last two ones occur later.

The quantities of dicalcium phosphate formed during this first stage are not very large. As a consequence, this compound is not easy to detect either by X-ray diffraction or by infrared spectroscopy. The effect of the formation of dicalcium phosphate can easily be correlated with the addition of small amounts of phosphoric acid: the first stage is shortened with the addition of acid (Figure 3). Also, the special tablet-like shape of the DCPD crystals(7), is a clear indicator of the very early formation of this compound which bridges neighboring particles and causes hardening of the paste (Figure 4).

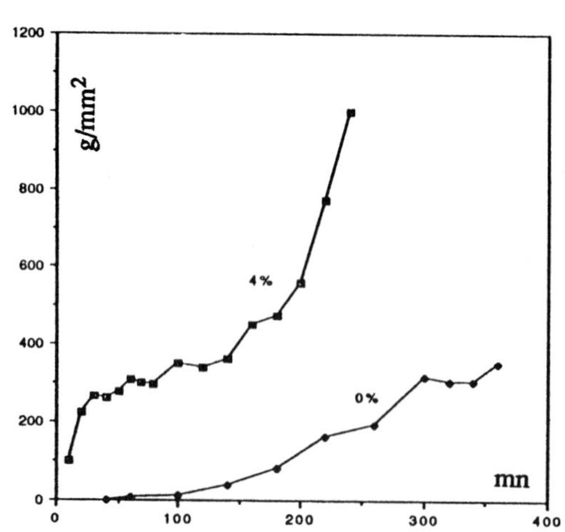

Figure 3.
Effect of the addition of phosphoric acid on the setting time.

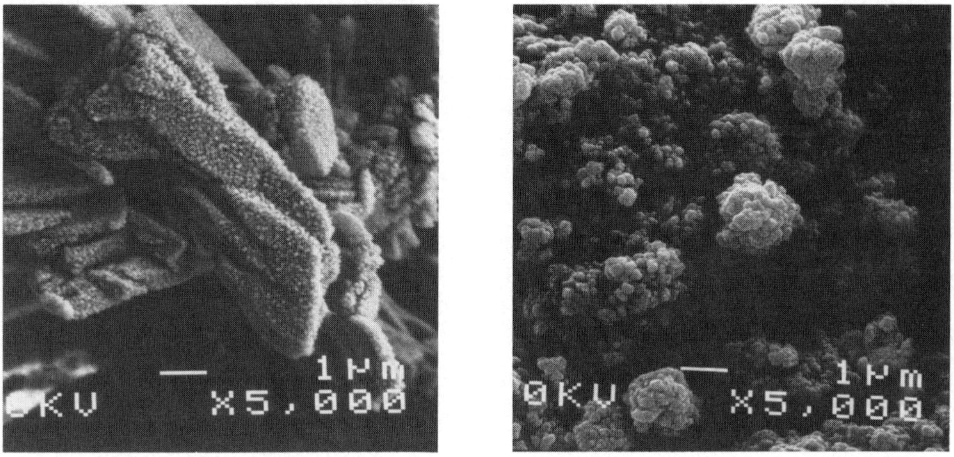

Figure 4. S.E.M of cement at 10 mn and 24 hours.

One hour after the start of setting, we can observe the disappearance of DCPD and the formation of a quite well crystalized compound which is apatite.

C. CONCLUSIONS

A mixture of dicalcium phosphate, tricalcium phosphate and tetracalcium phosphate, in convenientproportions and with an overall atomic calcium to phosphorus ratio equal to 1.67, when added to water, is a self-setting cement which forms hydroxyapatite.

Two different reactions take place. The first one is the formation of DCPD (5–60 minutes) which corresponds to setting. The second one is the formation of hydroxyapatite (2–48 hours) which corresponds to the hardening of the cement.

The setting time can be controlled and the quantity of TTCP can be reduced using an appropriate choice of the relative proportions of the three phosphate compounds of the initial mixture. Nevertheless, small amounts of TCP remain which reduce the compressive strength.

REFERENCES

1. A. C. Sugarawara, L. C. Chou, S. Tagaki, and H. Chohayeb, In vitro evaluation of the sealing ability of a calcium phosphate cement when used as a root canal filler, J. Endodon. 16:162–164 (1990).
2. L. C. Chow, Development of self-setting calcium phosphate cements, J. Ceram. Soc. Jap. 99(10):954–963 (1991).

3. W. E. Brown and L. C. Chow, A new calcium phosphate setting cement, J. Dent. Res. 62:672 (1983).
4. A. A. Mirtchi, J. Lemaitre and E. Munting, Biomaterials 11:83-88 (1990).
5. K. Ciesla and R. Rudnicki, Synthesis and transformation of tetracalcium phosphate in solid state, Part II., Polish J. Chem 62(31):31-39 (1988).
6. J. L. Lacout and E. Mejdoubi, Procédé d'obtention d'hydroxyapatite phosphocalcique, application au comblement osseux ou dentaire, ou au moulage de pièces et produits utilisés, Fr. patent 92.O9019.
7. W. M. M. Heijnen and P. Hartman, Structural morphology of gypsum, brushite and pharmacolite, J. Crystal Growth 108:290-300 (1991).

SYNTHESIS OF DAHLLITE: THE MINERAL PHASE OF BONE

Ira C. Ison, Mark T. Fulmer, Bryan M. Barr, and Brent R. Constantz
Norian Corporation
Mountain View, CA

ABSTRACT

Apatites are of substantial interest in medicine since dahllite, an apatite containing 4% to 6% carbonate by weight, is a major constituent in bone, teeth, and some invertebrate skeletons. While apatitic preforms, powders, and cements are currently being considered and used in a number of dental and orthopedic applications, carbonated apatites have been largely overlooked or ignored. Carbonated apatites may be promising in dental and medical applications as bioactive materials due to enhanced dissolution and increased osteoclast mediated resorption.

Apatitic solids may be produced by several different processes, and the amount of carbonate that may be incorporated into the solid lattice varies depending upon its processing history. In this study, various formulations were processed as low temperature cementitious reactions of acidic and basic calcium phosphates.

Formulations without calcite acquired less than 1 percent carbonate from the curing environment while those containing calcite were found to incorporate more than 3 percent carbonate by weight in the final product. Only the cements with the unique formulations incorporating both a reactive acid and calcite were found to contain greater than 4 percent carbonate by weight in the final product thus qualifying the product as dahllite. The crystallinity of this synthetic dahllite was found to resemble bone mineral more closely than did sintered hydroxyapatite.

Calcium phosphates, particularly thermally processed ceramic hydroxyapatites, have found very limited application in orthopedics because of their low fatigue properties relative to bone. Implants constructed of dahllite facilitate bone remodeling thus replacing the implant with living bone and creating an implant/bone composite. Replacement of dahllite implants by living bone may result in a more durable weight-bearing construct.

INTRODUCTION

Dahllite, an apatite containing 4% to 6% carbonate and less than 1% fluoride ion by weight, is a major constituent in bone, teeth, and some invertebrate skeletons.[1-7] The synthesis of apatitic materials which closely resemble bone is important for medical and dental applications.[8] While

0-8493-4750-5/94/$0.00 + $.50

apatitic preforms, powders, and cements are currently being used or considered in a number of dental and orthopedic applications, carbonated apatites have not received much attention.

In carbonated apatite, carbonate ions substitute in either the phosphate or the hydroxyl sites of the hydroxyapatite [$Ca_{10}(PO_4)_6(OH)_2$, or HAp] structure. Apatite products formed at low temperature generally acquire some carbonate substituted in the phosphate sites and are designated as type B carbonated apatite.[9,10] Since the carbonate ion is smaller than the phosphate ion, a decrease in the a-axis results.[5,11,12] In most high temperature apatites, the carbonate ion replaces two hydroxyl ions in the vicinity of the six fold axis. These are designated as type A carbonated apatites.[9,13] In this case the carbonate ion is larger than the hydroxyls, hence an increase in the a-axis of apatite occurs.[5,9,13,14]

The presence of carbonate in phosphate sites alters the mineral phase which is related to the following: a reduction in crystallite size and crystallinity; changes in the morphologies of the mineral phase from needles to rods to equi-axial crystals (spheroids); contraction of the a-axis, as well as an expansion in the c-axis; and internal strain.[5,11] These factors lead to increased solubility of carbonate-substituted HAp.

The purpose of this study was to produce the crystallinity and carbonate content found in bone mineral via a cementitious reaction. The data presented reports on a number of cement formulations which react to yield carbonated hydroxyapatite. These cements are compared mineralogically with each other, as well as with sintered and hydrothermally processed apatites, and bone mineral.

MATERIALS AND METHODS

Raw materials used to produce the cements include: tetracalcium phosphate [$Ca_4(PO_4)_2O$ (hilgenstockite)] of two different mean particle diameters, 2µm and 10µm; calcium carbonate [$CaCO_3$ (calcite)]; dibasic calcium phosphate, anhydrate [$CaHPO_4$ (monetite)]; dibasic calcium phosphate, dihydrate [$CaHPO_4{\cdot}2H_2O$ (brushite)]; monobasic calcium phosphate, monohydrate [$Ca(H_2PO_4)_2{\cdot}H_2O$]; and, orthophosphoric acid [H_3PO_4]. The lubricants used include deionized water (DI water), dilute sodium phosphate solution (SP sol'n), and dilute ortho-phosphoric acid (oPA sol'n).

Cement formulations were produced at both Ca/P ratios of 1.67:1 (Stoichiometric HAp) and 1.5:1 (Ca deficient HAp). Formulas containing calcium carbonate have greater than 8 percent by weight calcite. The formulations used in this study along with the results are summarized in Table 1. The first column of Table 1 identifies the formulas numerically. The second column indicates the solid reactants used in each formulation. Reactant quantities shown are normalized to form 1 mole of non-substituted apatite (either 1.5:1 or 1.67:1 Ca/P ratio). The third column shows the intended Ca/P ratio of each formulation. The fourth column gives the size of tetracalcium phosphate used in each reaction. The fifth column shows which solution was utilized for each reaction.

Each cement was mixed to a paste consistency using a mortar and pestle. These pastes were cured at 37°C in a sealed centrifuge tube containing approximately 30 ml of bovine serum treated with sodium azide to minimize microbial activity. After a 2-week curing period, the samples were placed into liquid nitrogen and lyophilized overnight. Non-cementitious products analyzed in this study (hydrothermally processed, coralline HAp, sintered HAp, and bone) were ground into a fine powder prior to analysis.

TABLE 1

EXPERIMENTAL METHOD					2 WEEK RESULTS	
#	Reactants	Ca/P	$Ca_4(PO_4)_2O$ dia. (mm)	Solution	Apatite (%)*	CO_3 (%)**
1a.	$2CaHPO_4 + 2Ca_4(PO_4)_2O$	1.67	10	DI water	~5%	0.28
1b.	" "	" "	10	oPA sol'n	~15%	0.32
1c.	" "	" "	2	DI water	~30%	0.35
1d.	" "	" "	2	oPA sol'n	~30%	0.46
2a.	$3CaHPO_4 + 1.5Ca_4(PO_4)_2O$	1.5	2	DI water	~75%	0.45
2b.	" "	" "	2	oPA sol'n	~75%	0.45
2c.	$3CaHPO_4 + 1.5Ca_4(PO_4)_2O$	1.5	10	DI water	~15%	0.35
2d.	" "	" "	10	oPA sol'n	~15%	0.29
3.	$3CaHPO_4 + 1.5Ca_4(PO_4)_2O + CaCO_3$	1.67	10	DI water	~60%	3.57***
4a.	$2CaHPO_4 \cdot 2H_2O + 2Ca_4(PO_4)_2O$	1.67	10	DI water	~96%	0.47
4b.	" "	" "	10	oPA sol'n	~96%	0.47
4c.	" "	" "	2	DI water	~98%	0.59
4d.	" "	" "	2	oPA sol'n	~98%	0.67
5.	$3CaHPO_4 \cdot 2H_2O + 1.5Ca_4(PO_4)_2O + CaCO_3$	1.67	10	DI water	~98%	4.65
6a.	$0.67Ca(H_2PO_4)_2.H_2O + 2.33Ca_4(PO_4)_2O$	1.67	10	DI water	~95%	0.33
6b.	" "	" "	2	DI water	~98%	0.46
7a.	$Ca(H_2PO_4)_2.H_2O + 2Ca_4(PO_4)_2O$	1.5	10	DI water	~96%	0.68
7b.	" "	" "	2	DI water	~97%	0.19
8.	$Ca(H_2PO_4)_2.H_2O + 2Ca_4(PO_4)_2O + CaCO_3$	1.67	10	DI water	~97%	3.83
9a.	$1.5H_3PO_4 + 2.25Ca_4(PO_4)_2O + CaCO_3$	1.67	10	SP sol'n	~98%	4.53
9b.	" "	" "	2	SP sol'n	~99%	4.83
10.	$H_3PO_4 + 2.5Ca_4(PO_4)_2O$	1.67	10	SP sol'n	~95%	0.53

* % apatite quantities are estimates for qualitative comparison, based upon XRD and FTIR data.

** Measured by carbon coulometry with acidification (several formulations were analyzed by different labs, and the differences averaged 0.10 weight percent and were no greater than 0.25 weight percent).

*** ~5% retained calcite accounts for CO_3^{2-} content.

All samples were analyzed by X-ray powder diffraction (XRD) (some by synchrotron diffraction), Fourier transform infrared spectroscopy (FTIR), and carbon coulometry using acidification for total inorganic carbon analysis. Direct current plasma spectroscopy was performed on selected samples, as described below.

RESULTS AND DISCUSSION

The results of this study are given in Tables 1, 2, and 3, and Figures 1 through 5. The last two columns of Table 1 summarize mineralogical data of the final products formed by the cement formulations studied. The sixth column of Table 1 gives qualitative estimates of the extent of completion of each reaction based upon mineralogical data taken from XRD and FTIR spectra. The last column provides the amount of total inorganic carbonate measured for each reaction in weight percent CO_3^{2-} of the total weight of the material.

TABLE 2

Material	CO_3^{2-} (% by weight)	Scherrer Crystal Size (nm)	Ca/P measured
Cement #4d	0.67	49.4	1.60
Cement #9b	4.83	40.8	1.66
Coral-derived Apatite	3.2	81.5	1.58
Sintered Hydroxyapatite	<0.005	135.9	1.67
Bone	4.65	37.1	1.71[3]

TABLE 3

Sample	AgO ppm	Al_2O_3	BaO	CuO	Fe_2O_3	K_2O	MgO
Cement #9b	<5	160	20	30	130	70	1070
Coralline HAp	10	40	<5	20	<5	30	2300
Sintered HAp	10	60	20	20	<5	30	30

Sample	MnO	Na_2O	PbO	SiO_2	SrO	ZnO
Cement #9b	40	6500	<5	680	100	10
Coralline HAp	<5	4300	30	<5	8900	10
Sintered HAp	<5	110	<5	760	230	<5

XRD and FTIR show that the formulations with either ortho-phosphoric acid, monobasic calcium phosphate (monohydrate), or brushite tend to react nearly to completion within a two week period. Formulations containing brushite tend to react slightly less as trace quantities of the initial reactants are more apparent. Cementitious compositions which utilized monetite failed to react to completion in the allotted two week curing period.

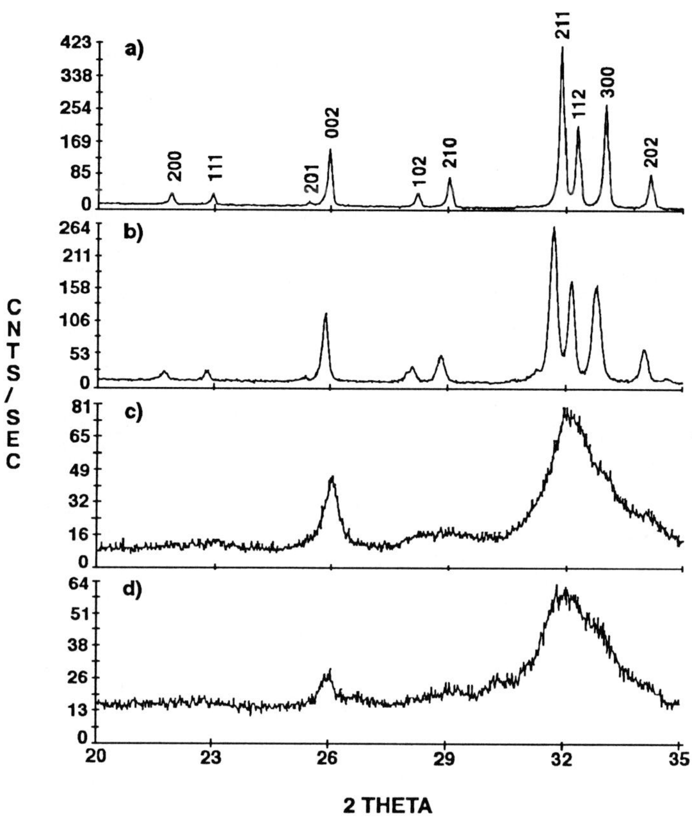

Figure 1. XRD comparison of (a) sintered hydroxyapatite, (b) coral-derived apatite, (c) formulation #9b (dahllite cement), and (d) mammalian bone.

Carbon coulometry using acidification for total inorganic carbon analysis revealed that formulations without calcite acquired less than 1 percent carbonate from the curing environment. This is consistent with previously reported results for open systems which allow atmospheric carbon dioxide to dissolve and participate in the reaction.[15] Formulations containing calcite were found to incorporate more than 3 percent carbonate by weight into the resultant apatite. Only the cements with the unique formulations incorporating both calcite and a highly reactive acid (such as formulations 5, 8, and 9) were found to contain greater than 4 percent carbonate by final weight in the synthetic apatite, thus qualifying such products as dahllite. For example, formulations 4a and 5 are very similar with the exception that #5 contains calcite. Consequently, formulation 5 resulted in a carbonated end product while #4a contained less than 0.5% carbonate by weight. A similar comparison can be made between the similar formulations 9a and 10. Of the two, only #9a contains calcite and in turn contains a significant quantity of carbonate in the final apatite product.

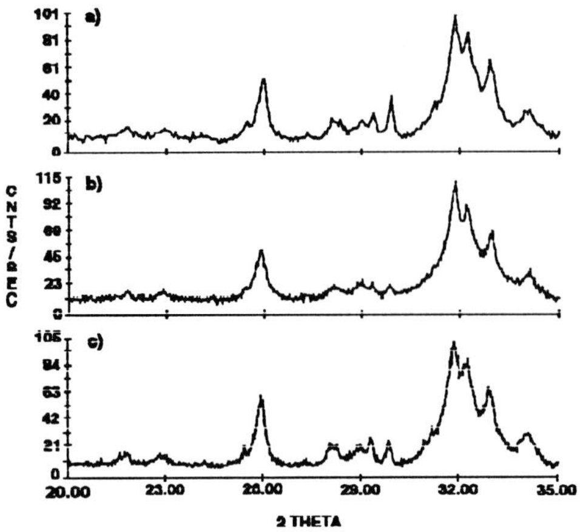

Figure 2. XRD comparison of (a) formulation #10; (b) formulation #9a (dahllite cement); and (c) formula-

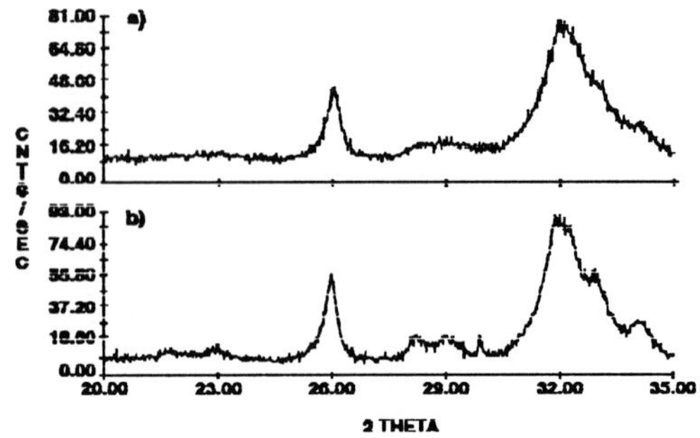

Figure 3. XRD comparison of (a) formulation #9b (dahllite cement) and (b) formulation #4d.

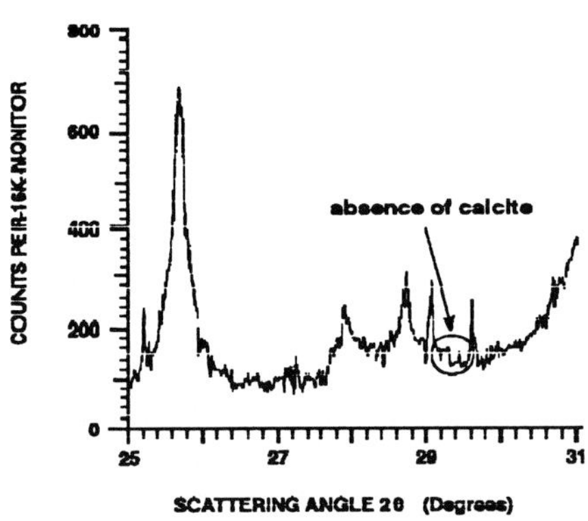

Figure 4. Synchrotron diffraction pattern of formulation #9a showing no detectable calcium carbonate phase in the carbonated apatite cement.

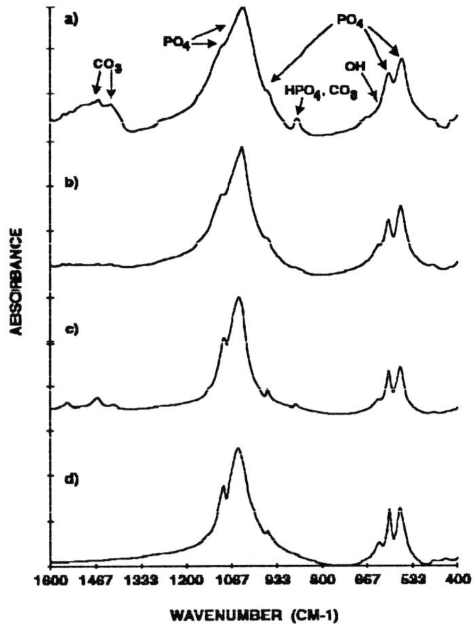

Figure 5. FTIR comparison of (a) formulation #9b; (b) formulation #4d; (c) coral-derived apatite; and (d) sintered hydroxyapatite.

Table 2 provides data from other apatitic materials for comparison with the cement formulations. Two representative cement formulations, 4d and 9b, are listed numerically in the first column and correspond to the reaction numbers in Table 1. The second column provides data for carbonate content. In addition, comparisons of the Scherrer perfect crystallite size (distance between crystal defects) were estimated using the Scherrer formula[16] and are provided in the third column of Table 2. Although the crystallite sizes are measured without compensating for strain and instrumental broadening, the values are indicative of the relative crystallinity of the materials examined. Finally, calcium to phosphate molar ratios are provided in the fourth column as measured by direct current plasma spectroscopy (DCP). Note that some values for bone are obtained from published values. The various Ca/P molar ratios observed may be due to the tendency for simultaneous loss of Ca, P, and $(OH)_2$ coincident with the formation of HPO_4 acid phosphate ions[6,13,17,18] as well as the tendency for cations, such as sodium, to substitute for calcium.[19,20] Of all the cement formulations evaluated in this study, formulation 9b seems to resemble bone the closest.

Those materials which were analyzed elementally via DCP spectroscopy are listed in Table 3 with corresponding quantities (in weight percent) of various elements reported as metal oxides. The only elemental oxides exceeding 0.1% in any of the materials are MgO and Na_2O in Cement #9b and the coral-derived HAp, and SrO in the coral-derived material alone. These elemental contaminants are commonly found in apatites including bone[17,19,21-23] and are likely to substitute into the calcium sites of the apatite lattice. The low quantities measured are probably biologically insignificant.

Figures 1 through 5 show diffraction and spectroscopic data as labeled. Figure 1 provides a comparison between the X-ray diffraction patterns for some of the apatites studied. Pattern 1a corresponds to sintered hydroxyapatite. The Miller indices are labeled on this pattern for clarification of the peaks. The sharp, distinct peaks from the sintered material correspond well to hydroxyapatite[24] and indicate a high degree of crystalline order. Pattern 1b corresponds to coral-derived, hydrothermally processed apatite. This pattern in conjunction with the data in Table 2 indicates that it is a carbonated apatite. The decrease in intensity and the slight broadening of the peaks is characteristic of lattice strain and defects most likely due to the incorporation of carbonate during processing. A 0.1 degree 2q peak shift observed between the 002 and 300 peaks in the hydrothermally processed material indicates ionic substitution in lattice sites resulting in an increase of the a-axis. Such a peak shift may correspond to strontium substitution for calcium or carbonate substitution in the hydroxyl site (characteristic of type A carbonated apatite). Pattern 1c corresponds to cement formulation #9b which, in conjunction with Table 2, is identified as a carbonated apatite. The lower crystalline order is readily apparent in the lower intensity, broader peaks. Finally, the pattern 1d corresponds to mammalian bone which has the lowest crystalline order of the patterns shown.

Figure 2 shows a comparison between three cement formulations characteristic of all cements utilizing the tetracalcium phosphate with a mean diameter of 10μm. At this mean diameter, particle size seems to be the predominant factor affecting crystallinity as all three cements have very similar crystal order. However, as shown in Figure 3, cements utilizing tetracalcium phosphate with a mean diameter of 2μm, tend to show slightly different crystallinity. The carbonated cement formulation #9b has lower crystalline order than the non-carbonated cement formulation #4d. This may be indicative of lattice strains and defects due to either the incorporation of carbonate in the apatite lattice or reaction rate. Also, Figures 2a and 2b (which correspond to formulations 10 and 9a, respectively), represent the general observation that for similar formulations those containing calcite tend to react faster and more completely than the counterparts without calcite. Column 6 of Table 1 gives further examples of this in the comparisons between 4a and 5 as well as 6a and 8.

Figure 4 shows a high resolution diffraction pattern of formulation #9a using synchrotron radiation. While a small amount of tetracalcium phosphate from precursor material is indicated, the absence of the calcite peak at 29.4 degrees 2q confirms that there is no calcium carbonate remaining in the apatite lattice in excess of the 1 percent detection limit. Therefore, the carbonate measured by coulometry and presented in Tables 1 and 2 is not present as calcite and is likely to be structurally incorporated in the apatite lattice; however, the carbonate may be adsorbed on the apatite surface.[10,17]

Figure 5 shows a FTIR comparison between apatite cement formulations #9b, #4d, coral-derived apatite, and sintered hydroxyapatite. The predominant absorption bands[10,17,20] are labeled. Of the spectra shown, only the cement formulation #9b contains carbonate bands of significant intensity with no indication of the band corresponding to calcium carbonate at about $712cm^{-1}$. Crystallinity is again shown by less distinct peaks of lower order for the cements than for the apatites produced at higher temperatures. Also, detailed comparison between cement #9b and the coral-derived apatite indicates a band shift near $874cm^{-1}$ which supports the assertion that the coral-derived material is Type-A carbonated apatite whereas cement #9b is Type-B dahllite.[10]

Cements in this investigation were cured *in vitro* in bovine serum at 37°C in order to mimic *in vivo* response in a controlled fashion. Similar cements to those reported here have been implanted *in vivo*, and the resulting explant samples taken from histology specimens have displayed similar chemical composition.[25] Thus, while there are obvious dissimilarities between this model and a true biological system, the cement reaction in biological fluids *in vitro* is expected to behave similarly to that which occurs *in vivo* .

Little can yet be reported regarding the mechanisms of the cement reactions and the reasons for the differing reaction rates. Further research needs to be performed to address these issues using solution chemistry techniques such as reported by Fulmer and Brown.[26]

CONCLUSIONS

The results indicate that the crystallinity of the synthetic dahllite of reactions similar to #9b more closely resemble bone mineral than do either thermally processed apatites or other cement formulations. The incorporation of carbonate within the apatite lattice of cements, such as formulation #9b, may contribute to reduced crystallinity as it seems to induce broad and diffuse peaks.

Calcium phosphates, particularly thermally processed ceramic hydroxyapatites, have found limited application in orthopedics because of their low fatigue properties relative to bone. By designing calcium phosphate implants of dahllite (carbonated apatite), enhanced native bone remodeling may occur replacing the implant with living bone and creating an implant-bone composite.[25,27-32] Replacement of dahllite implants by living bone may result in a progressively durable weight-bearing construct.

REFERENCES

1. Posner, A.S., The Mineral in Bone, *Clin. Ortho. and Rel. Res.*, 200, p. 87-99, 1985.
2. Shumizu, H., et al., The Effect of Substrate Composition and Condition on Resorption by Isolated Osteoclasts, *Bone and Mineral*, 6, p. 261-275, 1989.
3. Biltz, R. and E. Pellegrino, The Nature of Bone Carbonate, *Clin. Ortho. and Rel. Res.*, 129, p. 279-292, 1977.
4. LeGeros, R., N. Balmain, and G. Bonel, Structure and Composition of the Mineral Phase of Periosteal Bone, *J. Chem. Research*, S, p. 8-9, 1986.
5. LeGeros, R.Z. and J. LeGeros, Phosphate Minerals in Human Tissues, Chapter 12, in *Phosphate Minerals*, J.O. Nriagu and P.B. Moore, Eds., Springer-Verlag: NY, 1984.
6. McConnell, D., The Crystal Structure of Bone, *The Structure of Apatite*, 25, p. 253-268, 1962.
7. Bills, P.M. and E.J. Wheeler, Bone - A Composite Material, *Journal of Educational Modules for Materials Science and Engineering*, 4(3), p. 399-445, 1982.
8. Ducheyne, P., Bioceramics: Material Characteristics Versus *In Vivo* Behavior, *J. Biomed. Mater. Res.: Applied Biomaterials*, 21, p. A2, 219-236, 1987.
9. Skinner, H.C.W., Low Temperature Carbonate Phosphate Materials or the Carbonate-Apatite Problem: A Review, *Origin, Evolution, and Modern Aspects of Biomineralization in Plants and Animals*, Plenum Press, New York, p. 251-264, 1989.
10. Rey, C., et al., The Carbonate Environment in Bone Mineral, *A Resolution Enhanced FTIR Study*, 1969.
11. LeGeros, R., et al., Solutions-Mediated Transformation of OCP to Apatite, *Scanning Microscopy*, 3(1), p. 129-138, 1989.
12. Chickurer, N., M. Tung, and W. Brown, A Mechanism for Incorporation of Carbonate Into Apatite, *Calcif. Tiss. Int.*, 35, p. 55-62, 1980.
13. Nordstrom, E. and K. Karlsson, ed. Carbonate-doped Hydroxyapatite, *J. Materials Sci.: Materials in Medicine*, Chapman & Hall Ltd., p. 182-184, 1990.
14. Brown, W.E. and L.C. Chow, A New Calcium Phosphate Setting Cement, ADARF Research Unit, NBS, Gaitherburg, MD, p. 352-379, 1986.
15. Posner, A., N. Blumenthal, and F. Betts, Chapter 11, Chemistry and Structure of Precipitated Hydroxyapatites, in *Phosphate Minerals*, J.O. Nriagu and P.B. Moore, eds. Springer Verlag: New York. p. 330-349, 1984.
16. Cullity, B., *Elements of X-Ray Diffraction, Second Edition*, Addison-Wesley Publishing Co., Inc., Menlo Park, CA, p. 99-106, 1978.
17. Nelson, D. and J. Featherstone, Preparation, Analysis, and Characterization of Carbonated Apatites, *Calcif. Tissue Int.*, 34, p. S69-S81, 1982.
18. Arends, J. and W. Jongebloed, Apatite Single Crystals. Formation, Dissolution and Influence of CO_3^{2-} ions, *Recl. Trav. Chim. Pays-Bas*, 100, p. 3-9, 1981.
19. Featherstone, J. and D. Nelson, The Effect of Fluoride, Zinc, Strontium, Magnesium and Iron on the Crystal-Structural Disorder in Synthetic Carbonated Apatites, *Aust. J. Chem.*, 33, p. 2363-2368, 1980.

20. LeGeros, R., et al., Carbonate Substitution in the Apatite Structure, *Bulletin De La Societe Chimique De France*, p. 1712-1718, 1968.
21. LeGeros, R., et al., Two Types of Carbonate Substitution in the Apatite Structure, *Experientia Specialia*, 25/15, p. 5-7, 1969.
22. Nelson, D., et al., Effect of Carbonate and Fluoride on the Dissolution Behaviour of Synthetic Apatites, *Caries Res*, 17, p. 200-211, 1983.
23. Nelson, D., The Influence of Carbonate on the Atomic Structure and Reactivity of Hydroxyapatite, *J. Dent. Res.*, 60(c), p. 1621-1629, 1981.
24. Powder Diffraction File, Set 9, Card 348, Joint Committee on Powder Diffraction Standards, Swathmore, PA, 1979.
25. Constantz, B.R., *et al.*, Evaluation of Bioactive Cements Using a Rabbit Femoral Canal Model, 38th Annual Meeting, Orthopaedic Research Society. Washington, D.C, p. 370, 1992.
26. Fulmer, M. and P. Brown, Effects of Na_2HPO_4 and NaH_2PO_4 on Hydroxyapatite Formation, *J. Biomedical Materials Research*, 27, p. 1095-1102, 1993.
27. Baker, J.T., L.A. McKinney, and S. Gunasekaran. An *In Vivo* Evaluation of Artificial Bone Constructs, 38th Annual Meeting, Orthopaedic Research Society. Washington, D.C., p. 575, 1992.
28. Constantz, B.R., *In Situ* Calcium Phosphate Minerals - Method & Composition, in U.S. Patent #4,880,610, November 14, 1989.
29. Constantz, B.R., *In Situ* Calcium Phosphate Minerals - Method, in U.S. Patent #5,047,031, September 10, 1991.
30. Constantz, B.R., B.M. Barr, and K. McVicker, Intimate Mixture of Calcium and Phosphate Sources as Precursor to Hydroxyapatite, in U.S. Patent #5,053,212, October 1, 1991.
31. Constantz, B.R., Storage Stable Formulations for *In Situ* Prepared Calcium Phosphate Minerals, in U.S. Patent #5,129,905, July 14, 1992.
32. Constantz, B.R., K. McVicker, and B.M. Barr, Intimate Mixture of Calcium and Phosphate Sources as Precursor to Hydroxyapatite, in U.S. Patent #5,178,845, January 12, 1993.

DEPOSITION OF HYDROXYAPATITE COATINGS BY LASER ABLATION

G. Sardin, M. Varela and J. L. Morenza
Universitat de Barcelona, Departament de Física Aplicada i Electrònia
Av. Diagonal 647, E-08028 Barcelona (Spain)

This work is directed toward establishing the conditions for the deposition of hydroxyapatite (HA) coatings by pulsed laser deposition (PLD). Depending on the application different resorbable or non-resorbable bioceramics may be desired, so within this scope, layers of hydroxyapatite have been deposited on Ti substrates. By means of an ArF excimer laser beam, a rotating HA pellet is ablated within a deposition chamber with a low pressure atmosphere. Among the main technological parameters it has been selected: the influence of the atmosphere nature during deposition, the effects of its saturation with water, the use of water alone, the influence of the atmosphere pressure and of the deposition temperature. The characterization techniques used are x-ray diffractometry, FTIR spectroscopy, scanning electron microscopy and secondary ion mass spectrometry. Pure, crystalline HA coatings have been obtained using an atmosphere of water vapor.

I. INTRODUCTION

Hydroxyapatite (HA), which is the prime constituent of bone and the most biocompatible ceramics, presents moreover the essential advantage of establishing biological bonding with bone.[1-3] However large prosthetic devices of bulk HA could not be fabricated because sintered HA is not a strong enough ceramic. Therefore the search has centered on developing coatings for usual metallic structures, adding to their strength, durability and formability, the attractive biological profile of HA, for both dental and orthopedic implants.

Diverse means of coating HA have been developed. These include electrophoretic deposition, RF sputtering and plasma spraying, the latter having currently evolved the most, due to its advantage of providing in a short time thick coatings of large scale. However, shortcomings appear related to the durability and biocompatible performances.[2,4,5] These may arise from both the composition and the structure, since calcium phosphate coatings may additionall form the α and β phases of tricalcium phosphate (TCP). Crystallinity may also be poor. Such factors may influence the coating's biological performances, i.e. biological bonding and affinity.

Pulsed laser deposition (PLD) constitutes an attractive technique for the deposition of complex materials, since the target stoichiometry is quite easily preserved in the coating. Recently PLD has been applied to the formation of HA coatings.[4,6,7] The present work has been centered on determining the parameters

0-8493-4750-5/94/$0.00 + $.50

of the technique that determine each phase and fix its structure and composition, with the objective of determining the ones that optimize the HA content of the coatings. The main technological parameters to be assessed are the pressure, the temprature of deposition, the laser beam parameters, the distance between target and substrate, the sintering conditions of HA pellets and the substrate nature and surface. Of prime importance among all these parameters is the atmosphere used.[4,6,7] Atmosphere is determinant of the coating stoichiometry and crystalline structure. Therefore, our prime objective has been to further explore the influence of different atmospheres at diverse pressures and deposition temperatures.[7]

II. EXPERIMENTAL

A pellet made from HA powder (Aldrich-Chemie) pressed at 6×10^8 Pa pressure at room temperature is ablated by means of an ArF excimer laser beam with 193 nm wavelength. The beam, with an incident angle of 45°, is focused on a rotating HA target which is hence eroded all along a ring, the ejected material being deposited on a heated substrate placed near the target. In the deposition chamber a selected low pressure atmsophere is maintained in order to favor the HA coating composition. The laser was set at the following parameters: pulse energy of 200-250 mJ, pulse energy density of 2-3 J/cm^2, pulse lifetime of 23 ns and pulse frequency of 10 Hz. A total of 20,000 pulses was set for the deposition leading to a coating thickness of the order of the micron.

The substrates, made of Ti thick disks, have been located at 3.5 cm from the target and have been maintained during deposition at a temperature within the range of 400°C to 550°C, by means of a 100 W halogen lamp with a reflector focused on the substrate back. The temperature is measured with a thermocouple in pressed contact on the substrate deposition side. Diverse types of atmosphere have been tried, i.e. Ar and Ar/H_2O, O_2 and O_2/H_2O, and H_2O at pressure ranging from 6×10^{-3} to 1.2 mbar, a set of 4 to 9 samples being deposited for these three types of atmospheres.

The characterization techniques used are x-ray diffractometry (Siemens D-500), scanning electron microscopy (Hitachi S-2300), FTIR spectroscopy (Nicolet 5ZDX) and secondary ion mass spectrometry (Atomika A-DIDA 3000-30).

III. RESULTS AND DISCUSSION

A. X-RAY DIFFRACTOMETRY

Regarding x-ray diffractometry, deposition of HA coatings on Ti substrates, which is appropriate for close relationship with prostheses, is quite annoying since in addition to the Ti background diffraction peaks are often added ones from some of the many Ti oxides (e.g. rutile and anatase). These oxides are formed during deposition in presence of an oxidizing atmosphere. Because some of those peaks coincide with those of HA or TCP, the identification of the compounds present becomes difficult. Tests on Si substrates solve this difficulty since the SiO_2 layer is instead very thin and does not affect the XRD analyses. However, an SiO_2 substrate may not adequately simulate that of a prosthesis since the interfacial TiO_2 layer may significantly influence coating nucleation and growth. Three reference coatings, using a sole Ar atmosphere, have been deposited at a fixed temperature of 550°C and at pressure from 6×10^{-3} to 1.2 mbar. For a set of 6 samples, the saturation of Ar with H_2O, for a pressure range from 6×10^{-3} to 6×10^{-1} mbar and with the same deposition temperature, was shown to enhance the HA coating composition, lowering the presence of TCP. Figure 1 shows the XRD pattern of a coating obtained from an Ar atmosphere saturated with water. Even though the presence of water has improved the coating's HA composition, at these deposition conditions some TCP is still present. The higher pressures have also strengthened the HA composition, lowering however mechanical resistance to abrasion.

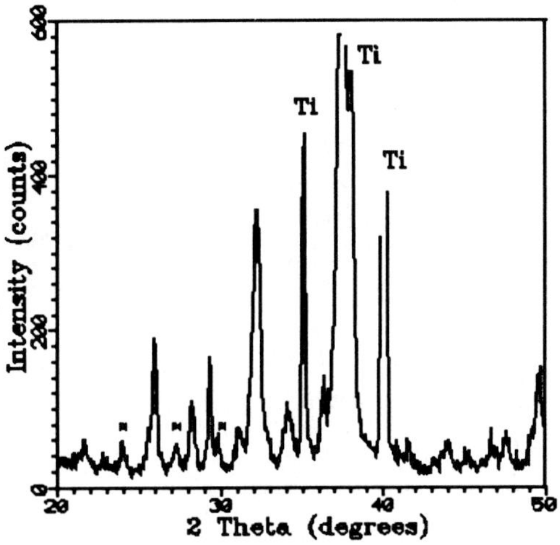

Figure 1. XRD pattern of a coating deposited in an Ar/H_2O atmosphere at 0.6 mbar and at 550°C. The main XRD peaks are those of HA, with some TCP designed with*.

A reference coating, using a sole oxygen atmosphere of 0.3 mbar pressure and a deposition temperature of 550°C, has shown some crystalline HA pattern with traces of TCP. The addition of water to the oxygen atmosphere caused the formation of a deeply oxidized Ti substrate and to lead to amorphous coatings, at least within the pressure range of 6×10^{-2} to 3×10^{-1} mbar and deposition temperature of 550°C. The XRD patterns of the samples show Ti and TiO_2 with none from HA or TCP, corresponding to a deep oxidation of only rutile in the case of O_2/H_2O and a weak oxidation of both rutile and anatase in the case of O_2 alone.

We have also examined the use of an atmosphere of water vapor, through a set of 7 samples, within a pressure range of 6×10^{-3} to 6×10^{-1} mbar and a temperature range of 400° to 550°C. Relative to the effect of pressure on the coatings, it has merged that the XRD patterns from HA are enhanced with increased pressure. This trend is typified in Figs. 2a and 2b showing the x-ray diffractograms of two samples obtained at water vapor pressures of 1.5×10^{-1} and 3×10^{-1} mbar and a deposition pressure being higher.

Regarding the effect of deposition temperature, coatings have been deposited at 400°, 450°, 500° and 550°C. The lower temperatures have shown a trend to enhance the HA composition. Figure 3 shows the diffractogram of a coating deposited at a pressure of 0.15 mbar and a temperature of 550°C. Contrasting it with the one of Fig. 1b provides evidence that the lower temperature of 400°C has favored the coating of HA composition, removing visible traces of other phosphate.

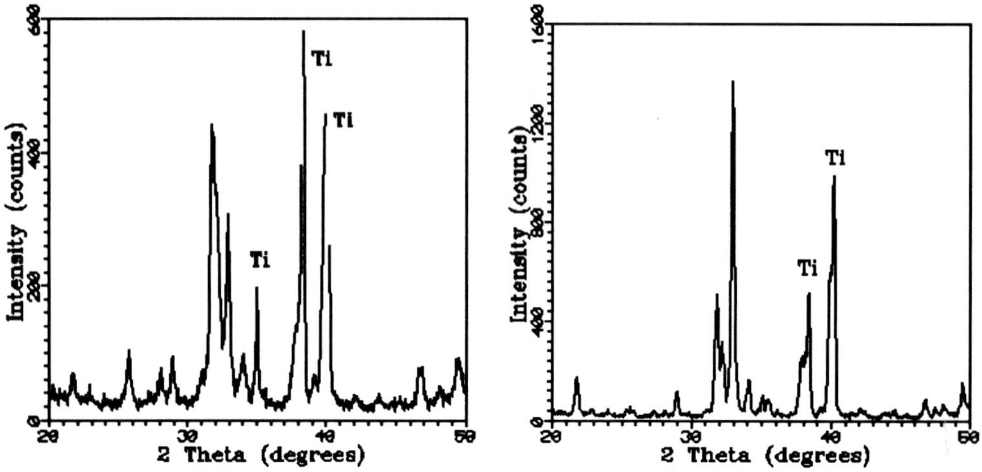

Figure 2. XRD patterns of two coatings deposited at 400°C in an H_2O atmosphere at (a) 0.15 mbar and (b) 0.3 mbar. Both show only HA patterns.

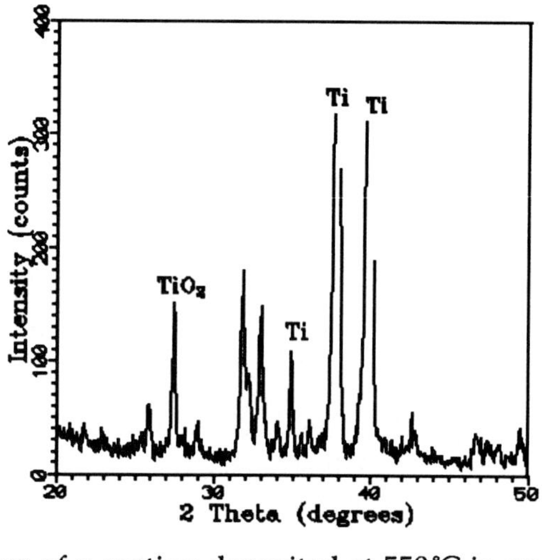

Figure 3. XRD pattern of a coating deposited at 550°C in an H_2O atmosphere at 0.15 mbar.

B. SCANNING ELECTRON MICROSCOPY

The morphologies of two coatings, both deposited at the same temperature of 550°C and pressure of 0.6 mbar, are compared in Fig. 4. These show a compact agglomeration of crystal-like grains of about 0.1–0.5μm in the case of a pure Ar atmosphere, and more increased compactness in the case of water-saturated Ar. Regarding the H_2O atmosphere, the effect of pressure on the coating morphology for an atmosphere of water vapor from two samples deposited at the same temperature of 400°C are contrasted. A disordered and very compact crystal-like granular structure appears at the higher pressure of 0.3 mbar, while at the lower one of 0.15 mbar the morphology is still much more compact and smooth.

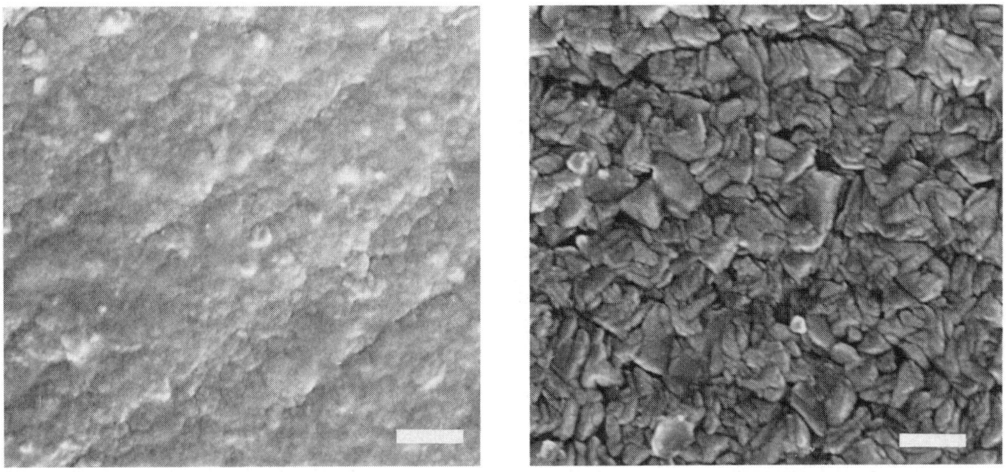

(a) (b)

Figure 4. Scanning electron micrographs from two samples deposited at 400°C using an H_2O atmosphere, at (a) 0.15 mbar and (b) 0.3 mbar (scale bar 1 μm).

It should be noted that these films do not exhibit the typical round-shaped PLD particulates and their morphologies appear instead to be made up by crystal-shaped grains. In fact, all through the diverse deposition conditions, our films have very scarcely presented a few of these particulates, in contrast with those of other researchers.[4,5] We have observed, along with the distinct deposition conditions, a shape diversity of the crystal-like grains and that some coatings do not show any granular structure.

C. INFRARED SPECTROSCOPY

A typical transmittance spectrum from the HA coatings, corresponding to a sample deposited at 550°C and an H_2O atmosphere pressure of 1.5×10^{-1} mbar is shown in Fig. 5. The IR spectra of the coatings show mainly three typical absorbance bands, one at about 3600 cm^{-1} from the O-H group and two others around 1060 cm^{-1} and 600 cm^{-1} from the P-O group. According to the coating deposition conditions, the stretching vibrational mode of the O-H group may exhibit two different types of absorbance band, a wide one alike the powder one, or instead a very narrow peak. The narrow peak, only 50 cm^{-1} large, can be fitted with a gaussian, while the wide band, about 800 cm^{-1} large, can be deconvoluted into two gaussians.[7] Samples deposited in an O_2/H_2O atmosphere have presented the wide band type, revealing some hydration of these coatings, through the incorporation of bulk water in hydrated crystals or intergrain phase. All other samples have shown only the narrow peak, without any visible presence of the corresponding large band from water, indicating thus no appreciable retention of water from these coatings.

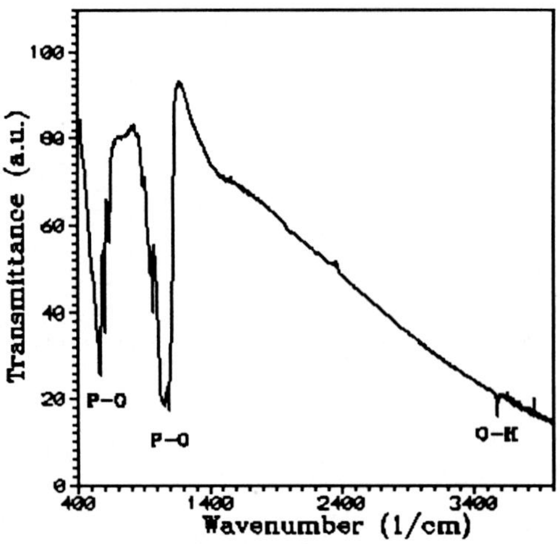

Figure 5. FTIR spectrum of a coating deposited at 550°C and 0.15 mbar in an H_2O atmosphere.

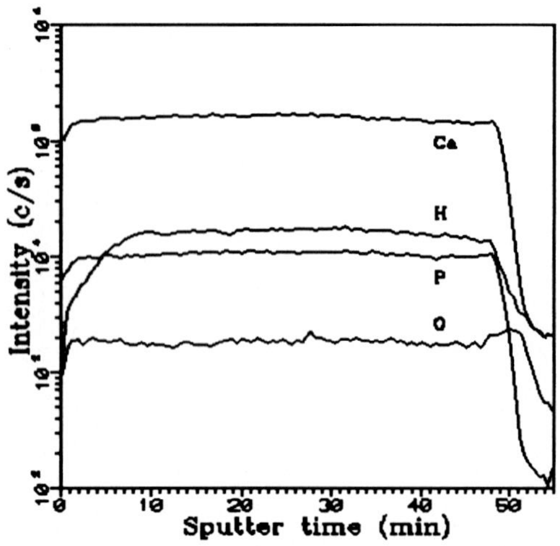

Figure 6. SIMS profile of a coating deposited within an H_2O atmosphere at 0.15 m bar and 400°C.

D. SECONDARY ION MASS SPECTROMETRY

The SIMS profile shown in Fig. 6, of a coating deposited within an H_2O atmosphere at 0.15 mbar and at 400°C, demonstrates a homogeneous depth stoichiometry of Ca, P, O and H throughout the coating up to the interface with the Ti substrate. The eventual appearance in some samples of a hump from Ti near the substrate reveals the presence of a TiO_2 interfacial layer, that we have identified by XRD as composed of rutile and anatase.

IV. CONCLUSION

As a conclusion it could be highlighted that PLD can be used to form compact, highly crystalline films with a maximized HA composition, importing to them a high resistance to body dissolution which could thus reveal to be efficient biocompatible protective barriers. This goal may, in view of the expectant results obtained, offer to HA-PLD suitable perspectives and justify further studies of this novel type of HA coatings. Let us also point out our finding that the use of an atmosphere of sole water can provide pure and crystalline HA coatings.

REFERENCES

1. M. Jarcho, J. F. Kay and K. Gumaer, J. Bioeng. 1:79-92 (1977).
2. J. F. Kay, Mat. Tech. 8(1/2):26-29 (1993).
3. A. Ravaglioli and A. Krajewski (eds.), *Bioceramics and the Human Body*, Elsevier Applied Science (London), 1992.
4. C. M. Cotell, D. B. Chrisey, K. S. Grabowski, J. A. Sprague and C. R. Gossett, J. Appl. Biomater. 3:87-93 (1992).
5. L. L. Hench and J. Wilson, MRS Bulletin, pp. 62-74 (September 1991).
6. C. M. Cotell, Appl. Surf. Sci. 69:140-148 (1993).
7. G. Sardin, F. Sánchez, M. Varela and J. L. Morenza, E-MRS, November 1992 (submitted).

GRAFTING OF PHOSPHORYLATED MOLECULES ON APATITE SURFACE

A. Lebugle, M. Subirade, V. Delpech
Laboratoire des Materiaux
Institut National Polytechnique
118, route de Narbonne
F-31077 Toulouse Cedex, France

A. INTRODUCTION

Much research has dealt with the improvement of the mechanical properties of bone cements by incorporating various fillers such as carbon fibres, Kevlar, polyethylene fibres or metal wires. Sometimes, these fillers are made of hydroxyapatite[1,2] with the aim of giving biological properties to the cement. Unfortunately, these fillers do not increase the mechanical properties to a great extent. On the contrary, a decrease is often observed. This is probably due to the lack of adequate bonding between filler and matrix.

Such a bond can be obtained by using a mixture of monomers, including a monomer able to complex the calcium ions of the filler.[3] Another approach consists of grafting an unsaturated molecule onto the filler, which is able to bond by copolymerization to the main polymer chain. Work has already be done in this last area. We have shown it is possible to graft a phosphorylated organic molecule onto an apatite surface by coprecipitation, the bond being obtained during the formation of apatite.[4-6] Organic phosphate molecules are grafted on apatite through their ionized phosphate group which is located at the apatite tunnel end. The carbon chain of the phosphorylated molecule is sited outside the mineral lattice, and keeps its reactivity. This configuration leads to the formation of crystallites with thicknesses ranging between 20 and 30 Å. These crystallites are similar in size and shape to the apatite plaquettes observed in the mineral component of calcified tissues. The nature of the organic chain can be chosen according to the required properties. For example, grafting an unsaturated molecule onto apatite such as hydroxyethylmethacrylate phosphate, allows the linkage by copolymerization with a monomer, methylmethacrylate, of the apatite to the polymer chain. Applications of such modified apatite include the reinforcement of acrylic bone cement. Another application concerns the modifications of surface properties of apatite. Grafting phosphorylated tensioactive molecules onto apatite, should give hydrophobic properties to the solid.

In this paper, we will discuss the influence of these two organic molecules (unsaturated or tensioactive chain), on the mechanical properties of P.M.M.A. bone cement, and on the dispersion of the filler in the P.M.M.A. matrix.

0-8493-4750-5/94/$0.00 + $.50

B. SYNTHESIS OF GRAFTED APATITES

1. Phosphorylated Molecules Synthesis

Phosphorylated molecules were synthesized as follows:

1. The reaction of hydroxyethylmethacrylate with phosphorus pentoxide in dichloromethane, at 40°C, gives a mixture of mono and diester.[7]

$$3\ R\text{-}OH + P_2O_5 \text{-----} H_2PO_4R + HPO_4R_2$$

In the case of dodecanol, it is necessary to hydrolyse the obtained organic pyrophosphate with water to get the mono and diester mixture.

2. The monoester is separated by precipitation as barium salt. Then, it is regenerated with sulfuric acid. In these conditions, pure hydroxyethylmethacrylate phosphate or dodecanolphosphate were obtained.

$$H_2PO_4R + BaCl_2 + 2\ NH_3OH \rightarrow BaPO_4R + 2NH_4Cl + 2H_2O$$
$$BaPO_4R + H_2SO_4 \rightarrow BaSO_4 + H_2PO_4R$$

2. Modified Apatite Synthesis

A mixture of a mineral phosphate (such as diammonium phosphate) and a previously obtained monoester phosphate are coprecipitated by a calcium salt, at 37°C, in a medium of low dielectric constant (mixture water-ethanol 50/50 % vol.).

More accurately, for example, in the case of HEMAphosphate-grafting, a solution containing 10 mM of calcium nitrate $Ca(NO_3)_2{\cdot}4H_2O$ in 30 ml of water and 30 ml of ethanol was added to a solution containing 6.5 mM of diammonium phosphate $(NH_4)_2HPO_4$ and 3.5 mM of HEMAphosphate in 80 ml of water, 15 ml of NH_4OH solution and 95 ml of ethanol. After formation, the coprecipitate is filtered, then washed with a solution containing 60 ml of water, 10 ml of NH_4OH solution and 70 ml of ethanol. After filtering and drying at 80°C for a night, Modified Apatite is obtained.

C. INFLUENCE OF GRAFTING ON THE MECHANICAL PROPERTIES OF THE CEMENT

The unsaturated organic phosphate grafted onto apatite was used as filler in a PMMA bone cement.

1. Preparation of Bone Cement

The preparation of an orthopaedic cement consists of mixing powdered PMMA (about 11 g) containing benzoid peroxide, with a monomer, MMA (about 6 ml) containing paratoluidine. The polymerization occurs and leads to the cement. In our case, part of the prepolymer (3 g) was replaced by Modified Apatite, the sum always being equal to 11 g. The polymerization is then carried out as previously. In order to demonstrate the influence of the grafted molecule, a parallel study was carried out in the same conditions but using an unmodified apatite.

2. Study of the Mechanical Properties

It is interesting to compare the physical properties of cements made of pure PMMA and those made of PMMA with MAp or unmodified apatite as filler.

The compressive strength and the Young's modulus were measured and are reported here. As seen in Table 1, a fall in the compressive strength, results from incorporating ordinary apatite. Using Modified Apatite however gives a slight increase of these properties.

Table 1
Compressive Strength and Young Modulus of Cements.

	PMMA	Apatite	Modified Apatite
R (MPa)	105	82	112
E (GPa)	2.2	1.8	2.4

The influence of apatite grafting on the fracture mechanisms were studied by XPS and SEM. These two techniques show that fracture occurs in the polymer with Modified Apatite in the cement, and in the filler or at the interface with ordinary apatite.

This can be seen in Figure 1, representing the fracture surface of cement containing ordinary apatite. The filler is uncovered and visible. However, the filler cannot be seen on the fracture surface of cement containing MAp.

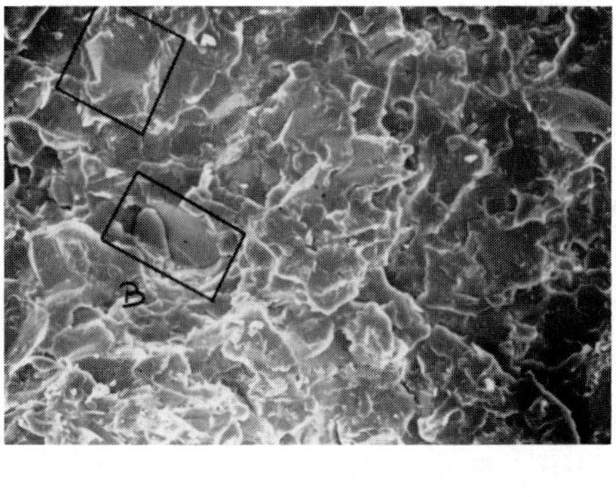

Figure 1. SEM fracture of a cement containing apatite.

100 μm

Other techniques reveal the influence of grafting on the cement behavior. Indeed, it was possible to show by thermo-stimulated currents, that the phases are segregated in a cement containing Apatite, whereas there is a stiffening of the polymer chains in cement containing modified apatite.[8]

The increase of the mechanical resistance of the cement is limited by the lack of dispersion of modified apatite in PMMA leading to a low amount of filler. Besides, there is an aggregation of the modified apatite grains in cement. The size goes from 50 μm to 150 μm as seen in Figure 2.

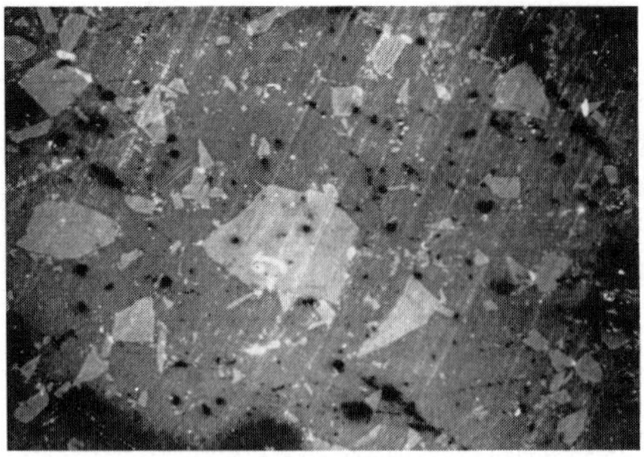

Figure 2. SEM of cement containing apatite modified with HEMAphosphate.

100 μm

D. INFLUENCE OF GRAFTING ON FILLER DISPERSION IN PMMA CEMENT

It is well known that the surface energy of a solid depends on the length of the grafted carbon chain.[9] In Figure 3, the variation of the energy of modified silica is reported vs the carbon atom number. After, an initial fall, the change is very small after 12 carbons.

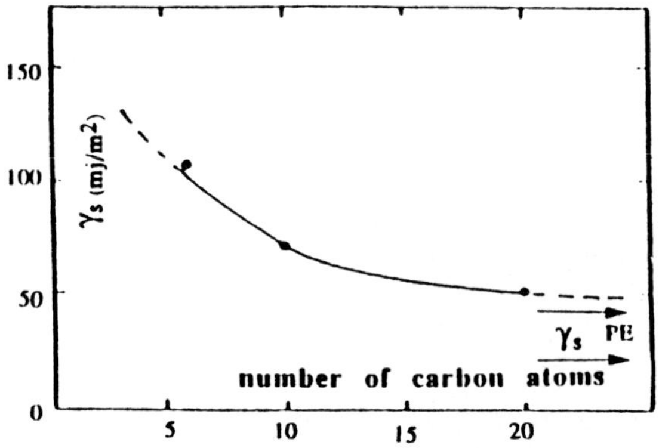

Figure 3. Variation of surface energy of modified silica vs grafted chain length.[9]

Therefore, the influence of dodecylphosphate grafting on the surface properties of apatite was examined. The Modified Apatite was obtained in the same way as unsaturated molecule grafting (cf. B. 2.), but by using dodecylphosphate instead of HEMAphosphate.

The grains of apatite modified with dodecyl phosphate have the same size order as grains of apatite modified with HEMAphosphate. But, dispersion of dodecylphosphate grafted apatite in MMA gives grains at least ten times smaller, than previously, between 2 μm and 10 μm, as seen in Figure 4.

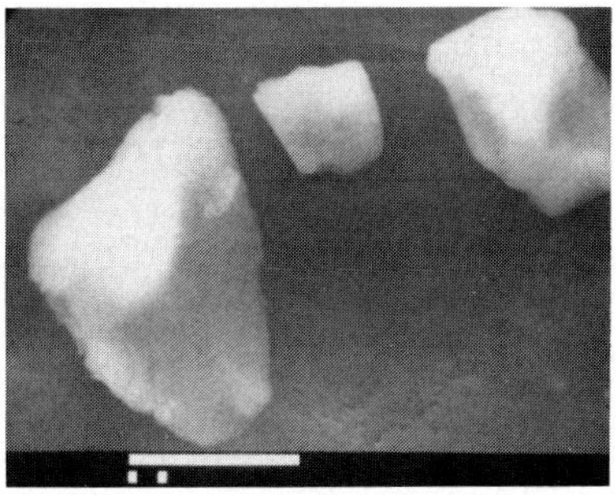

Figure 4. Dodecylphosphate modified apatite grains after dispersion in MMA.

----
10 µm

After polymerization, SEM of polished cement containing apatite modified with dodecyl phosphate shows no aggregation as in the case of HEMA phosphate. Furthermore, x-ray mapping reveals the very good dispersion of the calcium phosphate filler in the cement (Figure 5).

Figure 5. X-ray mapping of calcium in a cement containing Apatite Modified with dodecyl-phosphate.

----
10 µm

E. CONCLUSIONS

Grafting of unsaturated phosphorylated molecules onto apatites, by coprecipitation, gives a tight bond between the filler and the polymer in a polymethylmethacrylate cement. Compared to the usual PMMA cement, the mechanical properties are slightly increased in grafted apatite-PMMA cement, whereas they fall when the filler is an unmodified apatite. This increase can be enhanced by improving the dispersion of the particles ; of filler in the matrix (the proportion of filler cannot be brought above 17% owing to problems of wettability). However, if tensioactive molecules are also attached the filler particles, this drawback can be overcome. So future composites of this type having both a tensioactive moiety and an acrylic group, whether separately, or both on the same long aliphatic chain, should have greatly improved mechanical properties.

REFERENCES

1. Castaldini, A. and Cavallini, A., Setting properties fo bone cement with added synthetic hydroxyapatite, Biomaterials, 6, 55, 1985.
2. Castaldini, A. and Cavallini, A., Creep behaviour of composite bone cement, Biological and Biomedical Performance of Biomaterials, ed. P. Christel, A. Meunier and A. J. C. Lee, Elsevier Science Publishers, Amsterdam, 525, 1986.
3. Wilson, A. D., Prosser, H. J., and Powis D. M., Mechanisms of Adhesion of Polyelectrolyte cements to Hydroxyapatite, J. Dent. Res., 62(5), 590, 1983.
4. Subirade, M., Elaboration d'une liaison minéral-organique entre un phosphate de calcium et un monomère phosphorylé, Thesis, INP, Toulouse, 1986.
5. Montel, G., Bonel, G., Lebugle, A. and Subirade, M., Sur la fixation d'ions de grandes dimensions par le réseau cristallin des apatites, et ses conséquences biologiques, C.R. Acad. Sci., 309, 1155, 1989.
6. Subirade, M. and Lebugle A., Etude d'une liaison minéral-organique entre un phosphate de calcium et un monomère phosphorylé, Ann. Chim., 1993, sous presse.
7. Swart, J. G., Am. Ceram. Soc. Symp. Ser., 31, 151, 1976.
8. Dandurand, J., Delpech, V., Lebugle, A., Lamure, A., and Lacabanne, C., Study of the mineral-organic linkage in an apatitic reinforced bone cement, J. Biomedical Materials Research, 24, 1377, 1990.
9. Kessaissia Z., Papirer E. and Donnet J.B., Surface energy of Silicas, Grafted with Alkylchains of increasing Lengths as Measured by Contact Angle Techniques, J. Colloid Interface Sci., 82, 526, 1981.

INFLUENCE OF THE CRYSTALLINITY OF PLASMA SPRAYED HA-COATINGS ON THEIR OSSEOINTEGRATION

P. Frayssinet, P. Conte, F. Tourenne, N. Rouquet
Bioland
132 Rte. D'Espagne
31100 Toulouse, France

ABSTRACT

HA-coating crystallinity may affect the proliferation of isolated cells grown on the coating. We have implanted in rabbit femurs, metal cylinders coated with HA ceramic having high (100%) or low (40-48%) crystallinity. The surface in contact with bone tissue, the density of the bone close to the coating and the coating thickness were evaluated depending on time. No difference could be shown between the values of these parameters for each type of coating. In this study the coating crystallinity did not have an influence on the osseointegration.

INTRODUCTION

Plasma-sprayed HA-coatings are used as orthopaedic biomaterials in order to enhance the biocompatibility of the metal on which they are deposited. They allow the formation of a prosthesis having the mechanical properties of metal with the biological properties of HA.[1]

Depending on plasma spray parameters, the coatings can have very different characteristics (Table 1). Coating crystallinity is a very important characteristic because it affects the solubility of the ceramic coating and it makes it difficult to determine the presence of other calcium phosphate phases in the amorphous phase.

Bone formation at the interface with HA-coatings is due to the protein synthesis activity of differentiated osteoblasts adsorbed on the coating.[2] Therefore, the influence of coating characteristics on cell functions determines the ability of bone tissue to be formed in contact with the ceramic coating.

It has been suggested that coating characteristics could influence both basic cell functions (proliferation, cell adhesion on the material) and specific cell functions (bone specific protein synthesis). We have demonstrated that some of the cell functions and particularly the cell proliferation at the HA-coating contact was affected by the coating crystallinity,[3] the cell growth being inhibited when the crystallinity of the coating on which they were grown was high (100%). The cell growth rate was not affected on HA-coatings in which crystallinity was less than 70%. However, the membrane alkaline phosphatase activity was not altered on 100% crystalline coating.

0-8493-4750-5/94/$0.00 + $.50

Table 1. Characteristics of the HA-coating tested.

Plasma sprayed powder	HA >97%
Crystal structure	majority of HA ($Ca_{10}(PO_4)\wedge OH_2$ other compound tolerated: TCP (traces), CaO (traces), amorphous phase
Crystallinity	two kinds of specimen: CR40-48:40-48%; CR100: 100%
Coating thickness	120±30µm
Trace elements	As<3ppm Cd<5ppm Hg<5ppm Pb<3ppm
Porosity	<4%

We have implanted HA-coated cylinders where the coatings had poor or high crystallinity, into rabbit condyles in order to evaluate the effect of the crystallinity on the osseointegration.

MATERIALS AND METHODS

HA-coated cylinders having 3-mm diameter were implanted into the external condyle of each leg of ten white New Zealand rabbits. Right legs were implanted with 40-48% crystalline HA-coated implant and left legs were implanted with 100% crystalline HA-coated implants. The crystallinity of the HA-coating had been checked using x-ray diffraction. X-ray diffraction patterns were recorded on a Phillips goniometer TW1050. X-ray emission was obtained by a cobalt anode (λ = 1.78892Å). Crystallinity was measured by the index I_x (I_x = ((integrated surface of the crystalline powder spectrum measured between 2θ=35 to 39°/integrated surface of the coating spectrum measured between 2θ=35 to 39°) x 100). The integrated surfaces were measured by diffract PC-AT software (Socabim-Lyon, France). Two animals were killed after periods of two weeks, 1, 2, 4 and 6 months. The condyles were retrieved, fixed in 10% buffered formaldehyde for 24 hours, dehydrated in increasing ethanol and embedded in methylmethacrylate. Sections of the implanted materials were made using a low speed cooled diamond saw (cuto 1 Jean Wirtz, Germany) and were polished using a polisher (Lam Plan MM 823, Italy) equipped with silicon carbide discs up to a thickness of 100 µm. Sections were stained using the Von Kossa method and were examined using a light microscope (Polyvar-Reichert) coupled with an image analysis software (AES Image-Toulouse, France) in order to determine the percentage of the implant perimeter in contact with bone. The density of bone trabeculae in close proximity to the coatings were evaluated by the percentage of a virtual line parallel to the HA coating and located at a distance of 2 mm from the coating surface which was cutting bone trabeculae. The coating thickness was measured at each period of time.

RESULTS

Immature bone formed in the gaps between the HA-coatings and the implanted bone after a two-week implantation period. After an implantation period of one month, bone trabeculae were shown at the interfaces with both HA-coatings. No morphological difference was noted on sections of coatings having both crystallinities at all periods after implantation (Figs. 1 and 2).

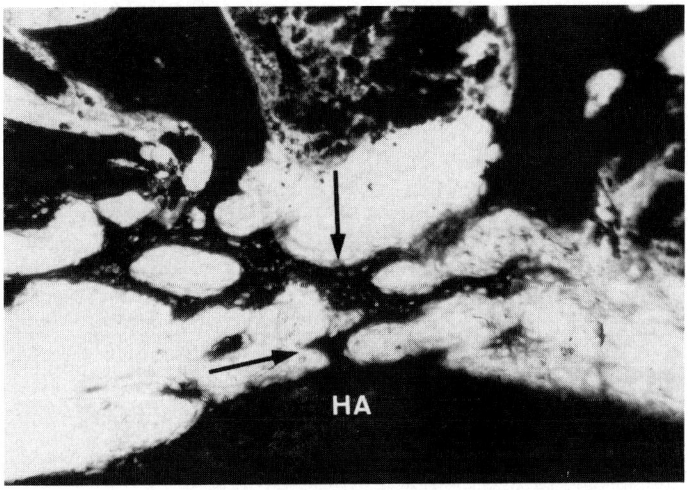

Figure 1. Forty percent crystalline coatings implanted 2 weeks. Immature bone (↑) formation is visible at the HA-coating (HA) surface. Von Kossa x400.

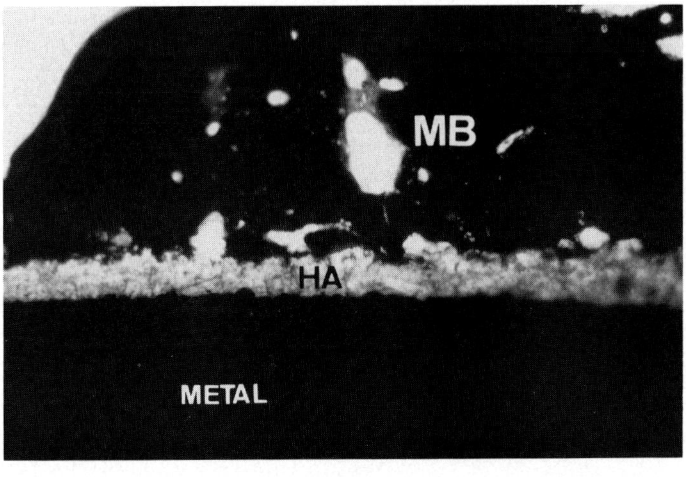

Figure 2. One hundred percent crystalline coating implanted 1 month. A mature bone (MB) is in contact with the HA-coating (HA). Von Kossa x 200.

The percentage of the implant perimeter in contact with the bone tissue did not vary significantly on poorly or highly crystalline coatings (Fig. 3).

The density of bone trabeculae close to the coating surfaces was nearly the same on both types of coating at all implantation periods (Fig. 4), although it decreased after one month of implantation regardless of the crystallinity. The mean thickness of HA-coatings after the implantation decreased faster on the highly crystalline than on the poorly crystalline coatings (Fig. 5).

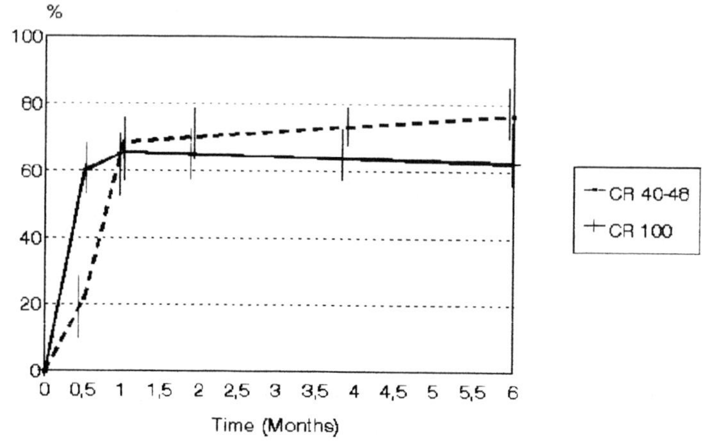

Figure 3. Percentage of the implant surface in contact with bone tissue.

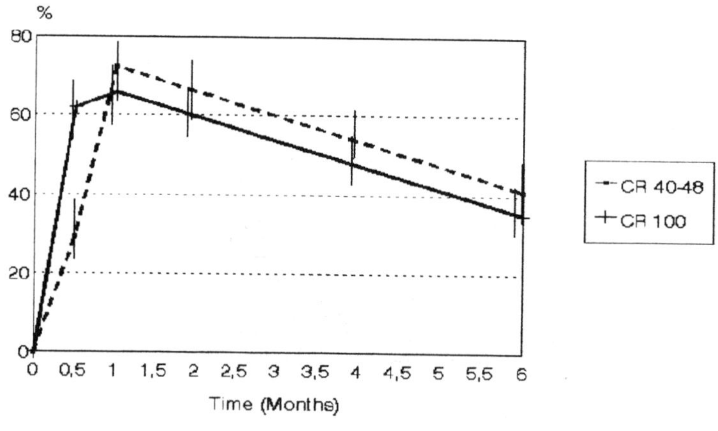

Figure 4. Density of the bone trabeculae close to the implant surface.

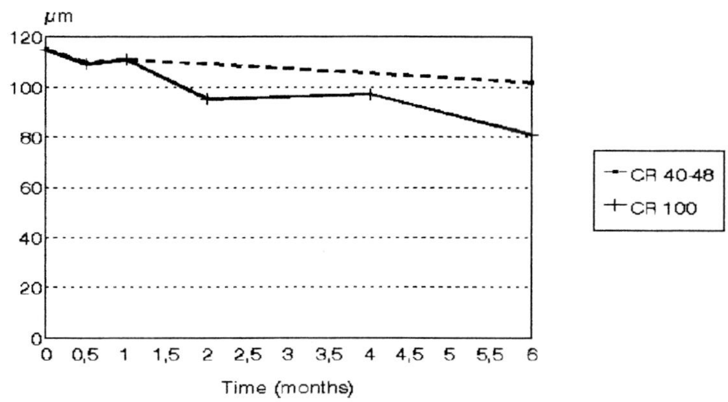

Figure 5. Mean thickness of the HA coating once implanted.

DISCUSSION

Although the crystallinity of HA-coatings may have biological effects on isolated cells *in vitro*, we could not observe an influence of this characteristic on the osseointegration of HA-coatings when they were evaluated *in vivo*.

Poorly crystalline coatings have proved to be more soluble at a physiological pH than 100% crystalline coatings,[3] although Maxian et al.[4] have reported that amorphous coatings showed significantly less resorption than poorly crystallized coatings. We showed in this study that, at least in short periods of time (less than 6 months), highly crystalline coatings may be resorbed more rapidly. That could be due to the larger size of the HA-grains in the highly crystalline coating. The cellular removal[5] of larger HA-grains due to the amorphous phase dissolution could explain the apparent higher degradation during this period of time.

It has been suggested that coating dissolution plays an important role in enhancing bone attachment strength.[6] This effect was not observed in this study in which osseointegration of both kinds of coatings were the same although the dissolution of a poorly crystalline coating has been shown to be greater in previous experiments.

The density of bone at the interface with coatings decreased after a few weeks of implantation and no fibrous tissue interposition was noted. This decrease in the bone density is due to the remodeling of bone tissue after bone healing. In the early time of healing, immature bone is formed at the surface of the coating and after a period of remodeling while immature bone is replaced by mature bone, the mature bone trabeculae are less dense.

CONCLUSIONS

The effect of the HA-coating crystallinity detected using cell culture had no influence on the osseointegration of HA-coating evaluated *in vivo*. The mechanism of the *in vitro* effect of coating crystallinity on cell proliferation is still unclear. In this study we could not determine whether or not the cell proliferation on the coating surface was affected.

REFERENCES

1. M. Jarcho, "Calcium phosphate ceramics as hard tissue prosthetics," *Clin. Orthop. Rel. Res.*, 1981, 157:257-278.
2. P. Frayssinet, D. Hardy, N. Rouquet, B. Giammara, A. Guilhem, and J. Hanker, "New observations on midle term hydroxyapatite coated titanium hip prostheses," *Biomaterials*, 1992, 13:668-674.
3. P. Frayssinet, F. Tourenne, N. Rouquet, P. Conte, C. Delga, and G. Bonel, "Comparative biological properties of HA-plasma sprayed coatings having different crystallinities," *J. Mat. Sci., Materials in Medicine* (in press).
4. S. H. Maxian, J. P. Zawadsky, and M. D. Dunn, "In vitro evaluation of amorphous calcium phosphate and poorly crystallized hydroxyapatite coatings on titanium implants," *J. Biomed. Mater. Res.*, 1993, 27:111-117.
5. P. Frayssinet, J. L. Trouillet, N. Rouquet, E. Azimus and A. Autefage, "Osseointegration of macroporous calcium phosphate ceramics having a different chemical composition," *Biomaterials*, 1993, 14:423-429.
6. P. Ducheyne, J. Beight, J. Cuckler, J. Evans, and S. Radin, "Effect of calcium phosphate coating characteristics on early post operative bone tissue ingrowth," *Biomaterials*, 1990, 11:531-540.

IN SITU TEM OBSERVATION OF RADIATION INDUCED AMORPHIZATION OF CRYSTALS WITH APATITE STRUCTURE

L.M. Wang,* M. Cameron,** W.J. Weber,† K.D. Crowley†† and R.C. Ewing*

Temperature dependence of amorphization doses for 1.5 MeV Kr ion irradiated $Ca_{10}(PO_4)_6F_2$ and $Ca_2La_8(SiO_4)_6O_2$ were studied with *in situ* transmission electron microscopy. At low temperatures, $Ca_{10}(PO_4)_6F_2$ became amorphized at lower doses than $Ca_2La_8(SiO_4)_6O_2$. However, the critical amorphization dose increased much more rapidly for the former above 350 K than the latter. Compared to $Ca_2La_8(SiO_4)_6O_2$ at 475 K, $Ca_{10}(PO_4)_6F_2$ required a dose nearly five times higher to become amorphous. Based on the dose-temperature curves, activation energies for the crystal structure recovery process were determined to be 0.07 eV for $Ca_{10}(PO_4)_6F_2$ and 0.13 eV for $Ca_2La_8(SiO_4)_6O_2$ respectively. The lower critical amorphization dose and lower activation energy for recovery of $Ca_{10}(PO_4)_6F_2$ are attributed to the weaker P-O bond and the higher fluorine mobility in the structure.

INTRODUCTION

Radiation effects in crystalline phases with the apatite structure are of interest to the biomedical, geoscience and materials science communities. Natural apatites with variable halogen compositions $[Ca_{10}(PO_4)_6(F,OH,Cl)_2]$ are used by geoscientists to place constraints on the thermochronologic conditions under which portions of the Earth evolved.[1] Rare-earth-silicate isomorphs of these naturally occurring apatites may be actinide hosts in the ceramic nuclear waste forms.[2] Comparison of these materials with different compositions but the same crystal structure provides an excellent opportunity to investigate bond type/strength controls on radiation effects in the crystal structure. This will be the basis for ion beam modification of apatite in order to change its physical and chemical properties for technological and biomedical applications.

EXPERIMENTAL PROCEDURE

The two apatites studied are $Ca_{10}(PO_4)_6F_2$ and $Ca_2La_8(SiO_4)_6O_2$. The former is a naturally occurring apatite from Durango, Mexico and the latter is synthetic. Both samples were undamaged single crystals in the scale of a transmission electron microscopy (TEM) specimen before the ion irradiations.

* Department of Earth and Planetary Sciences, University of New Mexico, Albuquerque, NM 87131.

** Division of Earth Sciences, National Science Foundation,, Washington DC 20550.

† Department of Materials Science, Pacific Northwest Laboratory, Richland, WA 99352.

†† Department of Geology, Miami University, Oxford, OH 45056.

0-8493-4750-5/94/$0.00 + $.50

TEM specimens were prepared by ion milling the well polished thin sections with the c-axis parallel to the foil normal. Although $Ca_{10}(PO_4)_6F_2$ was readily damaged by electron beams[3], it never became amorphous under intense irradiation of 200 keV to 1 MeV electrons at room temperature in this study.

The TEM samples were irradiated with 1.5 MeV Kr ions at various temperatures, from near liquid helium temperature (15 K) to 680 K in the HVEM-Tandem Facility at Argonne National Laboratory[4]. The facility consists a high-voltage TEM linked with a tandem ion accelerator so that the radiation damage process induced by ion beams can be monitored with *in situ* TEM. The ion irradiations were performed at dose rates near $\sim 10^{12}$ ions/cm^{2}s (or 10^{-2} ions/nm^{2}s). During the ion irradiations, the sample temperature was continuously monitored and its increase due to beam heating was < 50 °C. The critical dose for the ion beam induced amorphization was determined by selected area electron diffraction at the point where all the diffraction maxima from the crystalline phase disappeared. A 300 keV electron beam was used for the *in situ* observation. Before and after ion irradiation at various doses, a group of $Ca_2La_8(SiO_4)_6O_2$ samples were also examined by high resolution TEM (HRTEM) with a TOPCON 002B electron microscope at the TOPCON demonstration center in Japan. The microscope was operated at 200 kV.

RESULTS AND DISCUSSION

All of the samples irradiated with 1.5 MeV Kr ions have been amorphized, but after various ion doses. The progressive amorphization process was evidenced by the changes in electron diffraction pattern. At first, a diffuse halo appeared, and its intensity increased with increasing ion dose. Concurrently, the diffraction maxima from the crystalline volume became progressively less intense and completely vanished at a critical amorphization dose. A typical series of electron diffraction pattern obtained during the *in situ* experiment is shown in Fig. 1.

Under HRTEM imaging, areas with mottled contrast of 2 to 3 nm in size (the size of a displacement cascade) first appeared in a otherwise perfect high resolution lattice fringe image after a very low dose of irradiation (Fig. 2 (B)). With increased dose, the size of these areas increased and the lattice fringes were disrupted within these regions manifesting the overlapping of the cascades in projection. Finally, the lattice fringes completely disappeared at even higher doses. It should be mentioned that the sensitivity of the HRTEM imaging to the amorphous volume within the specimen depends on the local sample thickness as demonstrated both theoretically[5] and experimentally.[6] Nevertheless, the series of the HRTEM images showed qualitatively the progressive amorphization process in near atomic scale.

Figure 3 presents temperature dependence of critical amorphization ion doses for both $Ca_{10}(PO_4)_6F_2$ and $Ca_2La_8(SiO_4)_6O_2$ under 1.5 MeV Kr ion irradiations. Because the composition and density of the target affect the nuclear stopping power or collision efficiency, it is more reasonable to compare the critical amorphization dose in the unit of displacement per atom (dpa) rather than compare the critical Kr dose directly. To do so, a threshold displacement energy, E_d, of 25 eV was first assumed since no data on this energy is available for either of the two materials. Computer code TRIM[7] was then used to calculate the damage production per 1.5 MeV Kr ion per unit length (nm) in these two materials. The results are plotted against the sample depth as shown in figure 4. Since the electron transparent thickness of a TEM specimen is about 200 nm, the damage production data at the 100 nm depth were used to be the average value for the observed sample thickness. Thus, the data in figure 3 were converted to amorphization dose in dpa versus temperature as shown in figure 5.

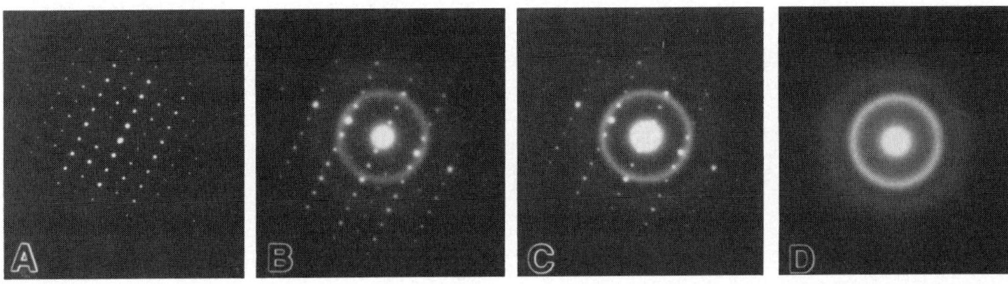

Figure 1. Electron diffraction patterns of $Ca_2La_8(SiO_4)_6O_2$ before and after 1.5 MeV Kr ion irradiation at 300 K. (A) Unirradiated, (B) 1.7, (C) 2.55, and (D) 4.25 ions/nm^2.

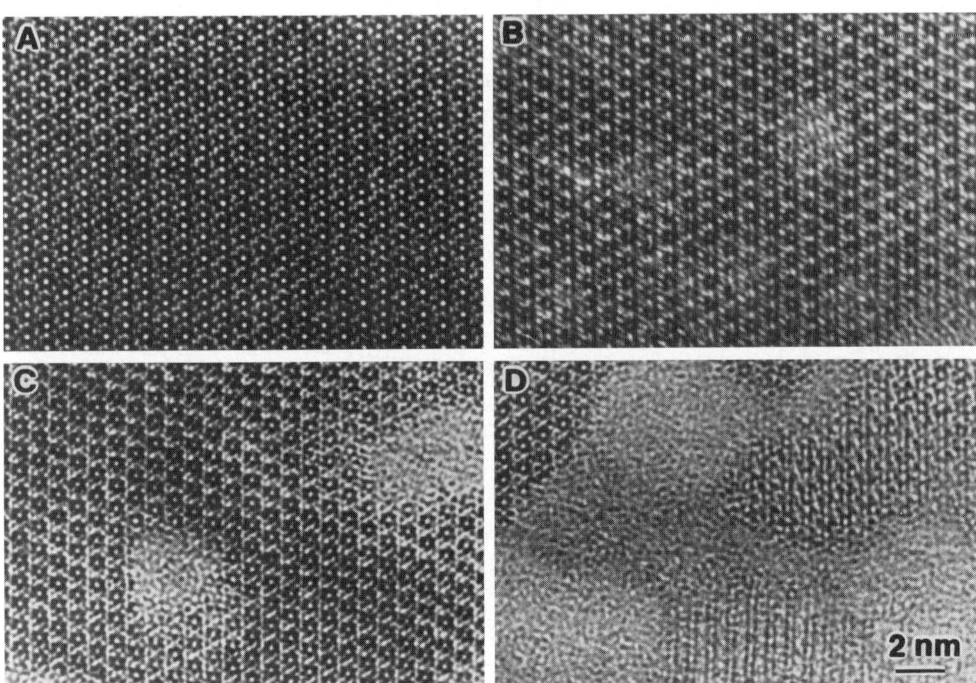

Figure 2. HRTEM micrographs of $Ca_2La_8(SiO_4)_6O_2$ before and after 1.5 MeV Kr ion irradiation at 300 K. (A) Unirradiated, (B) 0.25, (C) 0.51, and (D) 2.04 ions/nm^2.

A important observation of this study is that $Ca_{10}(PO_4)_6F_2$ became amorphized at lower doses than $Ca_2La_8(SiO_4)_6O_2$. at temperatures below 350 K, but the critical amorphization dose increased much more rapidly for the former than the latter at higher temperatures. At 475 K, $Ca_{10}(PO_4)_6F_2$ required nearly five times of higher dose to become amorphous than $Ca_2La_8(SiO_4)_6O_2$.

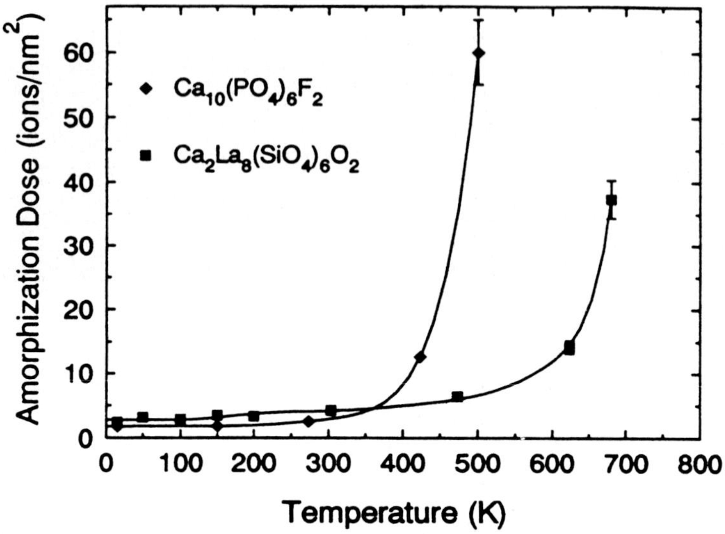

Figure 3. Comparison of temperature dependence of critical amorphization doses of $Ca_{10}(PO_4)_6F_2$ and $Ca_2La_8(SiO_4)_6O_2$ under 1.5 MeV Kr ion irradiation.

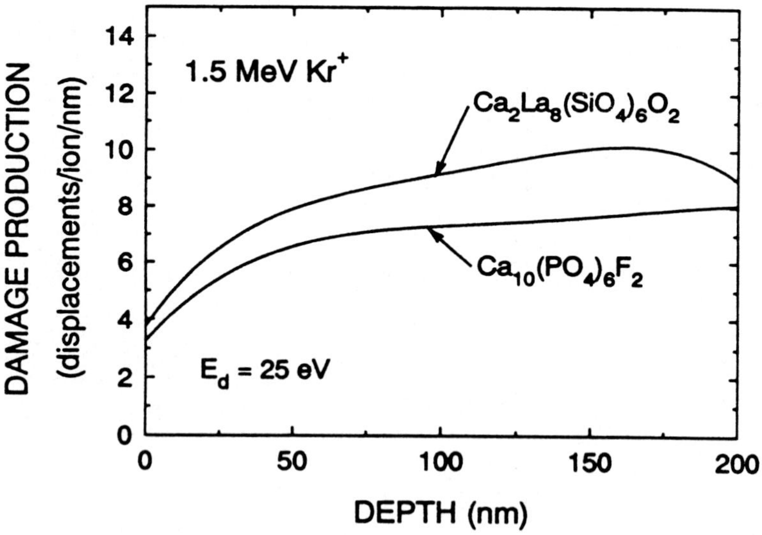

Figure 4. Damage production in 1.5 MeV Kr ion irradiated $Ca_{10}(PO_4)_6F_2$ and $Ca_2La_8(SiO_4)_6O_2$ calculated by the TRIM code[7]. A displacement energy of 25 eV was assumed for both materials.

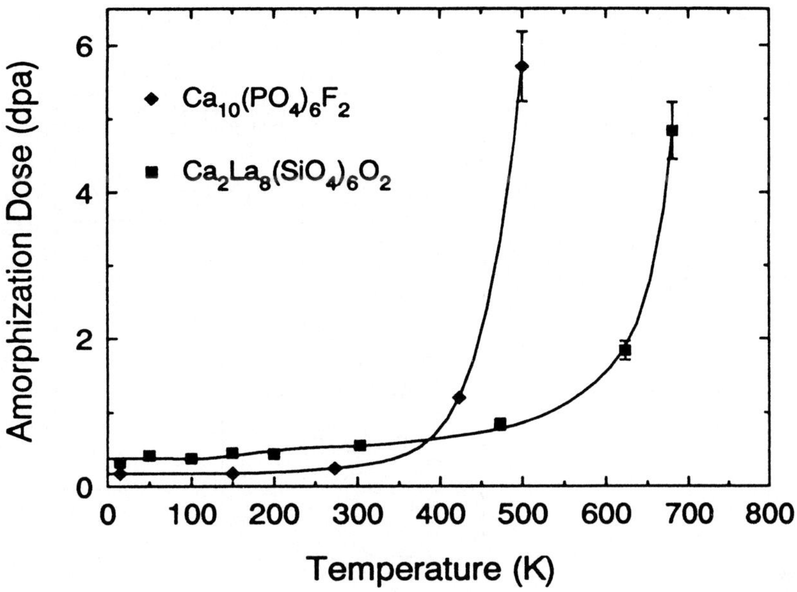

Figure 5. Comparison of temperature dependence of critical amorphization doses in displacement per atom (dpa) for 1.5 MeV Kr ion irradiated $Ca_{10}(PO_4)_6F_2$ and $Ca_2La_8(SiO_4)_6O_2$.

During ion beam irradiation of crystalline oxide ceramics, two competing processes, cascade formation and relaxation/annealing occur almost simultaneously. Although the recovery (or annealing) process is dominant at higher temperatures and can be enhanced by continued irradiation through irradiation enhanced diffusion, it is greatly suppressed at low temperatures. We assume annealing is completely suppressed at near 0 K, the two materials should become amorphous at the same displacement damage level. However, the data at 15 K in figure 5 show $Ca_{10}(PO_4)_6F_2$ and $Ca_2La_8(SiO_4)_6O_2$ amorphized at 0.17 dpa and 0.32 dpa respectively. This suggests that the E_d for the F-apatite has been overestimated for the TRIM calculation. The real value may be a factor of two less than that for $Ca_2La_8(SiO_4)_6O_2$.

Using a method of analysis described in detail by Weber[8], an activation energy, E_a, associated with the dynamic annealing process and a critical temperature, T_c, above which amorphization can not be completed can be determined from the amorphization dose-temperature curve. The relationship between temperature and dose required for complete amorphization is given by: $\ln(1-D_0/D) = C-E_a/kT$, where C is a constant dependent on dose rate and amorphization cross section, and D_0 is the amorphization dose at T=0 K. An Arrhenius plot of $\ln(1-D_0/D)$ versus $1/kT$ yields $-E_a$ as the slope (figure 6). Once C and E_a are determined, T_c can be obtained by: $T_c = E_a/kC$. Activation energies for recrystallization were determined to be 0.07 eV for $Ca_{10}(PO_4)_6F_2$ and 0.13 eV for $Ca_2La_8(SiO_4)_6O_2$, and the T_c were estimated to be 475 K for $Ca_{10}(PO_4)_6F_2$ and 711 K for $Ca_2La_8(SiO_4)_6O_2$.

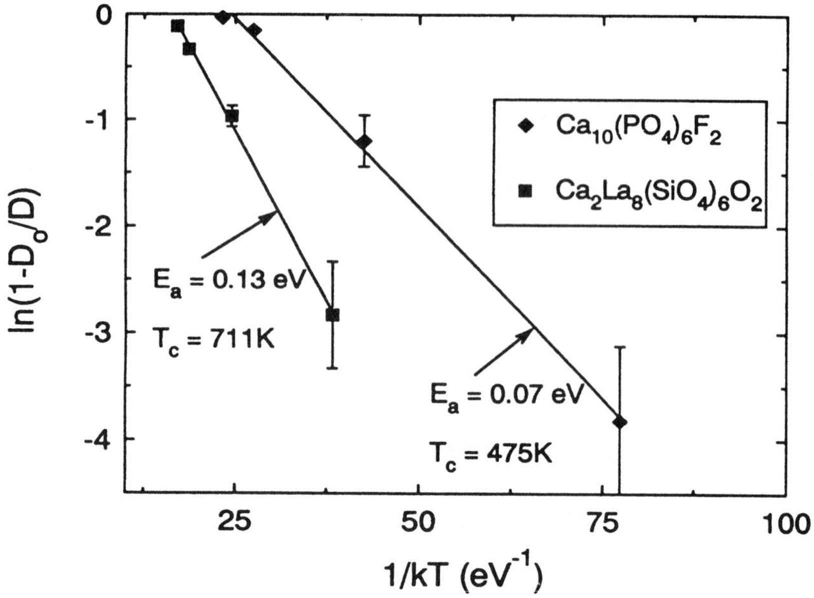

Figure 6. Arrhenius plot of ln $(1-D_0/D)$ versus 1/KT for 1.5 MeV Kr ion irradiated $Ca_{10}(PO_4)_6F_2$ and $Ca_2La_8(SiO_4)_6O_2$.

Since the two materials have the same apatite crystal structure, the difference in irradiation response must be attributed to the difference in crystal chemistry or the bond type/strength (differences in density and collision cross section have been addressed in the TRIM calculation). As a first approximation, we have examined the strength of the two diatomic bonds, P-O and Si-O. The bond energy for P-O and Si-O are 6.18 and 8.39 eV/molecule respectively. Apparently, the weaker the bond, the easier for displacement of the atoms (lower displacement energy, lower amorphization dose at 0 K). Also, earlier study on metamictization of minerals has shown that with the lower bond energy, the energy barrier to recrystallization during damage accumulation is also lower[9], thus the rapid increase of amorphization dose with temperature for $Ca_{10}(PO_4)_6F_2$ (lower activation for recovery, higher amorphization at high temperature) can also be attributed to the weaker P-O bond. In addition, Welch and Royce[10] have reported that the energies of motion for fluorine and oxygen ions in apatite are 0.77 eV and 2.0 eV, respectively. This high mobility of fluorine in $Ca_{10}(PO_4)_6F_2$ must contribute positively to the damage annealing process, so supports the observations in this study.

CONCLUSIONS

Both $Ca_{10}(PO_4)_6F_2$ and $Ca_2La_8(SiO_4)_6O_2$ have been amorphized by 1.5 MeV Kr ion irradiations. At lower temperatures (below 350 K), $Ca_{10}(PO_4)_6F_2$ amorphized at lower doses than $Ca_2La_8(SiO_4)_6O_2$ because of its low displacement energy. At higher temperatures, $Ca_{10}(PO_4)_6F_2$ required higher doses than $Ca_2La_8(SiO_4)_6O_2$ to be completely amorphized because it has a lower energy barrier to recrystallization. The lower displacement energy and lower activation energy for recovery (or recrystallization) in $Ca_{10}(PO_4)_6F_2$ are associated with the lower energy of the P-O bonds and the higher fluorine mobility. Activation energies for recrystallization under the irradiation condition were determined to be 0.07 eV for $Ca_{10}(PO_4)_6F_2$ and 0.13 eV for $Ca_2La_8(SiO_4)_6O_2$ respectively, and the critical temperatures above which complete amorphization can not be achieved were estimated to be 475 K for $Ca_{10}(PO_4)_6F_2$ and 711 K for $Ca_2La_8(SiO_4)_6O_2$.

ACKNOWLEDGMENTS

The authors thank the HVEM-Tandem Facility staff at Argonne National Laboratory for assistance during the ion irradiation, Shixin Wang of the University of New Mexico for TEM sample preparation, K. Moriyama of Topcon Inc. for assistance on HRTEM. This work was supported by the Division of Materials Sciences, Office of Basic Energy Sciences, U.S. Department of Energy under Contract DE-AC06-76RLO 1830 and Grant DE-FG04-84ER45099.

REFERENCES

1. K.D. Crowley et al., *Fission Track Analysis: Theory & Applications,* Geol. Soc. Amer. Shortcourse (1989).
2. W.J. Weber, J. Mater. Res. 6, 1334, 1991.
3. M. Cameron, L.M. Wang, K.D. Crowley and R.C. Ewing, Proc. 50th Annual Meeting of the Electron Microscopy Society of America, San Francisco Press, 1992, p. 378.
4. C.W. Allen, L.L. Funk, E.A. Ryan, and A. Taylor, Nucl. Instr. and Meth. B40/41, 553, 1989.
5. M.L. Miller and R.C. Ewing, Ultramicroscopy 48, 203, 1993.
6. L.M. Wang and W.J. Weber, Proc. 51th Annual Meeting of the Electron Microscopy Society of America, San Francisco Press, 1993, in press.
7. J.F. Ziegler, J.P. Biersack and U. Littmark, *The Stopping and Range of Ions in Solids* (Pergamon, New York, 1985).
8. W.J. Weber and L.M. Wang, Mater. Res. Sym. Proc. 279, 1993, in press.
9. R.C. Ewing, B.C. Chakoumakos, G.R. Lumpkin and T. Murakami, *MRS Bulletin,* May/June 1987, p. 58.
10. D.O. Welch and B.S.H. Royce, Phys. Stat. Sol. (b) 57, 193, 1973.

CARBONATE-CONTAINING EUROPIUM APATITE

J. L. Lacout and A. Taïtaï
Laboratoire des Matériaux - Physico-Chimie des Solides
ENSCT-INPT, URA 445 - 38, rue des Trente-Six Ponts
Fr - 31400 Toulouse, France.

ABSTRACT

It is possible to prepare by a gas-solid reaction europium-containing strontium apatite which contain, in the channels, up to two carbonate ions per unit cell. Above one ion per unit cell, the number of neighbouring carbonate ions increases and their distorsion can be seen by infrared spectrometry, especially by the distance of the V_3 band in the range 1420-1550 cm^{-1}.

A. INTRODUCTION

Apatites form a large family of calcium phosphate minerals isomorphous with hydroxyapatite $Ca_{10}(PO_4)_6(OH)_2$. They are most frequently found to be crystallized in the hexagonal system with a space group of $P6_3/m$. A characteristic of the apatitic structure is the existence of channels, containing the OH^- ions (1, 2).

It is well known that carbonate ions can be introduced into two sites of the apatitic structure: either replacing the PO_4 groups—these apatites are called B-type carbonated apatites (3) —or replacing OH^- anions in the channels. These apatites are called A-type carbonated apatites (4-5).

In the latter case it is quite easy to substitute one $CO_3^=$ ion for two hydroxyl ions. It was interesting to try to introduce more than one carbonate ion per unit cell and to observe the modifications of both the lattice and the carbonate ions.

In the channels in an apatite, just two negative charges exists. Of course, the introduction of more than one divalent ion (like the carbonate ion) into a channel increases the negative charge by more than 2, so the charge balance must be preserved. The chosen solution was to increase the positive charge by substituting a trivalent europium ion for a divalent cation.

In this paper only results obtained with strontium phosphate apatites will be described.

0-8493-4750-5/94/$0.00 + $.50

B. SYNTHESIS

The starting material was a europium-containing strontium oxyapatite previously prepared by a solid/solid reaction,

$$Sr_{10-x}\ Eu_x\ (PO_4)_6\ O_{1+x/2}\ \grave{O}_{1-x/2}\ ,$$

with x equal to 0.05; 0.10; 0.15 ; 0.20.

In these apatites trivalent europium balances the charge and it is possible to introduce up to two oxide ions into the channels (6).

Note that it has been proved that in these apatites, europium ions are located in the cationic sites around the channels, close to the oxide ions $O^{=}$ (7); in this configuration the charge is balanced in the smallest possible volume.

These apatites were prepared by a gas-solid reaction, at 900°C, under CO_2 for about 100 hours. This treatment was repeated until X-ray diffraction patterns and IR spectra became constant.

The expected reaction was:

$$Sr_{10-x}\ Eu_x\ (PO_4)_6\ O_{1+x/2}\grave{O}_{1-x/2} \text{ ------> }$$

$$Sr_{10-x}\ Eu_x\ (PO_4)_6\ (CO_3)_{1+x/2}\partial_{1-x/2}$$

C. RESULTS AND DISCUSSION

For all the compounds it was necessary to repeat the treatments three or four times. Of course, modifications of the starting materials were observed.

1. X-ray Diffraction

The patterns show that after treatment, all the solids were pure apatitic phases with no extra phases such as strontium oxide, europium oxides or carbonates. The lattice constants are reported in Table 1.

Table 1
a and c lattice constants A (± 0.003).

	Carbonated apatites		Oxyapatites	
Eu/(Eu+Sr)	a	c	a	c
0.20	9.892	7.219	9.658	7.185
0.15	9.887	7.212	9.675	7.207
0.10	9.899	7.233	9.692	7.214
0.05	M	M	9.720	7.221
0.00	M	M	9.713	7.243

At low europium content, x = 0.5, the apatitic structure is monoclinic. This is in aggreement with previous observations on carbonate apatite containing less than one carbonate ion (8). It is the same with just over one carbonate ion. On both sides of the value of 1 carbonate ion per unit cell i.e. in the concentration range 0.90 to 1.10, the carbonate ions and the vacancies have a definite order in the channels. Both parameters a and c increase from oxyapatite to carbonate apatite. The general rule for apatites that the substitution in the channels of an ion for a smaller one induces a decrease of parameter c and an increase of parameter a is not followed here. This remark can be correlated with the fact that parameter a remains almost constant in the carbonate series whatever the amount of europium or carbonate. These observations will be discussed later.

2. Carbonate content

The carbonate content (Table 2) was determined for each sample by thermogravimetric analysis up to 1350°C. These carbonate-containing apatites were especially stable; this fact has also been observed for other carbonate apatites prepared in a CO_2 atmosphere at high pressures.

Table 2
Carbonate content

Eu/(Eu + Sr)	0.20	0.15	0.10	0.05
Number of CO_3 ions (theoretical)	2.00	1.75	1.50	1.25
loss of weight (%)	4.69	4.22	3.48	3.26
Number of CO_3 ions (experimental)	1.81	1.58	1.38	1.15

After heating to 1350°C, carbonate ions disappear entirely from the structure so that the remaining solids are identical with the starting oxyapatites. Carbonatation is a reversible reaction.

3. Infrared spectra

The infrared spectra of carbonate apatites are reported in Figure 1. First, two PO_4^{3-} bands appear at 1105 cm^{-1} in the case of low europium content, that is to say low carbonate content. This is well-known for oxyapatite. It is correlated with the presence of vacancies in the anion sites in the channels. The most interesting observation can be made on carbonate ions: in the range 1400-1650 cm^{-1} appear four bands, which can be attributed to carbonate ions. A-type carbonate apatite presents only two bands for the totally degenerate ν_3 mode. AB-type carbonate apatite, which is an apatite containing simultaneously carbonate ions in the channels and the PO_4^{3-} sites, presents three bands in the range 1400-1600 (9). Also AB-type apatite presents two bands at 870 cm^{-1} whereas, here, just one band was observed. X-ray diffraction confirmed that only one pure apatitic phase was present and so the bands are not due to an extra phase.

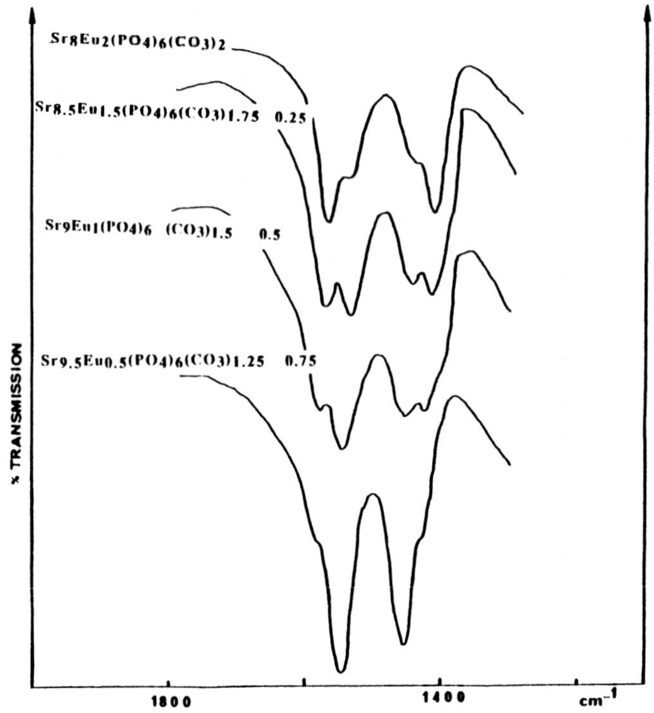

Figure 1. Infrared bands for various amount of carbonate.

Concerning these four bands, some other observations can be made. First, the inner bands (1460-1550 cm^{-1}) were in the same positions as in strontium carbonate apatite (10). Secondly the relative variation of the intensities of the four bands was correlated with the europium content (or the carbonate content): when the carbonate content increased, the intensity of the outer bands increased and the intensity of the inner bands decreased. At the limits, in the apatite $x = 0.5$ containing 1.15 carbonate ions per unit cell, the infrared bands were quite similar to the classical strontium apatite carbonate bands. However, when $x = 2$, the number of carbonate ions was 1.85, close to two ions per unit cell, the most intense bands were the outer bands and a simple shoulder occurred corresponding to the inner bands. It clearly appears that these four bands occur in two pairs.

Therefore, the existence of two kinds of carbonate in the channel can be proposed. And the explanation can be found with the modifications and the distortions of the carbonate ion, a large ion, in the channels.

Carbonate ions, formed by three oxygens placed in a plane around one carbon atom, are easily distorted. The distortions can be correlated to the distance between the two infra-red bands of the ν_3 mode. This is well-known for example in the case of arseniocalcium apatite and phosphocalcium apatite (11).

In the case of apatite which contains more than one carbonate ion per unit cell the increase of large carbonate ions in the channel induces their distortion. Three possibilities can exist: (i) a carbonate ion surrounded by two vacancies; (ii) a carbonate ion surrounded by one vacancy and another carbonate ion; (iii) a carbonate ion surrounded by two other carbonate ions. The two first situations can be found in carbonate apatite containing one or fewer carbonate ions per unit cell and the third situation can only exist in apatites which contain more than one carbonate ion per unit cell. This is in agreement with the increase of the outer bands, connected with the distorted carbonate, that is to say also with a high carbonate content. The distortion of the carbonate ions can also be correlated with the observations we have made about the lattice modifications. Parameter a remains constant and the volume of the unit cell also remains quite constant because the carbonate ions are distorted.

D. CONCLUSIONS

It is possible to prepare strontium apatite which contains more than one carbonate ion in the channels; it is of course necessary to preserve the charge balance, for instance by the substituion of trivalent europium for divalent strontium. In these conditions it is possible to introduce almost two carbonate ions by unit cell.

Apatitic structure is conserved ; the lattice constants, especially a, and the the unit cell volume do not significantly increase, because carbonate ions which are distorted and of course, the higher the carbonate content, the higher the number of distorted carbonates. Infrared can differentiate distorded and non-distorded carbonate ions.

REFERENCES

1. S. Naray-Szabo Zeitsch. Krist 75:323 (1930).
2. M. I. Kay, R. A. Young, and A. S. Posner, Nature 204:1050 (1964).
3. G. Bonel, Ann. Chim 7:127 (1972).
4. R. Wallaeys and C. R Coll, Intern. Chim. Münster Westph. 183 (1954).
5. A. N. Akhavan Niaki, Thèse, Paris (1959).
6. A. Taïtaï and J. L. Lacout, Ann. Chim. Fr. 18:31 (1993).
7. B. Piriou, D. Fahmi, J. Dexpert, A. TaïTaï and J. L. Lacout, J. Lum. 39(2):97 (1987).
8. G. Bonel and G. Montel, C. R. Acad. Sci. 263:1010 (1966).
9. R. Z. Legeros, O. R. Trautz, J. P. Legeros, and E. Klein, Bull. Soc. Chim. Fr. (Special Issue) 1712 (1968).
10. J. C. Trombe, Thèse, Toulouse (1972).
11. P. Roux, Thèse , Toulouse (1982).

APATITE CHANNELS AND ZEOLITE-LIKE PROPERTIES

Christian Rey
Laboratoire des Materiaux - Physico-chimie des Solides
ENSCT-INPT, URA CNRS 445,
38 rue des 36 ponts 31400 Toulouse, France

I. INTRODUCTION

Among the descriptions of the apatite structure, that suggested by Beevers and McIntyre,[1] showing channels aligned along the c axis, has received most attention. This description establishes an analogy between the apatite structure and that of zeolites. It explains some of the chemical properties of the apatite such as ion substitution reactions at high temperatures and ion exchange properties. However, another property of zeolites—the ability to trap molecules—was long to be discovered in apatites. This report is aimed at a description of apatite-containing molecules, their preparation conditions and some of their unusual properties. Let us first take a closer look at apatite channels.

II. GEOMETRY OF APATITE CHANNELS

A. DETERMINATION OF THE CHANNEL SIZE

Apatite channels are limited by the triangle of metallic cation II ions (Me) located at c/4 in the hexagonal structure and the distorted hexagon of oxygen III atoms belonging to the tetrahedral XO_4 groups located at c/2 (Figure 1).

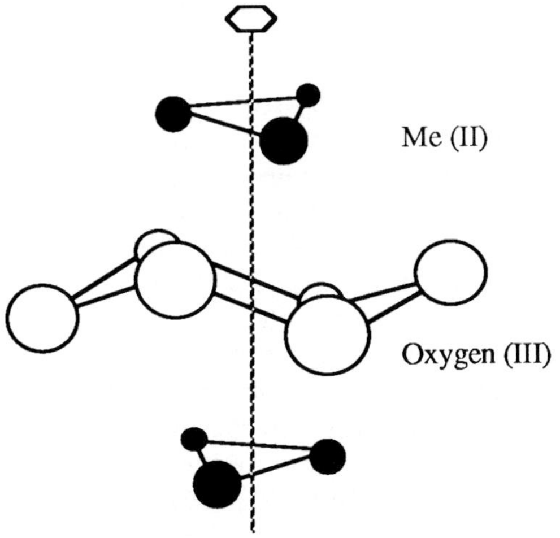

Figure 1. The apatite channels. The Me (II) triangles at c/4 and 3c/4 (where c is the unit-cell dimension along the hexagonal axis) and the oxygen (III) atoms, forming a distorted hexagon at c/2 determine the borders of the apatite channels

0-8493-4750-5/94/$0.00 + $.50

Several structural determinations have been made on apatites, and one notable property is that in most cases the distance of Me II ions and of oxygen III from the center of the channel is given with a good approximation by the following formula[2]:

Table 1
Channel dimensions of some apatites (Å).

Apatite (Me, X, Y)	c/2	c/4
Ca, P, F	2.97	2.61
Ca, P, OH	2.85	2.73
Ca, P, Cl	3.36	2.97
Cd, P, OH	2.89	2.69
Sr, P, OH	3.28	2.65
Ba, P, Cl	3.84	2.50

$$x\,(\text{Me II}) = 0.25\,a\ (\pm 0.01\,a) \qquad x\,(\text{O III}) = 0.31\,a\ (\pm 0.01\,a)$$

depending only on the a unit-cell dimension. Therefore it has been possible to evaluate the channel diameters of numerous apatites, knowing only the unit-cell dimensions.

The apatite channels can be described as a succession of ovoid cavities, with their largest diameters at c/2 and a neck at c/4 (Figure 2). Their size depends on the composition of the apatite; when the cation diameter increases the channels neck at c/4 narrows whereas the diameter at c/2 increases. When the dimension of the XO_4 group increases, both diameters increase. The monovalent Y anions, which are located in the channels, have only a weak influence on their dimensions, except for calcium-phosphate apatites.

Therefore it is possible to vary the channels dimensions in the apatite structure by appropriate substitution. Table 1 shows the channels dimensions of several apatites based on Shannon and Prewitt's ionic radii of atoms.[3] The channels appear quite narrow and only small molecules might be trapped.

B. AVAILABILITY OF THE CHANNEL SPACE

In stoichiometric apatites the channels are occupied by monovalent anions (Y) which leave no space for molecules, and it is only in non-stoichiometric apatites, presenting Y vacancies, that the trapping of molecules can be observed. Non-stoichiometry presents very different forms in apatites and vacancies in the channels are quite common in synthetic as well as in natural compounds. Such compounds may result from the substitution of a monovalent Y anion by a divalent one and a vacancy such as in type A carbonate apatite or in oxyapatite. More frequently, highly non-stoichiometric apatites can be obtained from the substitution of a trivalent XO_4 group by a divalent one, this leads to the loss of a negative charge which is then compensated by a complex defect consisting of a cationic vacancy and a monovalent Y anionic vacancy.[4] Bone mineral and most synthetic carbonate apatites satisfy closely this substitution scheme, and can present almost empty channels. If the cationic vacancies are located on cationic site II, apatites may then exhibit broad cavities in their lattice, available for molecule trapping. However, despite the presence of these empty spaces, small molecules cannot be incorporated into non-stoichiometric apatites using the techniques conventionally used for zeolites. This impossibility is due to the difficulty to reach the cavities from the outside of the crystals. In fact the Y ions, still present in the channels, are tangent to the cationic II triangle, as shown by structural determinations in numerous apatites.[2] These associations are very stable due to the electrostatic attraction of ions. Thus, the channels are in fact segmented by residual Y ions, acting like corks, and most of the space cannot be reached by diffusion.

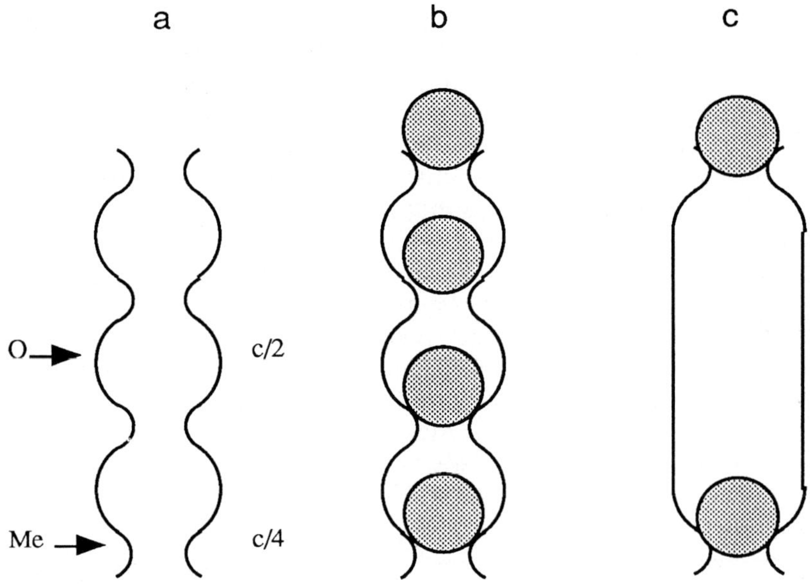

Figure 2. View of the apatite channels (a). In stoichiometric apatites all the channel space is occupied by the monovalent Y ions (b). In non-stoichiometric apatites large void cavities may exist in the structure due to the existence of Y and Me vacancies.

The portion of the channels which can be directly accessed from the outside of the crystals can be evaluated on a statistical basis. If y represents the ratio of anionic Y vacancies and if M is the average number of unit cells in a crystal along the c direction. Then the portion P of channels open to the outside is given by :

$$P = y/(1-y)M$$

A calculation based on a crystal of 100 unit-cells with 90% vacant Y sites shows that only 9 % of the empty space can be accessed. The elongated shape of apatites crystals along the c axis, is a further obstacle for the manifestation of their ability to trap small molecules. Despite these difficulties, such open spaces in the apatite structure, even if they are small, could be implicated in the adsorption ability of apatites and their role as catalyst support.

Although apatites cannot be considered to behave like zeolites, one may wonder if there is no possibility to trap molecules in the cavities of non-stoichiometric forms like in clathrates.

III. MOLECULE-CONTAINING APATITES (EXAMPLES)

Two types of process may lead to molecular trapping in apatites, the intracrystalline decomposition of unstable ions of the structure, the synthesis of apatites in solutions containing the molecules to incorporate. The first process is illustrated by molecular oxygen trapping in apatites; the second by glycine-containing apatites.

A. OXYGEN-CONTAINING APATITES

The trapping of molecular, oxygen, was reported for the first time by Simpson.[5] It was shown later that the trapping of molecular oxygen occurred from the decomposition of unstable peroxide ions inside the structure.[6]

Such intracrystalline decomposition was associated with the formation of hydroxide ions and the amount of oxygen trapped in the lattice was directly related to the vacant Y sites in the channels as shown in Figure 3. In this case the trapping capabilities of the structure are dependent on the proportion of the initial peroxide ions in the channels which varies with the composition of the apatite[2] and is roughly related to the channels dimensions (Figure 4). A rather spectacular feature of the oxygen-containing apatites is that the molecules are released at very high temperatures 600°-700°C when the non-stoichiometric structure itself begins to collapse. This temperature is at least a hundred degrees above the release temperature of water molecules (200°-500°C). This behavior can be related to the size of the molecules themselves and their diffusion capabilities in the narrow space of the channels.

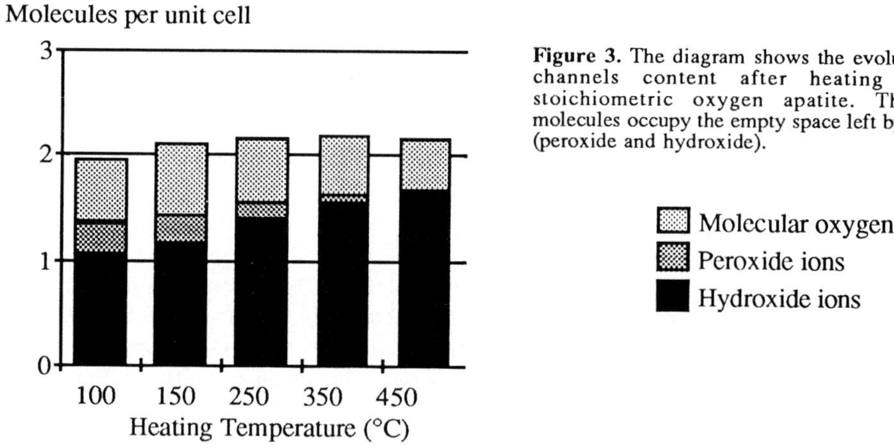

Figure 3. The diagram shows the evolution of the channels content after heating a nearly stoichiometric oxygen apatite. The oxygen molecules occupy the empty space left by the anions (peroxide and hydroxide).

The size of the crystals is also a parameter which determines the temperature of oxygen release. On apatites with increasing specific surface area, one can observe that the release temperature is lower for apatites with a high specific surface area (i.e. a small crystal size).[2] The trapping ability thus appears to be linked to the degree of confinement : small crystals with trapping sites in the vicinity of the outside are less efficient than large crystals with higher crystallinity and stronger cohesiveness.

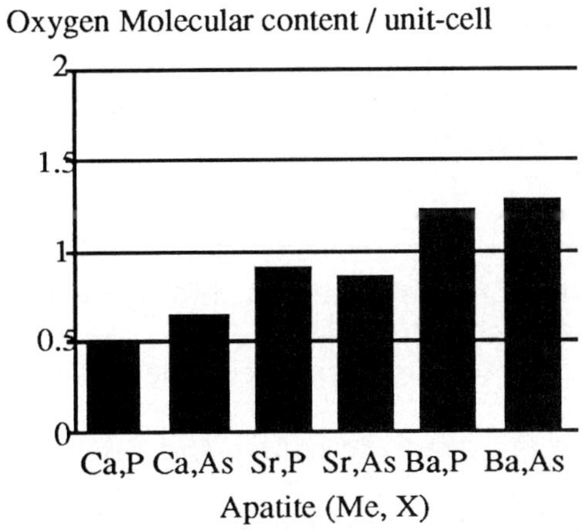

Figure 4. Oxygen uptake and apatite composition. The trapping of oxygen results from the decomposition of peroxide ions initially present in the structure and of the channels dimensions and occupancy. The amount of trapped molecules is roughly related to the size of the channels.

B. GLYCINE-CONTAINING APATITES

Another category of molecular trapping occurs during the formation of apatite crystals. The best example of these compounds is given by glycine apatites When the synthesis medium contains the smallest amino acid, glycine, it is possible to trap these smallmolecules in the apatites.[7] Glycine uptake seems more complex than that of oxygen: glycine is taken up under two ionic forms the glycinate ion and the bipolar ions. Y anionic vacancies are not sufficient to trap the molecule and it was shown that cationic vacancies were also needed[7] (Table 2).

Table 2
Influence of cationic and anionic vacancies on glycine uptake

Apatite	Me Vacancies	Y Vacancies	Glycine molar content
Lead, Non-stoichiometric	0.9	1.8	0.51
Lead, Nearly stoichiometric,	0.3	0.6	0.34
Lead, sodium	0.2	1.6	0.18

It was postulated that the anionic part of the molecule was located on a Y anionic site in the channel whereas the cationic part occupied a cationic site. As for oxygen, the uptake of glycine was shown to be related to the channel size: calcium apatites trapped only a very small amount of molecules while strontium and lead apatites could trap up to 0.58 glycine molecules per unit cell.[8]

CONCLUSION

The apatite channels may afford a high concentration of vacancies where molecules can be trapped. The existence of residual anions and the elongated shape of the crystals does not allow, however, the release or the exchange of these molecules and the manifestation of a zeolite-like behavior. The small proportion of channels open to the outside might, however, play a role in adsorption or catalytic properties of apatites which are still to be investigated. The synthesis of apatites in non-aqueous media, especially, is an interesting path to follow to prepare molecules-containing apatites.

REFERENCES

1. Beevers A., McIntyre D.B., Atomic structure of fluorapatite and its relation to tooth and bone materialn, *Miner. Mag.* 27, 254, 1947.
2. Rey C., Relations entre apatites et composés moléculaires, Thèse d'Etat, INPT, Toulouse 1984.
3. Shannon R.D., Prewitt C.T., Effective ionic radii in oxides and fluorides, *Acta Crys.* B25, 925, 1969.
4. Bonel G., Contribution à l'étude des apatites carbonatées, *Ann. Chim.* 7, 127, 1972.
5. Simpson D.R., Oxygen-rich apatite, *Amer. Miner.* 53, 432, 1968.
6. Rey C., Trombe J.C., Montel G.,Sur des apatites oxygénées contenant de l'oxygène à différents degrés d'oxydation, *C.R. Acad. Sci. Paris*, B 276, 559, 1971 .
7. Rey C., Trombe J.C., Montel G., Some aspect of glycine uptake in the apatitic structure, *J. Chem. Res.* S 188, M 2401, 1978.
8. Kodera M., Rey C., Trombe J.C., Montel G. A model for the mineral-organic bond in calcified tissues, *Proc. 5th International Workshop on calcified Tissues.* Elsevier, Amsterdam, 258, 1982.

PREPARATION OF CALCIUM PHOSPHATE POWDERS BY WATER EXTRACTION VARIANT OF SOL-GEL PROCESS

A. Deptuła,* T. Olczak,* W. Łada,* A. Borello,** C. Alvani,**
L. Lorenzini** and A. DiBartolomeo**
Institute of Nuclear Chemistry and Technology, Warsaw, Poland
*ENEA, C.R.E. Casaccia, Italy

ABSTRACT

The starting sols were prepared by ultrasonic mixing of concentrated solutions of calcium nitrate (5M), $Ca(OH)_2$ slurry or calcium acetate (1.7M) with 85% H_3PO_4 followed by emulsification in dehydrated 2-ethyl-1-hexanol. Drops of emulsion were solidified by extraction of water with this solvent. The process was carried out continuously. When starting from acetate sols spherical powders were obtained. Irregularly shaped powders were obtained from nitrate sols and $Ca(OH)_2$ slurry. In all cases, particle diameters were below 100 microns. The separated gel particles were calcined to calcium phosphates with molar ratio Ca/P from 0.8 to 2.8. This process was studied using differential thermal analysis (DTA), thermogravimetry (TG), x-ray diffraction analysis (XRD) and infrared spectrometry (IR). Hydroxyapatite was obtained from acetate Ca-P gels. However for Ca/P molar ratios higher than 2 the product contained CaO or even $CaCO_3$.

INTRODUCTION

Calcium-deficient hydroxyapatite is the main inorganic phase present in the bone.[1,2] Calcium phosphate ceramics, especially hydroxyapatite (HA) and tricalcium phosphate (TCP) are the most commonly used bone substitutes. These compounds are widely used as implants to repair hard tissues, generally in the form of dense shapes, porous bodies or coatings on metals devices.[3]

In a previous paper[4] it was reported that we had obtained HA spherical powders with diameters <100 microns by sol-gel process. Spherical powders of ceramics are very suitable for preparation of coatings by plasma-spraying technique.[5] However one of the present authors[6] has found that sintering of pellets prepared from this medium-sized spherical powder is poor, and the sintered bulk density is lower than 90% of the theoretical density (TD). Grinding of these powders before processing significantly improved the sintered density. However this operation is much more laborious for spherical powders prepared by the water extraction variant of sol-gel process described in Ref. 5 than for irregularly shaped powders.

This study was undertaken in order to prepare the irregularly shaped and spherical powders of calcium phosphates (with various Ca:P molar ratios) by the above-mentioned process.[5]

0-8493-4750-5/94/$0.00 + $.50

EXPERIMENTAL

In this study the IChTJ sol-gel process described in detail in Ref. 5 was used. Similarly as in the process of fabrication of the HA microspheres,[4] gel microspheres were formed from special "broth" solutions consisting of 1.7M calcium acetate aqueous solution and 85% H_3PO_4. Starting solutions with various Ca/P molar ratios were ultrasonically mixed. The organic solvent (2EH= 2-ethyl-1-hexanol with 1–2v% of SPAN-80) was saturated by contacting with the aqueous phase before the start of the run.

Irregularly shaped gel particles were prepared by gelation of ultrasonically mixed 5M solution of calcium nitrate or aqueous suspension of calcium hydroxide with 85% H_3PO_4.

After drying for 24 h at 50°C, gel powders were calcined at various temperatures. Pellets (diameter = 15 mm, h = 1.5 mm) were then prepared under a pressure of 2000 kg/cm^2. The bulk densities of both green and sintered compacts (3 h at 1200°C) were measured as geometric density.

The thermal decomposition of the gels (TG, DTA) was studied using a Hungarian MOM Derivatograph. X-ray diffraction measurements (using CoKα 1 radiation) were carried out with a positional sensitive detector (Ital Structure). Infrared-absorption spectra of ground samples, dispersed in KBr (1 mg/300 mg pellets) were recorded using a Perkin Elmer 983 IR-spectrophotometer. Carbonates were determined by the internal standardization[11] using $NaNO_3$ and measuring v_2 CO_3 bands 875 cm^{-1}.

RESULTS AND DISCUSSION

During emulsification of all starting "broths" the formation of regular spherical drops of an aqueous phase in 2EH was always observed. When gelating by extraction of water from emulsion drops the spherical shape was conserved only for acetate systems. Typical powders after calcination at 920°C are shown in Figure 1a.

For nitrate-containing systems and for $Ca(OH)_2$ suspensions, formation of irregularly shaped powders was observed (Fig. 1b). In the last case the lack of sphericity seems to be evident. For nitrate systems this can be due to high tendency for crystallization from the aqueous phase during solidification. This conclusion has not been proved in this work. However, one of the present authors observed the formation of irregularly shaped gel particles from alumina sols with NO_3^-/Al^{3+} molar ratios > 1.5.[7]

The results of thermal analysis of gels prepared from nitrate "broth" are shown in Figure 2. The significant weight loss that ends at approximately 180°C is connected with the loss of water.

The normal endothermic effect associated with this process is presumably masked by large exothermic effect (maximum temperature approximately 330°C) which indicates the formation of calcium phosphates. The weight loss in this range connected with the removal of nitrates and the partial removal of hydroxyl group, stops at about 480°C. The thermal analysis of the gel prepared from the $Ca(OH)_2$ slurry (Figure 3) is similar to that described above except that the stabilization of the sample weight is observed at higher temperatures.

This phenomenon can be connected with a higher content of hydroxyl groups, which are bonded very strongly in calcium phosphates.[4,8-10]

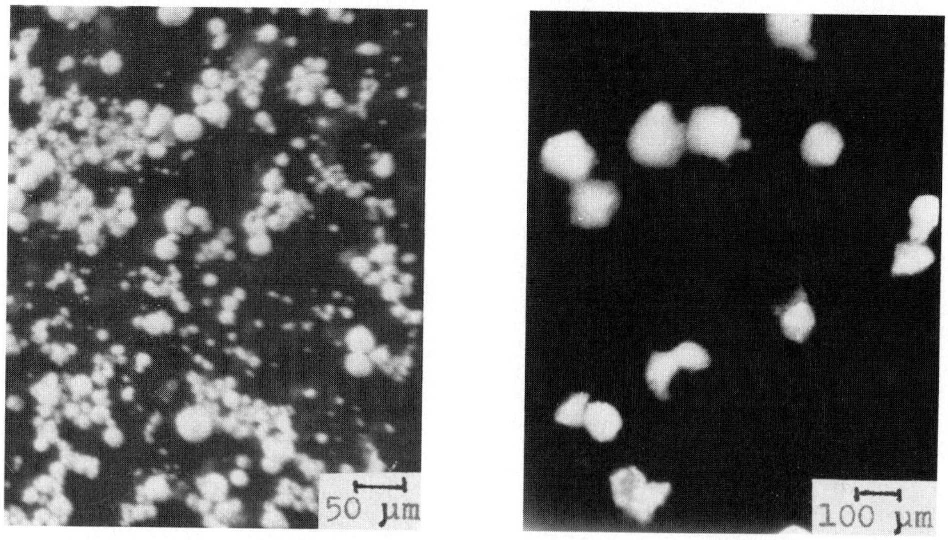

(a) (b)

Figure 1. Microphotographs of calcium phosphates prepared from calcium acetate (a) and from nitrate solutions or hydroxide suspension (b).

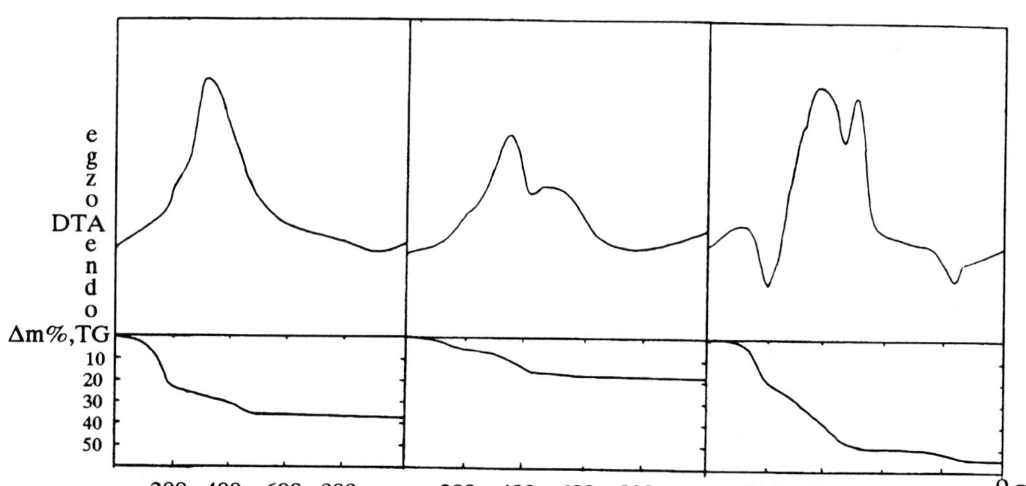

Fig.2. nitrate (No.1) Fig.3. $Ca(OH)_2$ slurry (No.2) Fig.4. acetate(No.5)

Figures 2, 3, 4. Thermal analysis of various Ca-P gels dried at 50°C.

Table 1. Characterization of Ca-P gels and derived products.

No.	Starting Ca^{2+} solution	Ca/P molar ratio in gel**	Calcination temp. ℃, h	Phases identified by XRD IR spectra***	CO_2 %	Shape*
1	nitrate	0.8-1.6		not examined	0	I
2	$Ca(OH)_2$ slurry	1.0		not examined	0	I
3	acetate	1.59	50,2 4	gel,$Ca(Ac)_2$,		S
			200, 24	gel,$Ca(Ac)_2$,$CaCO_3$		S
			400, 3	HA,$CaCO_3$		S
			600, 3	HA·CO_3, $CaCO_3$		S
			920 24	HA		S
4	acetate	2.08	50, 24	gel,$Ca(Ac)_2$		S
			200, 24	gel,$Ca(Ac)_2$,$CaCO_3$		S
			400, 3	Ha,$CaCO_3$, phosphates		S
			600, 3	Ha·CO_3,$CaCO_3$, CaO		S
			920, 24	HA, CaO		S
5	acetate	2.80	50, 24	gel, $Ca(Ac)_2$		S
			200, 24	gel, $Ca(Ac)_2$		S
			400, 3	$CaCO_3$,CaO, amorphous	21	S
			600, 3	$CaCO_3$, phosphates	23	S
			920, 24	HA, $CaCO_3$, CaO		

* I = irregularly shaped, S = spherical

** It was observed that the Ca/P molar ratios in gels were often slightly higher than those in the broth. This was due to extraction of H_3PO_4 by 2-EH despite saturation before the start of the run.

*** In all samples calcined at temperatures up to 400℃ hydroxyl groups engaged in OH---O bonding were observed. A sharp band of free OH appears at a temperature of 600℃ and is much more intense at 920℃.

The thermal decomposition behavior of gels prepared from acetate systems is more complex and similar for all the samples studied (Nos. 3, 4 and 5). The derivatogram of sample No. 5 is shown in Fig. 4. The endothermic effect at 150℃ with weight loss can be attributed to escape of water and partially acetates. Further weight losses accompanied by a large exothermic effect (with onset points 390° and 520℃) can be due to the oxidation of organics and formation of crystalline phases indicated in Table 1. The weight of the sample is stable from 400° till 750℃. The carbonate content for samples calcined at 400° and

600°C is practically the same despite different phase composition of the samples (Table 1, No. 4).

Above 750°C, the weight loss starts and is accompanied by endothermic effect with a maximum at 830°C. This is due to carbonate decomposition. Only for sample No. 5, with the highest Ca/P molar ratio, is the carbonate decomposition incomplete at 920°C.

It follows from the data presented in Table 1 that for acetate Ca-P gels with higher Ca/P molar ratios, the formation of all crystalline phases, especially HA, is strongly retarded. The excess of CaO seems to be bound by hydrogen bonds HO---O.

The morphologies of powders (Nos. 4 and 5) with an excess of calcium (Fig. 5) are very similar to that of HA shown in Ref. 4.

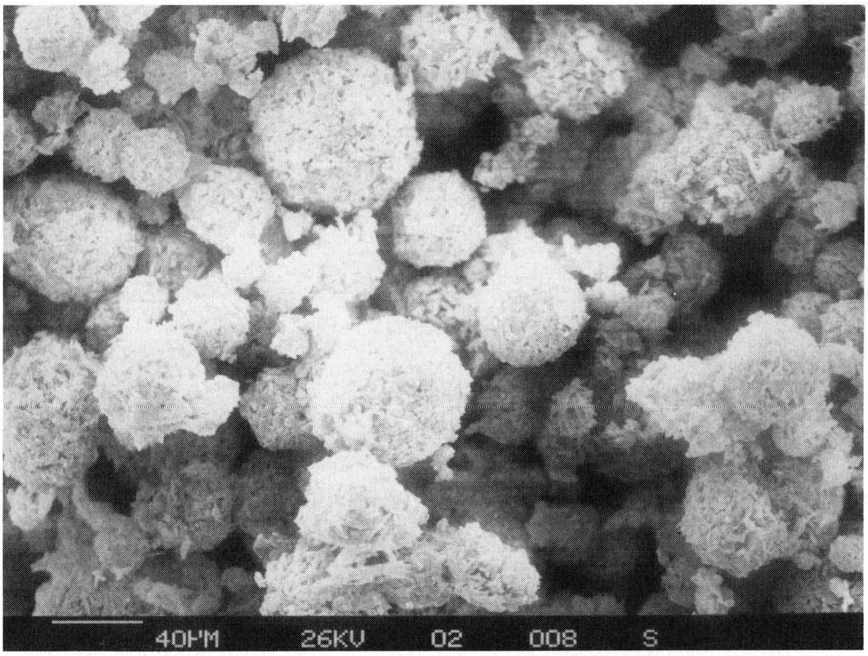

Figure 5. SEM micrograph of sample No. 5.

All powders consist of spherical grains which exhibit high porosity (pore diameters less than several microns). This means that the tissue cannot grow in, since this phenomenon occurs when the pore diameter is larger than about 100 microns.[2,3]

The spherical powder of HA (No. 3) after calcination at 850°C was pressed and the pellets obtained were sintered. The green and sintered pellets had a bulk density of 1.80 to 1.85 g/cm^3 and 2.54 (80.5%TD) to 2.68 (84.9%TD) g/cm^3, respectively. Commercial powders examined under the same conditions gave pellets with much higher (96.3%TD) bulk density. This means that, as was observed in our previous work,[6] medium-sized spherical powders without particle size reduction cannot be used for preparation of dense bodies. We hope that they can be used for the formation of macroporous bodies, while irregularly shaped powders (more suitable for particle size reduction by grinding) could be used for fabrication of dense bodies.

CONCLUSIONS

The water extraction variant of the sol-gel process was successfully applied to fabrication of spherical and irregularly shaped powders of calcium phosphates with various Ca/P ratios. During calcination of acetate Ca-P gels the formation of crystalline phases is retarded for higher Ca/P molar ratios. After final calcination of these powders at 920°C hydroxyapatite is formed. However for molar Ca/P ratios higher than 2 the presence of CaO and even $CaCO_3$ is observed. The spherical powders show high porosity. The sintered pellets prepared from these materials have bulk density lower than 85%TD.

Acknowledgements

This work has been done in the framework of Italian (ENEA)–Polish (PAA) scientific collaboration. The authors would like to thank Mrs. Będkowska, B. Goszczyńska and Mr. H. Hahn for their assistance in the experimental work.

REFERENCES

1. C. Lavernia and J. M. Shoenung, *Am. Ceram. Soc. Bull.* 70:95 (1991).
2. P. W. Brown and M. Fulmer, *J. Am. Ceram. Soc.* 74:934 (1991).
3. L. L. Hench, *J. Am. Ceram. Soc.* 74:1487 (1991).
4. A. Deptuła, W. Łada, T. Olczak, A. Borello, C. Alvani, and A. DiBartolomeo, *J. Non-Cryst. Solids* 147&148:537 (1992).
5. A. Deptuła, J. Rebandel, W. Drozda, W. Łada, T. Olczak, in *Better Ceramics Through Chemistry V*, M. J. Hampden-Smith, W. G. Klemperer and C. J. Brinker (eds.), Mat. Res. Soc. Symp. Proc. 270, Pittsburgh, PA, p. 277 (1992).
6. A. Deptuła, M. Carewska, F. Croce, B. Scrosati and C. Majani, in *Ceramics Today—Tomorrow's Ceramics*, P. Vincenzini (ed.), Elsevier Science Publisher V.B., p. 2253 (1991).
7. A. Deptuła, J. Rebandel, W. Drozda, III Ceramic Science Symposium, Cetniewo, Poland, Proceedings, p. 379 (1976).
8. A. Akoi, S. Ohno, T. Uhikoshi and Y. Muramatsu, *Phiosphorus Research Bulletin* 1:31 (1991).
9. J. Zhou, X. Zhang, J. Chen, S. Zeng and K. De Groot, *J. Mat. Sci. in Medicine* 4:83 (1993).
10. T. Kijma and M. Tsutsumi, *J. Am. Ceram. Soc.* 62:455 (1979).
11. A. L. Smith, *Applied Infrared Spectroscopy, Fundamentals, Techniques and Analytical Problem-Solving*, J. Wiley and Sons, NY, Chichester-Brisbane-Toronto, p. 251 (1969).

THERMAL STABILITY OF SYNTHETIC HYDROXYAPATITE

Y. Fang, D. K. Agrawal, and D. M. Roy
Intercollege Materials Research Laboratory
The Pennsylvania State University
University Park, PA 16802

ABSTRACT

The thermal stabilities of a variety of hydroxyapatite (HAp), $Ca_{10}(PO_4)_6(OH)_2$, samples prepared by different wet-chemical methods have been studied. The results show that the thermal stability of a HAp is intrinsically dependent on its stoichiometry and the crystal structure. The stoichiometry and crystal structure are, in turn, related to both the precursor and the synthesis conditions. The optimum thermal stability up to 1370°C (in air with 50% relative humidity) was observed in the HAp samples prepared by a hydrothermal method and by the hydrolysis of brushite followed by proper ripening.

INTRODUCTION

Synthetic hydroxyapatite (HAp), with a stoichiometric composition as $Ca_{10}(PO_4)_6(OH)_2$, has excellent biocompatibility with human tooth and bone, and thus making it very attractive for biomedical applications. The studies of HAp cements,[1-3] ceramics,[4-8] and composites,[9-12] for biomedical applications, have been well documented in the recent years.[13-17] As a biomedical material, HAp is mainly used in its ceramic forms fabricated by sintering the compacted powder of synthetic HAp at temperatures between 1000 and 1350°C.[18] The standards for HAp used for bone replacement[19,20] specify that the material must be in the ceramic state and exclude non-ceramic hydroxyapatite since non-ceramic HAp does not exhibit the biological/medical properties as ceramic HAp. Because of this, high thermal stability of starting HAp powder is very important for obtaining essentially pure HAp ceramics.

HAp can be prepared by various synthesis methods, including solid-state reaction (dry process) and wet-chemical methods.[15, 20-24] In general, the wet processes which have been widely adopted provide finer, more homogeneous and more reactive powders. Decomposition of HAp at high temperatures is frequently encountered during the fabrication of HAp ceramics. This inhibits the sinterability of the apatite ceramics and partly or completely transforms HAp into a mixture of tetracalcium phosphate (TetCP), $Ca_4(PO_4)_2O$, and tricalcium phosphate (TCP), $Ca_3(PO_4)_2$. TetCP and α-form of TCP can readily react with water. If such reactions occur in the bioceramics under the physiological conditions, the mechanical integrity of the ceramics would be deteriorated. In order to obtain ceramics of pure HAp, the decomposition of

0-8493-4750-5/94/$0.00+$.50

HAp during ceramic fabrication must be prevented. Since the dehydroxylation and decomposition of HAp are a process accompanied by the release of hydroxyl or molecular water from HAp, therefore the partial pressure of water vapor is an important factor affecting the thermal stability of HAp. Riboud[25] has showed the dependence of the decomposition temperature of HAp on the water vapor partial pressure. Also it has been shown[26] recently that the dehydroxylation and decomposition of HAp can be effectively suppressed by moisture sintering. The objective of this paper is to discuss various aspects related to the thermal stability (in air) of synthetic HAp powders prepared by wet-chemical methods, and investigate the influence of synthesis conditions on the thermal stability of HAp.

EXPERIMENTAL

MATERIAL PREPARATION

1. By hydrolysis of α-TCP, α-$Ca_3(PO_4)_2$

α-TCP was synthesized by a solid-state reaction method in the following way. Stoichiometric amounts of fine powders of $CaCO_3$ and $NH_4H_2PO_4$ (both Reagent Grade) were hand-mixed in acetone to obtain a homogeneous mixture. This mixture was air-dried and then heated at 300°C for 16 hours to remove NH_3 and H_2O, and then at 900°C for 24 hours to remove CO_2. The calcined product was once again ground to improve homogeneity, and finally fired at 1200°C for 16 hours to form α-TCP.

50 grams α-TCP powder (-325 mesh) in 2000 ml deionized water was hydrolyzed at 60°C to form HAp. The pH of the system was adjusted in the range of 7.6-8.5 with NH_4OH and kept relatively constant during the hydrolysis by using more NH_4OH as desired. The suspension was subjected to continuous stirring condition throughout the entire hydrolysis process which lasted about two hours. The product was then repeatedly washed three times with deionized water and dried at 90°C in a ventilated oven.

2. By hydrolysis of brushite plus ripening

Brushite ($CaHPO_4 \cdot 2H_2O$), also called dibasic calcium phosphate dihydrate (DCPD) (J.T. Baker Chemical Co., Philipsburg, NJ) was used as a precursor to prepare HAp by hydrolysis under the same conditions as employed for the α-TCP hydrolysis mentioned above. The powder thus obtained was washed with deionized water and dried, and then ripened. The ripening treatment was conducted under varying conditions as the following.

a. Adding 20% (by weight) calcium chloride dihydrate (CCD), $CaCl_2 \cdot 2H_2O$, under the same conditions as in the hydrolysis. The ripening was carried out three times repeatedly. The product was washed with deionized water and dried at 90°C after each ripening.

b. Instead of the above three-step treatment, ripening was alternatively carried out at 75±5°C using 60% CCD, with the initial pH at 8.87 and 11.00, respectively. This treatment lasted 24 h. The ripening of 20% CCD was also carried out at the same pH for 70 min. for comparison. After the ripening treatment, the powders were washed with deionized water and dried at 100°C. This simple one-step ripening will be referred as "SOR" hereafter.

3. Precipitation method

A precipitate was prepared by mixing stoichiometric amounts (Ca/P mol ratio =1.67) of $Ca(NO_3)_2 \cdot 4H_2O$ and $NH_4H_2PO_4$ solutions (both of 0.5 M) at room temperature and pH 11 (adjusted with NH_4OH). $NH_4H_2PO_4$ solution was slowly added to the $Ca(NO_3)_2 \cdot 4H_2O$ solution over an hour, and the mixture was subjected to constant stirring for 24 hours. The resultant white precipitate was centrifuged to a slurry. The slurry thus obtained was then dried at 60°C.

4. Hydrothermal method

A portion of the precipitate obtained in **(3)** was hydrothermally treated at 200°C in a Parr bomb under the estimated vapor pressure of about 1.5 MPa for 24 h. The powder obtained by the hydrothermal treatment was washed with deionized water and dried at 110°C.

CHARACTERIZATION

The morphologies of the HAp powders were examined by electron microscopy. The phase compositions were determined by powder X-ray diffraction (XRD) using a Scintag diffractometer (Scintag Inc., Sunnyvale, CA) and CuKα radiation. Lattice parameter refinement was conducted by XRD in conjunction with a computerized calculation program. Thermogravimetric analyses (TGA) were carried out on HAp powders at a heating rate of 10°C per min. The chemical analyses were performed on selected HAp samples using spectrochemical methods.

THERMAL STABILITY

The thermal stabilities of the above HAp samples were investigated by XRD analysis of the air-quenched samples after isothermal heating. The samples were heated at various temperatures in air with 50% relative humidity. The firing time for all samples at all temperatures was 1 h. The heated samples were ground to fine powders and the slides were made with acetone for XRD analysis. Thermal stability was characterized by the decomposition temperature of the specific HAp sample. Since the decomposition of HAp is always accompanied by the appearance of TCP (either β- or α-form), the minimum temperature at which the HAp sample was heated and TCP was detected by XRD from the sample was recorded as the decomposition temperature of that sample. A high decomposition temperature of the HAp implies good thermal stability, and low decomposition temperature, poor thermal stability. The appearance of diffraction peak at d=2.905Å (2q=30.8°) was used as the evidence of α-TCP and d=2.88Å (2q=31°) for β-TCP.

RESULTS AND DISCUSSION

MORPHOLOGY

Figure 1 shows the morphologies of the as-synthesized HAp powders. As can be seen, highly crystalline HAp whiskers were obtained from the hydrolysis of α-TCP (Fig. 1A). Typical grain size of these single crystals was about 0.2 x 5 mm. HAp obtained from the hydrolysis of DCPD was a mixture of finer grains and some non-uniform needle-shaped crystallites (Fig. 1B). The morphology of the HAp from precipitation was agglomerates of tiny particles (Fig. 1C). The HAp obtained by hydrothermal method was highly nanocrystalline, uniform in shape and particle size (Fig. 1D). The average particle size was about 0.025 x 0.1 mm. It is obvious from this study that the method of preparation and nature of precursors strongly influenced the morphology of HAp powders.

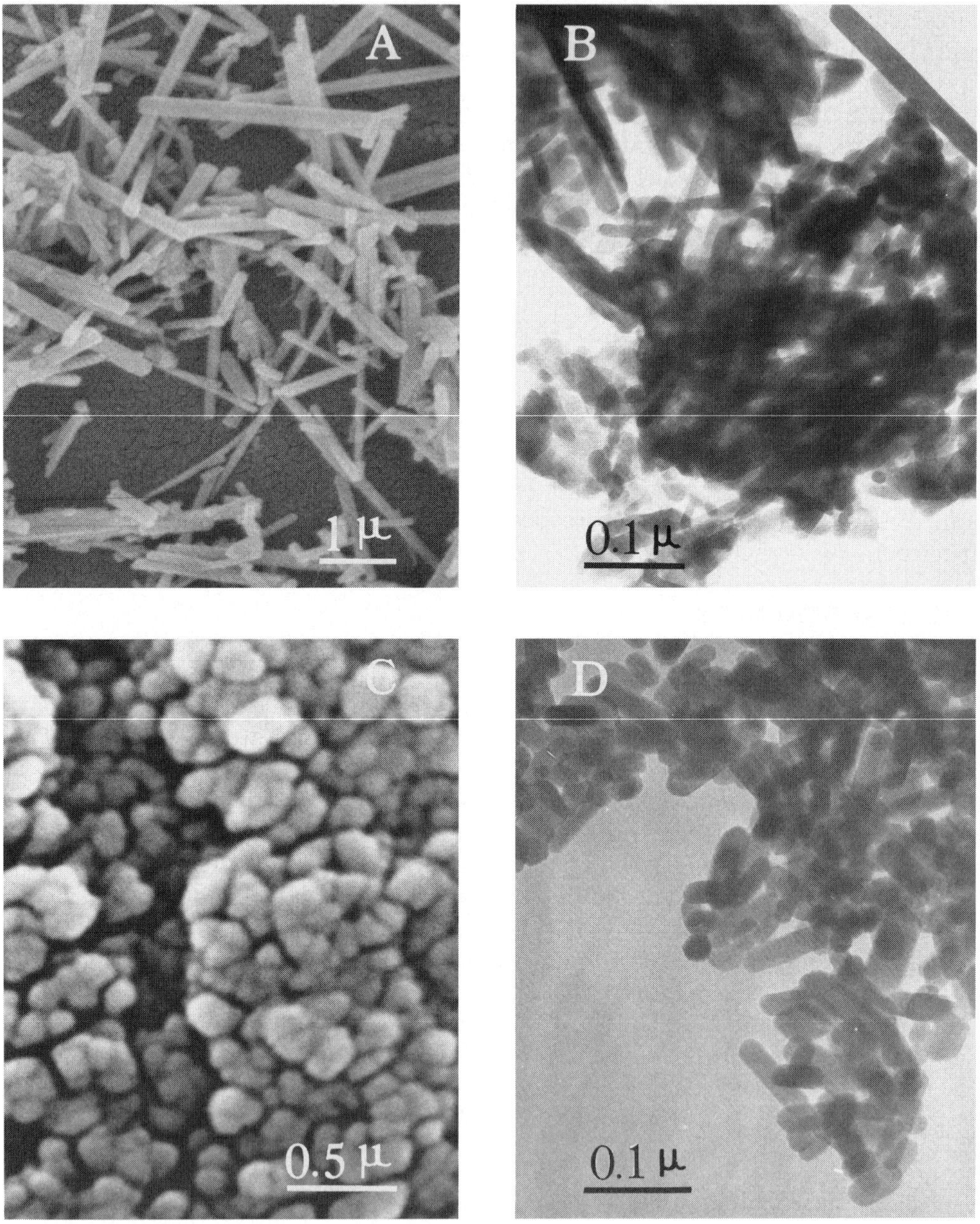

Figure 1. Electron micrographs showing morphology of HAp synthesized by (A) hydrolysis of α-TCP, (B) hydrolysis of DCPD followed by ripening, (C) precipitation, and (D) hydrothermal method.

CRYSTALLINITY

The crystallinity of the synthetic HAp can be evaluated from either electron micrographs or X-ray diffraction patterns. A XRD pattern containing strong and sharp peaks corresponds to high crystallinity, and that of broad and low intensity diffraction peaks corresponds to poor crystallinity. Figure 2 indicates that the crystallinity of the as-synthesized HAp prepared by the hydrolysis of α-TCP was very high; that from hydrothermal method was high; that from DCPD was poor; and that from precipitation was almost X-ray amorphous (Fig. 2A). Comparison of the crystallinity of the precipitate and the hydrothermally synthesized HAp samples indicated that the precipitate had undergone crystallization under the hydrothermal conditions. This made the hydrothermally synthesized HAp different from that obtained directly from precipitation. It was also noticed that ripening treatment did not significantly change the crystallinity of the product. Heating did promote the crystallinity of the HAp. For example, crystallinity of the precipitated HAp increased with the firing temperature (Fig. 3). Similar effect was also observed before decomposition in the HAp samples from the hydrolysis of DCPD followed by ripening.

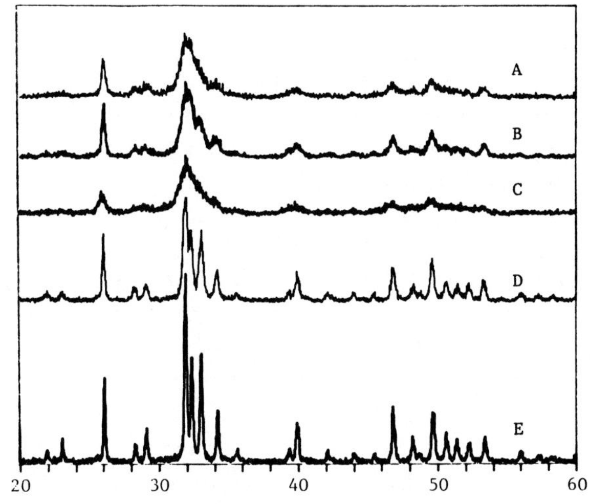

Two theta, degree

Figure 2. XRD patterns of the as-synthesized HAp by (A) hydrolysis of DCPD, (B) hydrolysis of DCPD plus triple ripening, (C) precipitation, (D) hydrothermal method, and (E) hydrolysis of α-TCP.

STOICHIOMETRY

The Ca/P molar ratios of the HAp samples determined by atomic absorption spectroscopy technique are presented in Table 1. According to the chemical formula, stoichiometric HAp should have Ca/P molar ratio of 1.67, therefore the HAp with Ca/P lower than 1.67 is characterized as calcium deficient, or nonstoichiometric. Although nonstoichiometry of HAp may also include hydroxyl deficiency, the latter will not be considered in this study. It was noticed that the HAp sample from α-TCP and the unripened sample from DCPD were both calcium-deficient, while the samples from precipitation and hydrothermal treatment were stoichiometric. The ripening treatment increased the Ca/P ratio of the treated sample from 1.52 to 1.68, thus stoichiometric HAp was obtained through ripening.

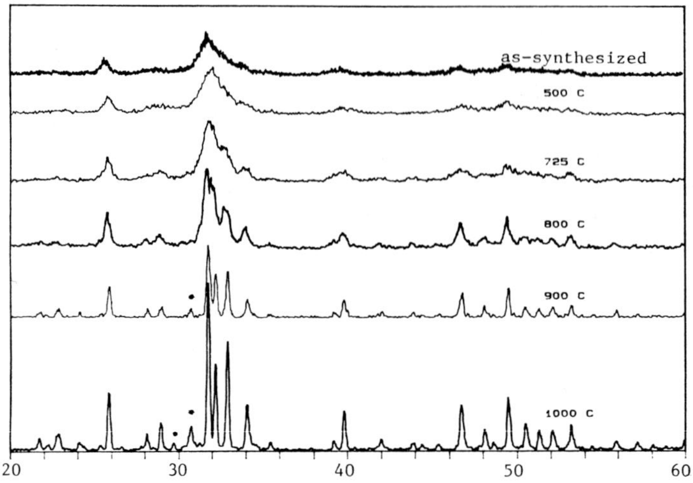

Two theta, degree

Figure 3. XRD patterns showing that the crystallinity of the precipitated HAp increased with heating temperature. Samples were heated at the specified temperatures for 1 h. (•) TCP; unmarked, HAp.

TABLE 1

Ca/P ratios of HAp samples determined by atomic absorption spectroscopy.

Method	Ca/P	Synthesis conditions
Hydrolysis of α-TCP	1.65	60 °C, 2 h, pH 7.6 - 8.5
Hydrolysis of DCPD	1.52	As hydrolyzed, 60 °C, 2 h, pH 7.6 - 8.5
Hydrolysis of DCPD	1.68	Ripened once, 60 °C, 2 h, 20% CCD
Precipitation	1.67	25 °C, 24 h, pH 11
Hydrothermal	1.67	200 °C, 1.5 MPa, 12 h, pH 11

In order to examine the HAp obtained after repeated ripening with calcium chloride, and to check whether it was chloroapatite or HAp, special chemical analysis of the powders was carried out by atomic absorption spectroscopic technique on the ripened samples, using an unripened sample as reference. The results are given in Table 2.

It should be noted that NO_3^- and SO_4^{2-} sources were never used nor introduced during the synthesis. Thus the fact that the amounts of Cl^- were at the same level as that of NO_3^- and SO_4^{2-}, could be considered either as the impurities present in the material, or as the instrument noise. The exceptionally high count of Cl^- in sample "C" might be due to incomplete washing after ripening, otherwise the Cl^- contents of sample "D," which was ripened one more time than sample "C," would be even higher. A simple calculation shows that if 1% OH^- in the HAp is substituted by Cl^-, the content of Cl^- would be about 700 ppm. If complete substitution occurred, the content of Cl^- should be 6.8%, or 68000 ppm. Further more, the incorporation of Cl^- in HAp would make OH^- stretching band in IR absorption pattern shift from 3573 to 3495 cm^{-1},[23] but the IR spectra of the samples ripened with $CaCl_2$ showed OH^- stretching at 3560 cm^{-1} which was very close to 3573 cm^{-1}. Apparently the substitution of Cl^- for OH^- to form chloroapatite did not, or not significantly, if any, occur in the ripening process under the current processing conditions.

TABLE 2

Spectrochemical analysis of chloride ions in HAp samples (in ppm).

Sample #	Cl^-	NO_3^-	SO_4^{2-}	Remarks
A	80	90	110	Before ripening
B	130	70	40	Ripened once
C	460	200	140	Ripened twice
D	130	70	50	Ripened thrice

TGA RESULTS

It was reported[27] that nonstoichiometric HAp decomposes via dehydration according to the following reactions:

$$Ca_{10-x}(HPO_4)_x(PO_4)_{2-x}nH_2O \xrightarrow{<700^\circ C} Ca_{10-x}(P_2O_7)_x(PO_4)_{6-2x}(OH)_2 + nH_2O(g) \quad (a)$$

$$\xrightarrow{700^\circ\text{-}800^\circ C} (1\text{-}x)Ca_{10}(PO_4)_6(OH)_2 + 3Ca_3(PO_4)_2 + xH_2O(g) \quad (b)$$

The resultants after thermal treatment are stoichiometric HAp and TCP. At temperatures higher than 900°C, further partial dehydration of HAp may take place as follows.

$$Ca_{10}(PO_4)_6(OH)_2 \xrightarrow{>900^\circ C} Ca_{10}(PO_4)_6(OH)_{2-2y}O_y + yH_2O(g) \quad (c)$$

According to above reactions one would observe a gradual wt. loss before 700°C, a sharp loss in 700°-800°C region, and a slight and gradual loss above 900°C in the TGA thermogram of a nonstoichiometric HAp sample. There should not be any sharp loss for stoichiometric HAp in its TGA curve. Thus stoichiometric and nonstoichiometric HAp samples can be easily distinguished by TGA.

The TGA thermograms of HAp prepared by the different methods are shown in Fig. 4. Among these only two samples, i.e., HAp prepared by the hydrolysis of α-TCP and DCPD (without ripening) showed sharp deflection (Figs. 4A, 4E) between 700°-800°C in the thermograms, and hence they were both nonstoichiometric. The rest of the samples did not show such a sharp loss, and therefore they were considered to be stoichiometric (Figs. 4B, C, D, F, G). The difference in the wt. loss below 300°C was due to the degree of drying before the TGA experiment. The substantial wt. loss of the precipitated HAp below 200°C indicated that this sample contained large amount of entrapped water. The DCPD-derived samples also showed moderate wt. loss, at low temperature range. The HAp from α-TCP hydrolysis showed the least wt. loss in the low temperature rang, because the near complete drying of this sample composed of relatively large crystals was much easier prior to TGA.

The whiskered HAp had good crystallinity but still showed wt. loss between 700° and 800°C (Fig. 4A) and was confirmed to be nonstoichiometric. This conclusion is in good agreement with what reported by Monma et al.[23] These results indicate that good crystallinity does not necessarily imply good stoichiometry, and vice versa. The precipitated HAp had poor crystallinity (broad XRD peaks, Fig. 2C) but did not show any sharp weight loss in the 700°-800°C region in the TGA curve (Fig. 4F).

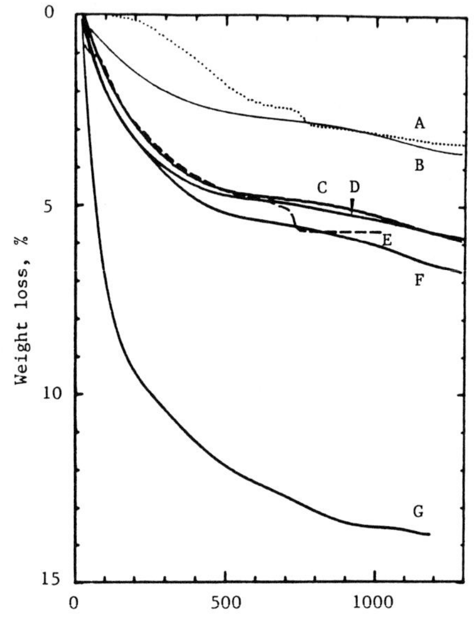

Figure 4. TG thermograms of HAp synthesized by (A) hydrolysis of α-TCP, (B) hydrothermal method, (C) DCPD hydrolysis, ripened twice, (D) DCPD hydrolysis, ripened thrice, (E) DCPD hydrolysis without ripening, (F) DCPD hydrolysis (ripened once), and (G) precipitation.

LATTICE PARAMETERS

The lattice parameters of the HAp samples determined by XRD are listed in Table 3. The reported values from the JCPDS file (9-432) was considered as references for stoichiometric HAp. Compared with the as-synthesized HAp by DCPD hydrolysis (sample A) it is seen that ripening reduced (sample C) both *a* and *c* slightly, as the Ca/P ratio was increased (Table 1). Compared with the values of the precipitate (sample D), it is obvious that hydrothermal treatment reduced both *a* and *c* through crystallization thus making the resultant HAp denser in crystal structure.

THERMAL STABILITY

The thermal stability is discussed with respect to the decomposition of the specific HAp sample. The precipitated HAp, which was chemically stoichiometric as observed in the previous section, was found to be stable up to about 900°C. The highest thermal stability, up to 1370°C, was found in the hydrothermally synthesized HAp (Fig. 5). It is evident that the crystallization of the precipitate under the hydrothermal conditions is a very effective maturing process to drive the amorphous precipitate of stoichiometric composition for HAp towards the highly thermally stable crystalline HAp. Although crystallization also occurred when heating the precipitate in air, the pressure of water vapor in air was low. Under the hydrothermal condition of high pH region, the atmosphere is saturated and the pressure is high, thus favoring the formation of fine, uniform, stoichiometric, and structurally dense crystalline HAp.

TABLE 3

Lattice parameters of the HAp samples synthesized in the current study, Å.

Sample No.	*a*	*c*	synthesis method
ref.	9.418	6.884	JCPDS file (9-432)
A	9.432	6.89	Hydrolysis of DCPD
B	9.430	6.878	Hydrolysis of α-TCP
C	9.428	6.875	"A" plus ripening
D	9.427	6.893	Precipitation
E	9.418	6.884	Hydrothermal

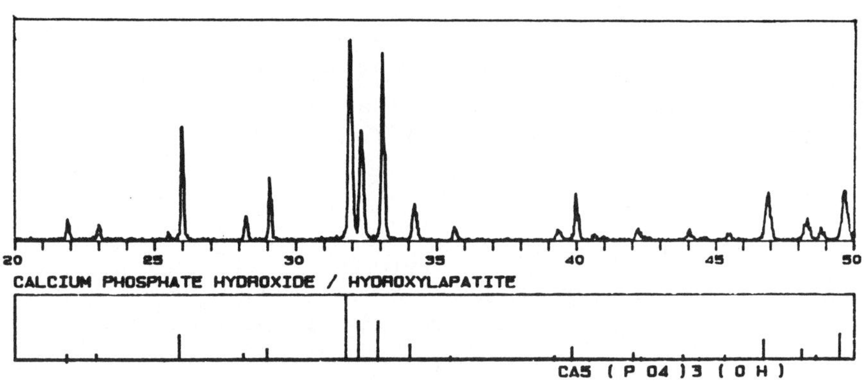

Figure 5. XRD showing that the HAp hydrothermally synthesized at 200°C, 1.5 MPa, remained undecomposed at 1370°C in air of 50% RH (11.88 mm Hg).

For the DCPD-derived HAp samples, ripening treatment really made difference. The as-synthesized HAp by DCPD hydrolysis was nonstoichiometric and completely decomposed into β-TCP at 733°C (Fig. 6), but the sample ripened once with 20% CCD remained undecomposed until 1000°C. Repeated ripening treatment (three times) further enhanced the decomposition temperature up to about 1200°C. Fig. 7 shows the effect of ripening on the thermal stability of HAp. The increase of Ca/P ratio of the HAp from 1.52 to 1.67 or 1.68 (Table 1) clearly showed that the stoichiometry was one of the key factors that controls the thermal stability of HAp. However, since both temperature and pressure in the ripening process were much lower than in the hydrothermal process, the repeated ripening did not achieve a result as good as by the hydrothermal method. On the other hand, increasing treatment time, increasing amount of CCD, and high pH, all favored the transformation of nonstoichiometric HAp towards stoichiometry. This is evident in the SOR samples. For example, the HAp ripened with 60% CCD at initial pH of 11 and treated for 24 h was stable up to 1370°C. The samples used for comparison, i.e., those treated at lower pH, less CCD, or shorter period of time, were stable up to 1300°-1350°C. Figure 8 shows the XRD patterns of the SOR HAp, heating at 1350°C and 1370°C for 1 h.

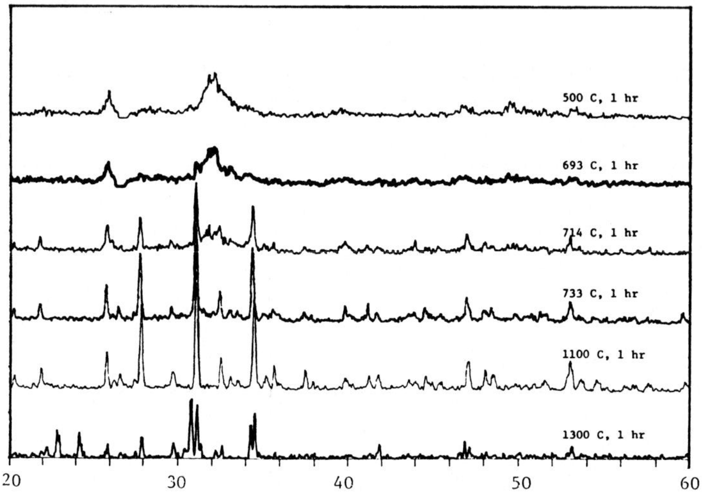

Figure 6. XRD patterns of the as-synthesized HAp by DCPD hydrolysis, heated at various temperatures. It is seen that the decomposition started at about 700°C. 714°C, β-TCP + HAp; 733, 1100°C, β-TCP. 1300°C; α-TCP + β-TCP.

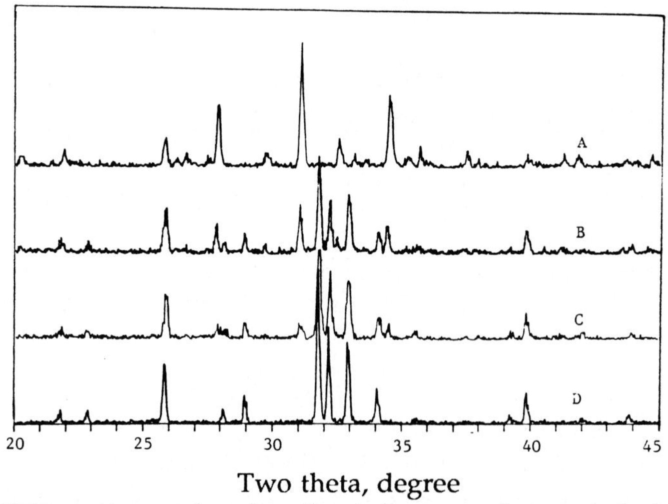

Figure 7. XRD patterns showing the influence of repeated ripening on the thermal stability of HAp obtained by DCPD hydrolysis. Samples were heated 1 h at 1100°C in air of 50% RH. (A) Without ripening: β-TCP. (B) Ripened once:

HAp+ β-TCP. (C) Ripened twice: HAp+β-TCP (tr.). (D) Ripened thrice: HAp only, no decomposition.

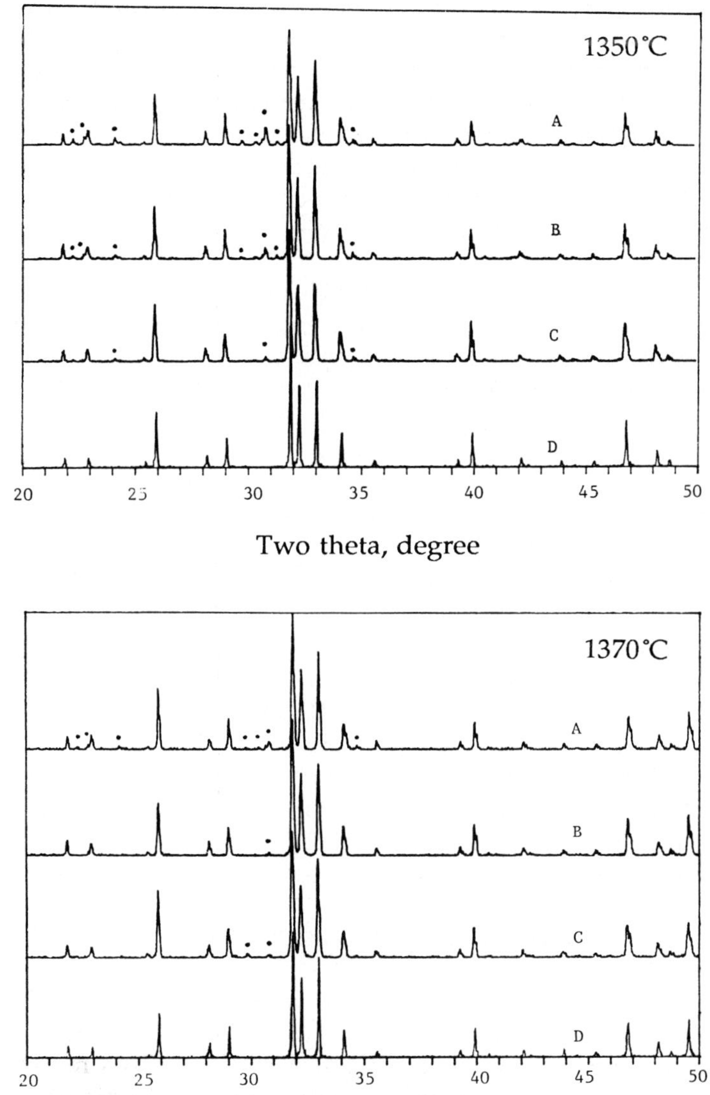

Figure 8. XRD patterns showing the phase composition of SOR (strengthened one-step ripening) heated 1 h at 1350°C and 1370°C, respectively. The ripening after the hydrolysis of DCPD was carried out at 75°C and (A) 20% CCD, 70 min., initial pH 8.87, (B) 60% CCD, 24 h, initial pH=8.87, (C) 20% CCD, 70 min., initial pH=11.0, and (D) 60% CCD, 24 h, initial pH=11. (•) α-TCP.

Table 4 summarizes the phase composition results of the HAp samples heated at various temperatures. It can be seen that the thermal stability of the synthetic HAp varied with both the nature of the precursor and the synthesis method. By the precipitation method, the hydrothermal treatment substantially enhanced the thermal stability. By hydrolysis of DCPD, one-step ripening offered good thermal stability. The as-synthesized HAp by hydrolysis of α-TCP began to decompose at 800℃ and remained as a mixture of HAp and TCP in a large temperature range. For the SOR samples, only thermal stability was studied. Comprehensive explanation on the behavior of these samples needs further study. It should be indicated that during heating in air, HAp might have at least partially transformed to so-called oxy-hydroxyapatite (OHA) by dehydroxylation. If this is considered, the HAp detected in the samples heated at high temperatures should be more accurately called OHA. To completely prevent the appearance of OHA, sintering of HAp should be conducted in the presence of moisture.[26]

TABLE 4

The main phase composition appearing in the HAp samples heated in air of 50% relative humidity at various temperatures.

T	Hydrolysis of	Hydrolysis of DCPD						
			Ripened					
(℃)	α-TCP	As is	I	II	III	SOR	PPT	Hydrothermal
700	H	H	H	H	H	H	H	H
800	H+β(tr)	β	H	H	H	H	H	H
900	H+β	β	H	H	H	H	H+α(tr.)	H
1000	H+β	β	H+β	H+β(tr.)	H	H	H+α(tr.)	H
1100	H+β	β	H+β	H+β(tr.)	H	H	H+α	H
1200	H+α	α	-	H+β	H+α(tr.)	H	H+α	H
1300	H+α	α	H+α	H+α	H+α	H	H+α	H

a,b—α- or β-TCP. H—HAp. PPT.—precipitated. I, II, and III indicate the number of ripening time. SOR—strengthened one-step ripening. (tr.)—trace amount, defined arbitrarily by relative intensity of XRD patterns.

SUMMARY AND CONCLUSIONS

Thermal stabilities of several synthetic hydroxyapatite samples prepared by wet-chemical methods have been studied. The HAp synthesized by the hydrothermal method was uniformly nanocrystalline. This material showed very high thermal stability, remaining undecomposed in air of 50% relative humidity up to 1370℃. The as-synthesized HAp by the hydrolysis of brushite showed poor thermal stability, starting decomposing at about 700℃. Repeated ripening with addition of calcium chloride enhanced the thermal stability up to about 1200℃. A one-step ripening treatment of this DCPD-derived HAp increased the decomposition temperature of the HAp up to 1370℃. The HAp obtained by the hydrolysis of α-TCP was highly crystalline but nonstoichiometric and began to partially decompose at about 800℃. The as-synthesized HAp obtained directly by precipitation was almost X-ray amorphous. The crystallinity of this HAp increased with temperature and it decomposed at about 900℃.

The results in this study indicated that the thermal stability of the synthetic HAp does not depend on the crystallinity but on the stoichiometry and crystal structure. In air of given relative humidity, the chemically stoichiometric and structurally dense HAp showed the best thermal stability. To avoid dehydroxylation and decomposition of HAp during ceramic preparation, a moist sintering technique should be adopted, or alternatively, high thermal stability HAp powder should be used. However, the combination of the both should enable to completely prevent the decomposition of HAp in the general sintering temperature range.

ACKNOWLEDGMENT

`This research is supported by the National Science Foundation under contract number DMR 8812824, and by the Consortium on Chemically Bonded Ceramics.

REFERENCES

1. Brown, W.E., Chow, L.C., Dental Restorative Cement Pastes, US Pat. No. 4518430, May 21, 1985.
2. Brown, W.E., Chow, L.C., Combinations of sparingly soluble calcium phosphates, in slurries and pastes as mineralizers and cements, US Pat. 4612053, Sep. 16, 1986.
3. Brown, P.W., and Fulmer, M., Kinetics of hydroxyapatite formation at low temperature, *J. Am. Ceram. Soc.*, 74(5), 934-940, 1991.
4. Heise, U., Osborn, J.F., and Duwe, F., Hdroxyapatite ceramic as a bone substitute, *International Orthopedics* (SICOT) 14:329-338, 1990.
5. Roy, D.M., Porous Biomaterials and Method of Making Same, US Pat. No. 3929971, 1975.
6. Fang, Y., Agrawal, D.K., Roy, D.M., and Roy, R., Rapid sintering of hydroxyapatite ceramics by microwave processing, *Ceramic Transactions*, Vol. 21, edited by D.E. Clark, F.D. Gac, and W.H. Sutton, American Ceramic Society, Westerville, Ohio, 1991.
7. Fang, Y., Agrawal, D.K., Roy, D.M., and Roy, R., Fabrication of porous hydroxyapatite ceramics by microwave processing, *J. Mater. Res.*, Vol. 7(2), 490-494, 1992.
8. Agrawal, D.K., Fang, Y., Roy, D.M., and Roy, R., Fabrication of hydroxyapatite ceramics by microwave processing, *MRS symp. proc. Vol.* 269, 231-236, MRS, Pittsburgh, PA, 1992.
9. Ioku, I., Yoshimura, M., Somiya, S., Hydrothermal synthesis of hydroxyapatite powders with zirconia dispersion, in *Biomedical materials and devices, MRS Sympo. Proc.*, Vol. 110, 445-450, 1989.
10. Wu, J.-M., Yeh, T.-S., Sintering of Hydroxyapatite-zirconia composite materials, *J. Mat. Sci.*, 23, 3771-3777, 1988.
11. Yoshimura, M., Ioku, K., and Somiya, S., Apatite ceramics with tailored microstructures from hydrothermally-prepared ultra-fine hydroxyapatite crystals, *Euro-Ceramics*, Vol. 3, edited by de With, G., Terpstra, R.A., and Metselaar, R., Elsevier, 3.17-3.20, 1989.
12. Fang, Y., Roy, D.M., Cheng, J., Roy, R., and Agrawal, D.K., Microwave sintering of hydroxyapatite-based composites", in *Ceramic Transactions*,

Microwaves: Theory and Application in Materials Processing II, Am. Ceram. Soc., Inc., Westerville, OH (1993).

13. Ducheyne, P., and Lemons, J.E., Eds. *Bioceramics: Material characteristics versus in vivo behavior*, Annals of the New York Academy of Sciences, Vol. 523, The New York Academy of sciences, New York, NY., 1988.
14. Hanker, J.S., Giammara, B.L., Biomedical Mat. and Devices, *MRS Symp. Proc.*, Vol. 110, MRS, Pittsburgh, PA, 1989.
15. Kanazawa, T., Ed., *Inorganic Phosphate Materials*, Elsevier, 1989.
16. Yamamuro, T., Hench, L.L., Wilson, J., Eds. *Handbook of Bioactive Ceramics, Vol. II, Calcium Phosphate and Hydroxylapatite Ceramics*, CRC Press, Boca Raton, FL 1990.
17. Hench, L.L., Bioceramics: from concept to clinic, *J. Am. Ceram. Soc.*, 74 (7), 1484-1510, 1991.
18. Willmann, G., Normbestimmungen fur hydrxyapatit als Knochenersatz (Standards for Hydroxyapatite used for Bone Replacement), *Sonderdruck aus Biomedizinische Technik*, 35(9), 205-207, 1990.
19. ASTM F1185-88, Standard specification for composition of ceramic hydroxyapatite for surgical implant, American Society of Testing and Materials, 1988.
20. Jarcho, M., Bolen, C.H., Thomas, M.B., Bobick, J., Kay, J.F., Doremus, R.H., Hydroxyapatite synthesis and characterization in dense polycrystalline form, *J. Mat. Sci.* 11, 2027-35, 1976.
21. Monma, H., and Kamiya, T., Preparation of hydroxyapatite by the hydrolysis of brushite, *J. Mat. Sci.* 22, 4247-50, 1987.
22. Monma, H., Takahashi, T., Ushio, H., Soeda, S., and Kiyosawa, T., Preparation and properties of porous apatite by the hydration and hardening method, Gypsum & Lime, 212, 25-28, 1988.
23. Monma, H., Ueno, S., and Kanazawa, T., Properties of hydroxyapatite prepared by the hydrolysis of tricalcium phosphate, *J. Chem. Tech. Biotechnol.*, 31,15-24, 1981.
24. Hattori, T., Iwadate, Y., Kato, T., Hydrothermal synthesis of hydroxyapatite from calcium acetate and triethyl phosphate, *Advanced Cer. Mat.* 3 (4), 426-428, 1988.
25. Riboud, P.V., Bull. Soc. Chim. Fr., *Spec. No. Cpmparaison de la stabilite de l'apatite d'oxyde de fer et de l'hydroxyapatite a haute temperature*, 1701-1703, 1968.
26. Wang, P.E., Chaki, T.K., Sintering behaviour and mechanical properties of hydroxyapatite and dicalcium phosphate, *J. Mat. Sci.: Mat. in Medicine*, 4, 150-158, 1993.
27. Yamashita, K., Kanazawa, T., Hydroxyapatite, in *Inorganic Phosphate Materials*, edited by Kanazawa, T., Elsevier, 1989.

HUMAN BONE MARROW CELL CULTURE-ANALYSIS OF CELL BEHAVIOUR AT BIOCOMPATIBILITY TESTING OF CERAMICS

A. Wilke, S.v. Hirschheydt, and J. Orth
Department of Orthopaedic Surgery
Philipps-University
Baldingerstraße, 3550 Marburg, Germany

I. INTRODUCTION

The most cell culture systems, which are used to test biomaterials are either of none human origin or are using cells, which in vivo are not in contact to orthopaedic implants [Goshima, 1991]. The objective of this study was to investigate the behaviour and the immunological properties of cultured human bone marrow cells on the surface of different biomaterials.

II. MATERIALS AND METHODS

Human bone marrow was harvested during first total hip replacement by removing a marrow containing cancellous bone block from the side of femoral osteotomy. Human bone marrow cells were isolated and freshly incubated.

One day after culture initiation the following growth factors were added: Il 3 and GM-CSF. Five to seven days later a monolayer had developed [Kalla, 1991]. Five million cells were seeded directly onto each tested biomaterial. After further 2 weeks the following techniques were used to investigate the adherent cells:

Episcopic light microscopy, episcopic fluorescence light microscopy, transparent light microscopy and SEM. The following materials were tested:

A. Ceramics: Porous bulk hydroxyapatite ceramic (Cerasiv),Bovine hydroxyapatite
ceramic (Endobon),Aluminiumoxid (Biolox).

B. Metals: Pure titanium (Ti), nitrited Ti6Al4V (Ti-ni), Ti6AI4V alloy, Ti 6Al7Nb (Protasul), stainless steel, cobalt chrome alloy (CoCrMb).

C. Polymere: Polysulfone (PS), Polyaryletherketon (PAEK), Polyethylen (UHMWPE), Loctite (Cyanmethacrylat). All samples were round shaped (26 mm in diameter, 2 mm thickness). The adherent cells on the different surfaces were investigated by different methods:

– Matrix production and adherent cells by SEM.

– Cell vitality with acridine-orange or toluidine blue staining in episcopic fluorescence
light microscopy and in episcopic light microscopy.

– Cell counts after Hämatoxilin staining by episcopic light microscopy.

– Cell differentiation:

0-8493-4750-5/94/$0.00 + $.50

1. after Pappenheim staining by episcopic light microscopy
2. after incubation with monoclonal antibodies against CD-antigen (2, 14, 15, 19) in episcopic fluorescence microscopy
3. after incubation with antibodies against cytoskeletal, intermediate filaments and alkaline phosphatase in episcopic light fluorescence microscopy
4. Analysis of the extracellular matrix after incubation with antibodies (fibronectin, laminin, collagen I, III) in episcopic light microscopy.

III. RESULTS

The controls demonstrated a physiological population of normoblasts, granulocytes and lymphocytes (Pappenheim staining , light microscopy).

By SEM analysis we could observe well attached cells, which spread out, proliferated and showed morphological signs of extracellular matrix (ECM) in case of the ceramics and the titanium specimens (Fig. 1).

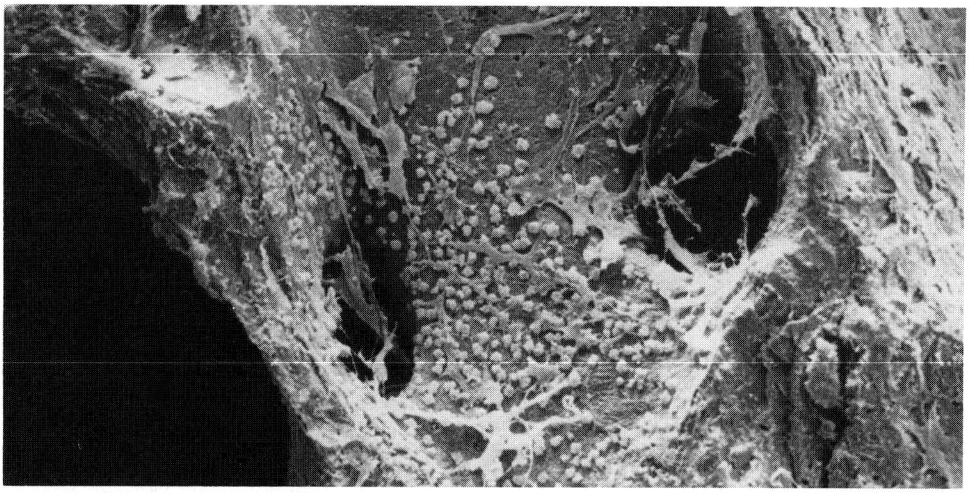

Figure 1. SEM picture of cells and extracellular matrix attached to bovine hydroxyapatite ceramic (Endobon) (magnification X 120).

The ECM was evaluated by use of antibodies against fibronectin, laminin, collagen I, III. The ceramics and the titanium specimens demonstrated high amounts of fibronectin. Laminin and collagen I and III could also be observed, but the amount were less compared to fibronectin. In contact to stainless steel, PS, PAEK (Fig. 2), CoCrMb there were less cells without extracellular matrix and in contact to UHWMPE we could not observe cell development.

By episcopic light microscopy of cells, which were stained (Pappenheim and CD-antibodies) on the material surfaces, no cytomorphological differences appeared to the controls in all samples with cell proliferation,especially in case of the ceramics and the titanium specimens. Cells, which adhered on these biomaterials demonstrated a physiological network of stressfibers after incubation with antibodies against cytoskeleton (esp.actin).

Also the incubation of the adhered cells (on the different biomaterials) with Toluidine blue demonstrated cell attachement by episcopic light microscopy.

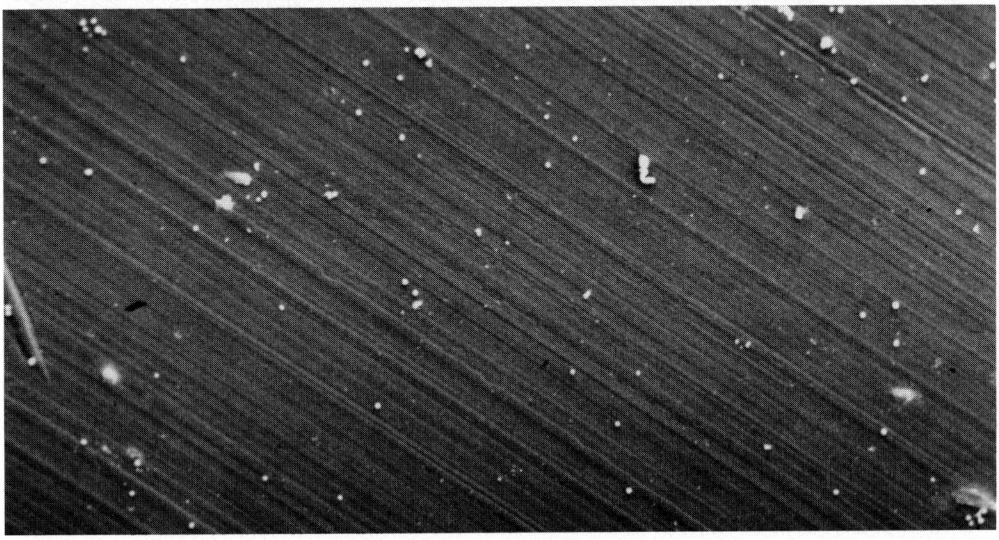

Figure 2. SEM picture of cells attached to polyaryletherketon (PAEK) surface (magnification X 80).

Using episcopic fluorescence light microscopy cell vitality also could be demonstrated after incubation with Acridine orange.As a specific sign of vitality we could see incorporated Acridine orange particles in lysosomes(esp.:in case of the ceramics and the Ti-specimens).

Concerning cell proliferation, cell attachment, cell vitality and segregation of extracellular matrix our results demonstrate striking differences between the tested materials with best results in the ceramics followed by Ti, ni-TI (Fig. 3), Ti6Al4V alloy, stainless steel, PS, Paek, CoCrMb and PE.

IV. DISCUSSION

Regarding the results in our cell culture system it is possible to differentiate the tested biomaterials into three groups:

- "good biocompatibility" in case of the HA-ceramics and Ti-specimens.
- "impaired biocompatibility" in case of stainless steel, CoCrMb , PS, PAEK and Loctite.
- "no biocompatibility" in case of UHMWPE [Wilke, 1992].

The results of our cell culture experiment correlate with the results of numerous animal experiments,which were performed in our laboratories in case of HA-ceramics, Ti alloys, stainless steel, Paek and Polyethylen [Orth, 1990].

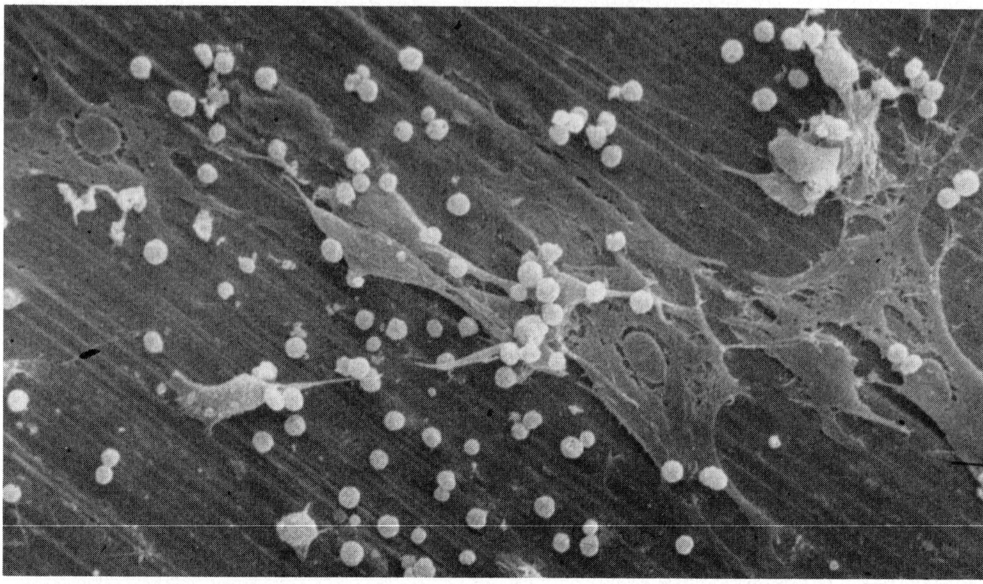

Figure 3. SEM picture of cells and extracellular matrix attached to Ti6Al4V-nitrited surface (magnification X 320).

The biocompatibility was defined by histological response to tested materials (for example, different behaviour concerning "osseointegration") in these animal experiments. Our experimental set up using human bone marrow cells provides to supply reliable results and replace animal experiments. In any way a material of well known histological behaviour should be used as material of reference.

REFERENCES

1. Goshima, J., V. M. Goldberg, and A. J. Caplan, "The osteogenetic potential of culture-expanded rat mesenchymal cells essayed in vivo in calcium phosphate ceramics blocks," Clin. Orthop., 262:298-311 (1991).
2. Kalla , P., P. Hinz-Obertreis, A. Wilke, P. Griss, F. R. Seiler, E. Rüde, and D. Krumwieh, "Bone marrow obtained during hip surgery: A novel source of hemopoisis in human long-term bone marrow culture (LTBMC)," Behring Inst. Mitteil., 90:93-98 (1991).
3. Orth, J., J. Kautzmann, P. Griss, "Bone tissue response to porous hydroxyapatite and wire meshs of stainless steel with and without coatings of hydroxyapatite and titaniumnitrite," in *Clinical Implant Materials, Advances in Biomaterials*, Vol. 9, G. Heimke, U. Soltesz and A. J. C. Lee (eds.), Elsevier Science Publishers, B.V. ,Amsterdam, pp. 283-287 (1990).
4. Wilke, A., J. Orth, H. Kienapfel, G. Schröder, P. Griss, "Sensitivity of different biomaterials," *Trans. 4 th World Biomaterial Congress*, April 24-28, 1992, Berlin, p. 162 (1992).

MINERAL-ORGANIC INTERFACIAL BONDING: EFFECT OF STRAIN RATE ON THE MECHANICAL PROPERTIES OF BONE

W.R. Walsh,*@ H. D. Kim,* D.P. Labrador* and N. Guzelsu#
*Biomechanics Laboratory, Department of Orthopaedics, Brown University School of Medicine, Rhode Island Hospital, Providence, RI 02903.
@Division Of Engineering, Brown University, Providence, RI 02912.
#University of Medicine and Dentistry of New Jersey–SOM Biomechanics & Rutgers University Biomedical Engineering, Piscataway, NJ 08854.

INTRODUCTION

The viscoelastic response of cortical bone to dynamic loads is important for bone's physiological function and has been well documented in tension[1,2] compression[3] and torsional loading.[4,5] An increase in the strength and stiffness has been found with an increase in strain rate. Cortical bone tissue is a hierarchical ceramic composite of organic (30%) and inorganic constituents (70%). The organic matrix is composed of type I collagen and non-collagenous proteins. The inorganic mineral fibers are a hydroxyapatite-like material (HA).[6] Similar to other composites, the mechanical properties of bone have been shown to be dependent upon constituent volume fraction (density) and microstructural organization. In addition, we have demonstrated that interfacial bonding between the constituents of bone play an important role in providing the tensile and compressive strength and stiffness[7-9] and ultrasonic properties of cortical bone.[10] Interfacial bonding between the mineral and organic phases of bone is due, in part, to the strong adsorption affinity of hydroxyapatite for organic material. Mineral-organic interfacial bonding interactions reflects the quality of bone can be modified using ions such as fluoride or phosphate causing a permutation in the mechanical properties. The present study explores the effects of fluoride ion treatment on the compressive properties of cortical bone at different strain rates.

MATERIALS AND METHODS

Adult bovine femurs were obtained from a local slaughterhouse immediately after death and stored frozen in 0.145 M NaCl in plastic bags until use at -20°C. This storage protocol does not alter the mechanical properties of bone tissue.[11] Forty adult bovine cortical bone cubes (5mmx5mmx5mm) were prepared from the medial and lateral quadrant of the central diaphysis by cutting on a low speed saw with a diamond disc blade (Buelher Ltd., Lake Bluff, IL) under dripping distilled water. The long bone (**Z**) axis was marked with a pencil. Samples remained completely wet through all stages of the experiment.

Samples were randomly separated into two treatment groups (20 samples/group). Dimensions were measured in triplicate and averaged using a

0-8493-4750-5/94/$0.00 + $.50

digital caliper. The detergent - ion treatment protocol developed by Walsh and Guzelsu[12] was used in this study. This protocol allows ions access to the mineralized bone matrix[12] and alter mineral-organic interfacial bonding.7-10 All treatments and testing were carried out at room temperature under constant shaking in solutions. Samples were treated in 0.1% Nonidet P40 (NP40) for 24 hours followed by 72 hours in ion treatment solutions: 2.0 M NaCl or 2.0 M NaF (pH 7.5). The pH of the ion treatment solutions were checked daily.

Unconfined uniaxial compression tests were carried out submerged in testing solutions (NaCl or NaF) at strain rates 2.65 x 10^{-3} s^{-1} and 2.65 x 10^{-4} s^{-1} (10 samples/group/strain rate). Samples were tested in the long bone (**Z**) axis. Sample density was determined after mechanical testing using the water displacement technique. Mineral content (ash fraction) was determined by placing the samples in acetone for three days and determining the dry weight followed by ashing in a muffle furnace at 650°C for 18 hours (ashed weight). The ash fraction was calculated by dividing the ashed weight by the dry weight. Fourier transform infrared spectroscopy (FT-IR) was also carried out on a few additional samples using a Perkin-Elmer 1725 IR System using KBr pellets. IR spectra were obtained between 4000 cm-1 and 400 cm-1 at a resolution of 2 cm-1.

Statistical differences between the groups were determined using Statistical Analysis Software (SAS, Cary, NC). Student's t-tests were used to determine the differences between physical properties (density, ash fraction) and mechanical properties of the NaCl and NaF treatments (ultimate stress, elastic modulus) at the different strain rates. Co-analysis of variance and post-hoc analysis using density and ash fraction as covariates.

RESULTS

The pH of the NaCl solution remained stable during the 72 hour treatment period. The pH of the NaF solution rose to near pH 10.0 by the end of the treatment as found in our previous work[6,7,10]. Sample densities and ash fractions did not differ between groups. IR spectra did not reveal any significant effects of treatment[7-9]. Sodium fluoride ion treatment significantly lowered the mechanical properties compared to NaCl controls at both strain rates ($p < 0.001$) (figures 1,2). The ten-fold reduction in strain rate also significantly lowered the mechanical properties of both groups ($p < 0.001$).

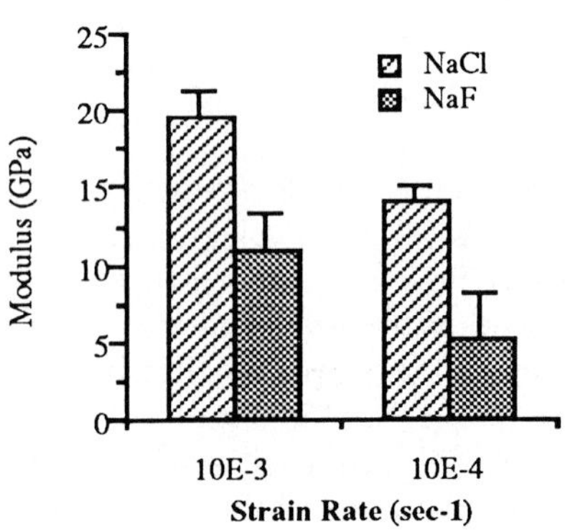

Figure 1. Elastic Modulus at 2.65e-3 s-1 is significantly greater than at 2.65e-4 s-1 in both NaCl and NaF ($p < 0.001$). Moreover, NaF treated samples exhibit a lower modulus than the control specimens ($p < 0.001$).

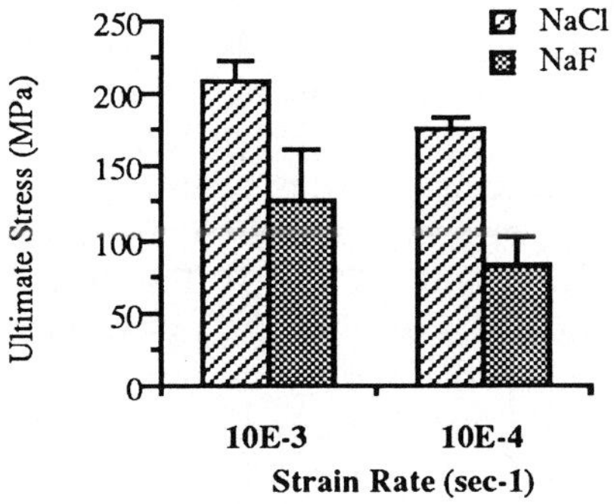

Figure 2. Ultimate stress at 2.65e-3 s-1 is statistically greater than at 2.65e-4 s-1 in both NaF and NaCl ($p < 0.001$). Note that the fluoride treated specimens have a lower ultimate stress than the specimens treated in NaCl ($p < 0.001$).

DISCUSSION

The detergent-ion treatment protocol used in the present study has been shown to alter bonding interactions between the mineral and organic phases of bone leading to an alteration in the mechanical properties.[7-10] This treatment regime does not demineralize or deorganify the bone but rather acts at the interface between the adsorbed organic phase on the hydroxyapatite mineral fibers. Our earlier work has shown that the mechanical properties of cortical bone tissue can be altered following phosphate or fluoride ion treatment. Electrokinetically, these ions are considered potential-determining and specifically adsorbed and can exert a fundamental control over the surface charge of the mineral phase.[12,13] Alterations in the electrostatic interactions (coulombic forces) will modify HA-organic interactions and the mechanical properties of the composite.[7-10]

Increasing the strain rate increases the ultimate stress and elastic modulus of bone when tested in tension or compression.[1-3] Alterations in the quantity of bone (i.e. density, mineral content) have a significant effect on the mechanical properties of bone tissue. Alterations in the quality of bone (mineral-organic bonding interactions) have also been demonstrated to play an important role in governing the strength and stiffness of cortical bone.[7-10] Considering the use of sodium fluoride treatment for osteoporosis and the wide range of loads bone is subjected to during daily living we sought to investigate the influence of a slow strain rate and alterations in mineral-organic bonding following fluoride ion treatment on the mechanical properties of bone.

In the present study, fluoride ion treatment significantly lowered the compressive properties of cortical bone at both strain rates tested (figures 1,2). In tension, *in-vitro* fluoride ion treatment caused a significant reduction in the ultimate stress and elastic modulus as well as an increased plastic deformation.[14] Possible mechanisms for the fluoride effect include a local increase in the pH at the interface between the mineral and organic constituents due to fluoride ion exchange for the hydroxyl ions of HA. The increase in pH to near 10.0, which is above the isoelectric point of collagen and hydroxyapatite, results in an electrostatically unfavorable condition between the constituents of bone; both will be negatively charged. Fluoride ion substitution into HA and possible conversion to fluoroapatite also lower the surface energy and decreases the affinity for organic material.[7,9,14,15] Our results suggest a number of forces are involved between the mineral and organic constituents of bone that contribute to the overall mechanical behavior of this calcified composite.

Modifications in electrostatic interactions along with other forces (van der Waals', hydrogen and hydrophic bonding)[16] and possible shifts in secondary and tertiary structures of the organic phase may also account for the alteration in the mechanical properties.

Alterations in mineral-organic bonding due to the action of fluoride ions significantly influences the viscoelastic properties of bone tissue. The bonds that are modified due to fluoride ion treatment seem to play a role in the dynamic response of bone tissue. Permutations in bone quality also play an important role in the strength and stiffness of bone tissue. This work may have implications considering the quality of bony tissue following clinical treatment regimes for osteoporosis. An increase in bone quantity (density) may not result in an increase in the mechanical properties due to a reduction in the quality or bonding interactions between the mineral and organic constituents.

REFERENCES

1. Wright, T.M. and Hayes, W.C., Tensile testing of bone over a wide range of strain rates: effects of strain rate, microstructure and density, *Medical and Biological Engineering*, 11:671, 1976.
2. Crowinshield, R.D. and Pope, M.H., The Response of Compact Bone in Tension at Various Strain Rates, *Annals of Biomedical Engineering*, 2:217, 1974.
3. McElhaney, J.H., Dynamic response of bone and muscle tissue, *Journal of Applied Physiology*, 21(4): 1231, 1966.
4. Burstein, A.H. and Frankel, V.H., The viscoelastic properties of some biological materials, *Ann. N.Y. Acad. Sci*, 46:158, 1968.
5. Panjabi, M.M., White, A.A. and Southwick, W.O., Mechanical properties of bone as a function of rate of deformation, *J. Bone Jt. Surg.*, 55A:322, 1973.
6. Posner, A.S., Betts, F., and Blumenthal, N.C., Bone mineral composition and structure, in *Skeletal Research: An Experimentral Approach*, Simmons, D.J. and Kunin, A.S., Eds., Academic Press, New York, 1979.
7. Walsh, W.R., Ohno, M., and Guzelsu, N., Bone composite behavior: effects of mineral organic bonding, *J. Material Science - Materials in Medicine*, in press, 1993.
8. Walsh, W.R. and Guzelsu, N., Mineral organic interfacial bonding and the mechanical properties of cortical bone tissue, *Biomimetics*, in press, 1993
9. Walsh, W.R. and Guzelsu, N., Compressive properties of cortical bone: mineral-organic interfacial bonding, *Biomaterials*, in press, 1993.
10. Walsh, W.R., Labrador, D.P, Kim, H.D and Guzelsu, N., Ultrasonic Properties of Cortical Bone Following In-Vitro Fluoride Ion Treatment, *Materials Research Society*, in press, 1993.
11. Sedlin, E.D and Hirsch, C., Factors affecting the determination of physical properties of femoral cortical bone, *Acta Orto. Scand.*, 37:29, 1966.
12. Walsh, W.R. and Guzelsu, N., Electrokinetic Behavior of Intact Wet Bone: Compartmental Model, *J. Ortho. Res.*, 9:683, 1991.
13. Chander, S. and Fuerstenau, D.W., On the dissolution and interfacial properties of hydroxyapatite, *Coll. Surf.*, 4:101, 1982.
14. Guzelsu, N., Ohno, M. and Walsh, W.R., Effects of fluoride ions on the mechanical properties of bone, *Bone*, submitted, 1993.
15. Young, R.A., Implications of atomic substitutions and other structural details in apatites, *J. Dent. Res.*, 2:(Suppl.) 193, 1974.
16. Pearce, E.I., Ion displacement following the adsorption of anionic macromolecules on hydroxyapatite, *Calcif. Tiss. Int.*, 33:395, 1981.

STRUCTURAL ANALYSIS OF THE HUMAN TOOTH ENAMEL BY TRANSMISSION ELECTRON MICROSCOPY

J. Reyes-Gasga* and C.M. Alcántara-Rodríguez**
Instituto de Física,* Facultad de Odontología,**
Universidad Nacional Autónoma de México,
Apartado postal 20-364, 01000 México D.F., MEXICO

1. INTRODUCTION

Human tooth enamel is formed by grains which, when observed with the electron transmission electron microscope, sometimes exhibit a line 1 to 1.5nm thick along their centers. This line has been called "dark line."[1-3] A distinctive feature of the line is that it appears dark in defocus, disappears when the image goes through focus, and is white bordered by two slightly darker fringes in overfocus. This line is observed in conjunction with the (100) lattice fringes of the hydroxyapatite when the grains are observed along the [010] zone axis and parallel to one of the {110} planes when the grains are observed along the [001] zone axis.[4] The occurrence of this line is of particular interest because it seems to go under preferential dissolution during early stages of caries.[5] However many questions remains unanswered as to what the central defect plane really is and what its role in the enamel structure is. In this work we present the results obtained on the human tooth enamel grains and on the dark line when techniques of transmission electron microscopy, x-ray diffraction, digital processing and image simulations are used.

2. EXPERIMENTAL PROCEDURE

Specimens of human tooth enamel from healthy teeth of 20 year old patients were prepared by ion milling technique as follow. The teeth were sectioned with a diamond wheel producing 0.3 x 0.3 cm slices of 250 to 500mm thick. These slices were polished to the thickness of approximately 100mm with No. 1000 silicon carbide paper and water. A slice was glued to a grinder holder and ground in a Fishione 2000 grinder machine to a thickness of 10 mm with periodic reversal to make the grinding uniform on both sides. Afterward the specimens were thinned in a Gatan ion mill until a small hole was produced (approximately 15 hours). The thin edges of the produced hole were thin enough for TEM observation. In addition to the ion milled samples, enamel powder was observed in TEM for comparison. In order to obtain these samples, the enamel was finely ground in a mortar and pestle, the powder dispersed in ethanol and deposited on a copper grid which had been previously coated with a carbon film. An x-ray diffraction pattern was also obtained from this enamel

0-8493-4750-5/94/$0.00 + $.50

powder using a Siemens D-500 diffractometer. The specimens were examined at 100 KV in a JEOL 100CX analytical electron microscope. In particular, techniques of bright field, dark field, lattice imaging and selected area electron diffraction were used. A JEOL 4000EX at 400 KV was used for the high resolution observations. Some images were computer processed using an Innovion system on-line with a 1178 VAX computer in order to enhance their contrast. Computer image simulations of some crystals were carried out using the McTempas image simulation program.

3. RESULTS

a. Electron microscopy

The contrast presented by the enamel in the transmission electron microscope shows small enlongated grains (Fig. 1). The enamel grains are sufficiently small that, when a selected area diffraction pattern is done, many of them contribute to the pattern. This selected area diffraction pattern shows several series of arcs (Fig. 2a) which indicate a textured sample formed by polycrystalline aggregates with a preferential orientation.[6] In this kind of diffraction patterns, along the diameter parallel to the preferential axis the arcs coincide with the original ring pattern whereas along the perpendicular diameter the original rings disappear and new ones appear because the tilting causes the sphere of reflection to cut the planes of the reciprocal lattice circles of higher order. When micro-diffraction patterns are taken from each of these

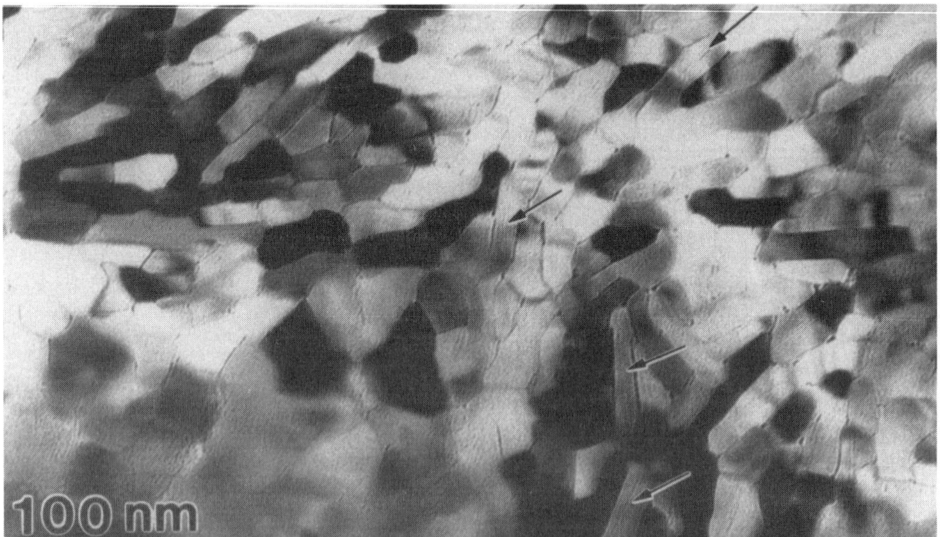

Figure 1. Bright field image of the human tooth enamel. The arrows indicate the black lines observed in some grains.

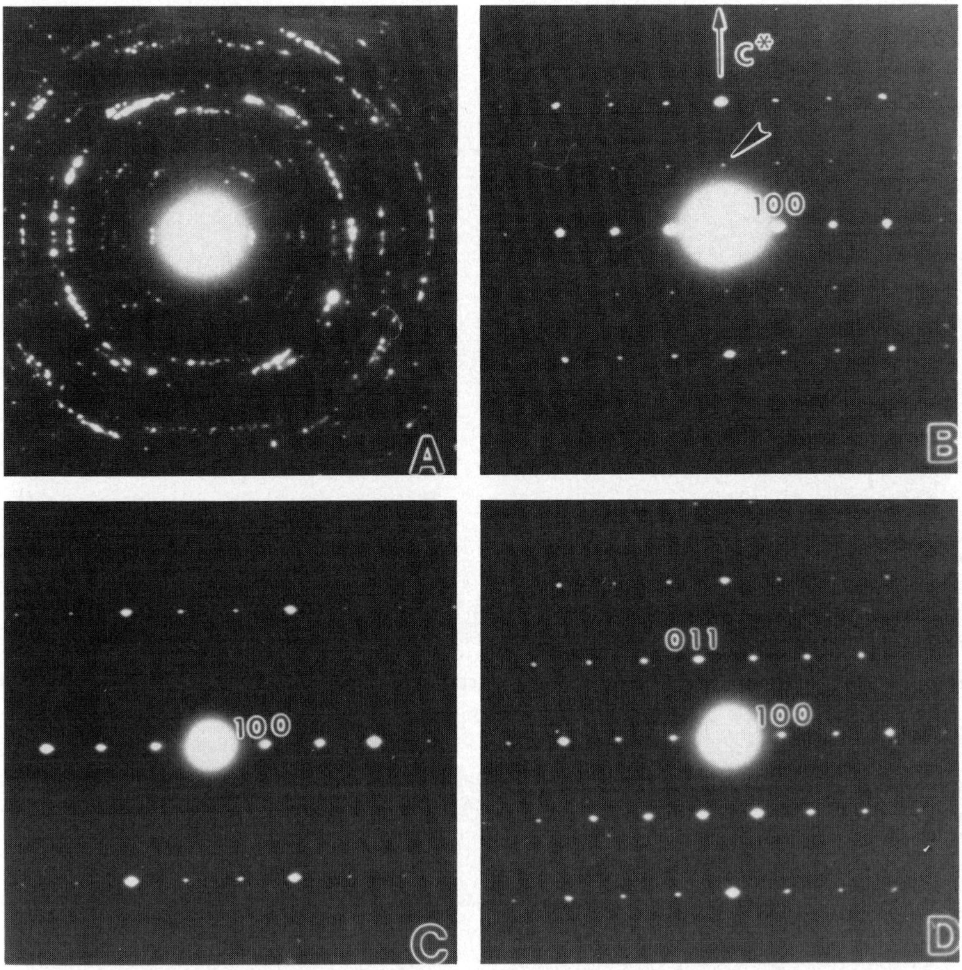

Figure 2. Electron diffraction patterns from the enamel grains. (a) Selected area diffraction patterns, (b-d) m-diffraction patterns: (b) [010], (c) [016], and (d) [011] of the hydroxyapatite unit cell.

grains monocrystalline diffraction patterns are obtained (Figs. 2b-d). The high resolution images of the enamel grains show the existence of amorphous material, surely remanent organic material, among the grains (Fig. 3). From these images we can note the absence of a shift or another feature across the dark line except the line itself.

b. Image simulations

In order to interpret the contrast observed in the high resolution images of the enamel grains image simulations of some apatite structures, such as fluorapatite,[7] chlorapatite[8] and hydroxyapatite,[9] were done. Those hydroxyapatite reproduce the experimental contrast very well. Figure 4 shows the [010] image together with some simulated [010] hydroxyapatite images.

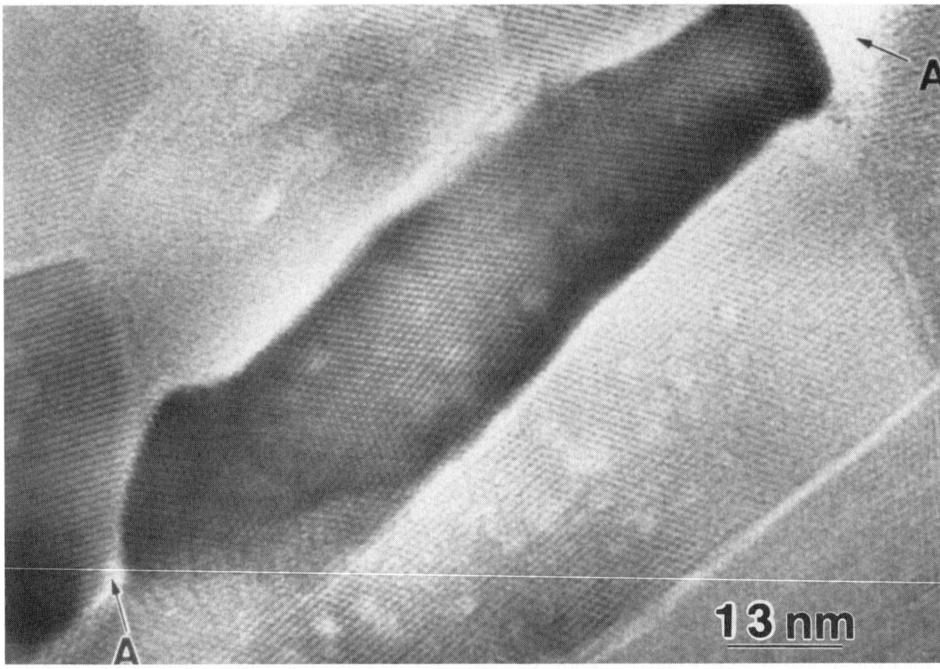

Figure 3. High resolution image of the enamel grains along the [001] zone axis. "A" shows the location of amorphous material.

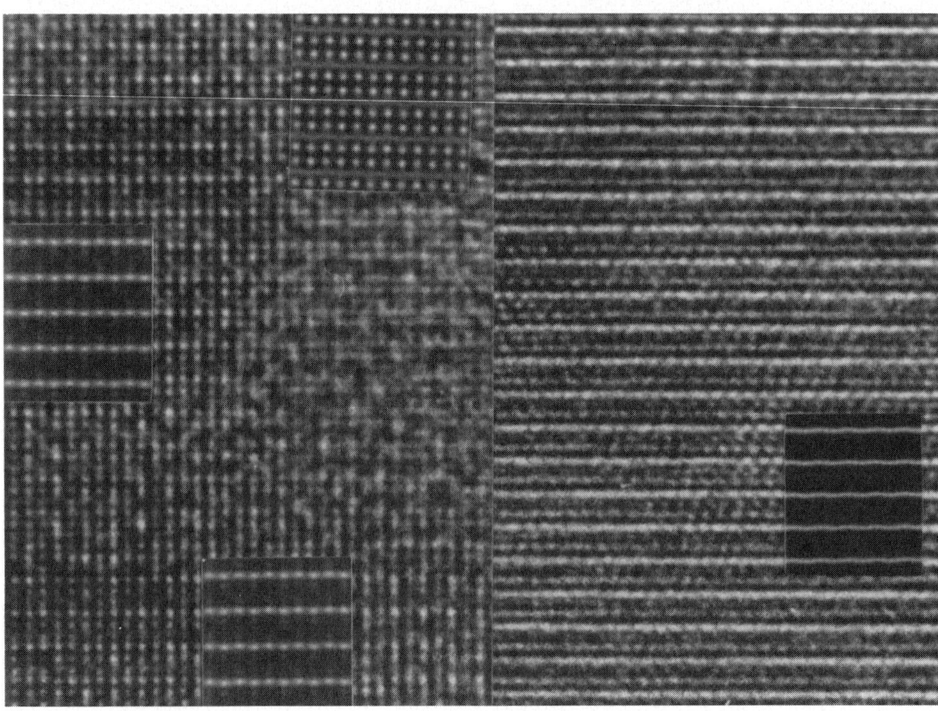

Figure 4. High resolution image along the [010] zone axis. The inserts show the simulated images of hydroxyapatite along this direction.

One of the advantages of the simulation technique is that the diffraction patterns of the structure along any direction are easily obtained. In Figures 5 and 6 the diffraction patterns along the [001], [010] and [011] for the hydroxyapatite and fluorapatite are shown respectively. They can be compared with the experimental ones shown in Figure 2. Immediately we observe some differences among them. First at all, the patterns of the fluorapatite shows several spots missing whereas the ones of the hydroxyapatite are very similar to the experimental ones, except for one missing spot (marked by an arrow in both patterns). It is highly probable that the existence of this spot in the experimental diffraction pattern is the result of a double diffraction phenomenon.

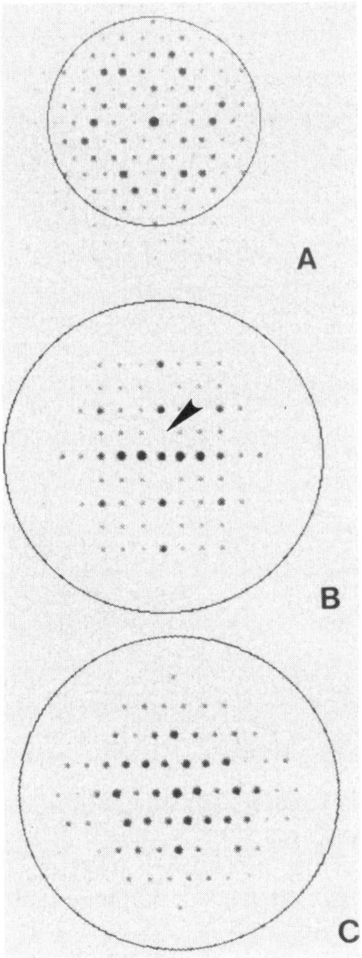

Figure 5. Simulated electron diffraction patterns from the hydroxyapatite unit cell along the [001] (a), [010] (b), and [001] (c) zone axes.

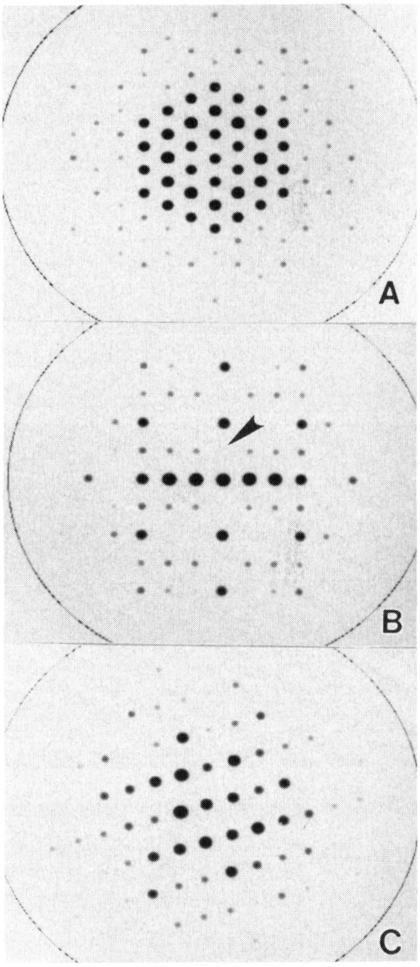

Figure 6. Simulated electron diffraction patterns from the luorapatite unit cell along the [001] (a), [010] (b), and [011] (c) zone axes.

c. Image processing

In order to improve the image contrast and to determine more about the dark line, several high resolution images of the enamel grains were digitally processed. Figure 7 shows one of them. In Figure 7a the original image is shown. From this image the Fourier transform shown in Figure 8 was obtained. Two important features are observed on this last figure: one is the diffuse line between the spots 1 and 4, and the other is the splitting showed by the spots 2 and 5. When all the spot and the diffuse line are allowed to form the processed image, the Figure 7b is obtained. However when only the spots pass through the filter, the Figure 7c is observed, i.e. the line disappears. If only the diffuse line is used to generate the image the figure 7d is obtained. Therefore the line produces both the diffuse line and the splitting of the spots.

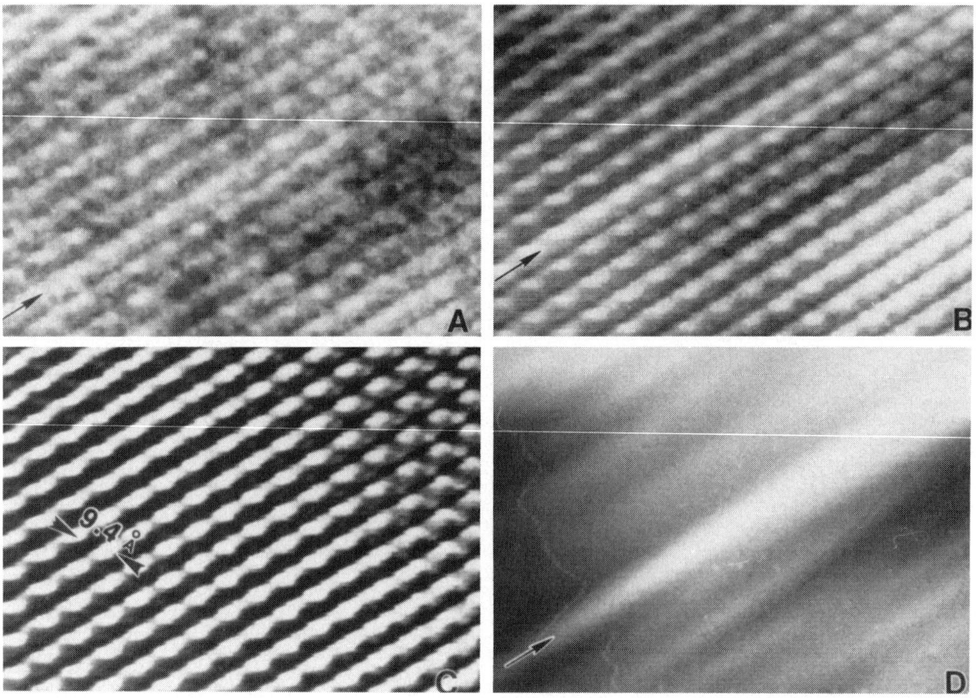

Figure 7. Enamel grain processed image. (a) original image, (b) image observed when all the Fourier transform (F.T.) features (Fig. 8) pass through the filter, (c) image observed when only the hexagonal array of the F.T. pass through the filter, and (d) image observed when only the diffuse line of the F.T. pass through the filter.

d. X-ray analysis

Taking in account the positions and intensities of the peaks, the x-ray analysis from the enamel powder showed that the enamel structure corresponds to the hydroxyapatite structure (Fig. 9a) as it is well known. However when bulk enamel samples are analyzed, depending on which zone of the tooth, the x-ray diffractograms shows important differences. Figures 9b and 9c show the diffractograms obtained from the cuspid and proximal areas of the tooth, respectively. As observed in these figures, there are some preferential orientations: in the proximal sample; the (122) peak is slightly higher than the (002) and the (320) peak is higher than the (402). In the cuspid sample the reverse situation is presented.

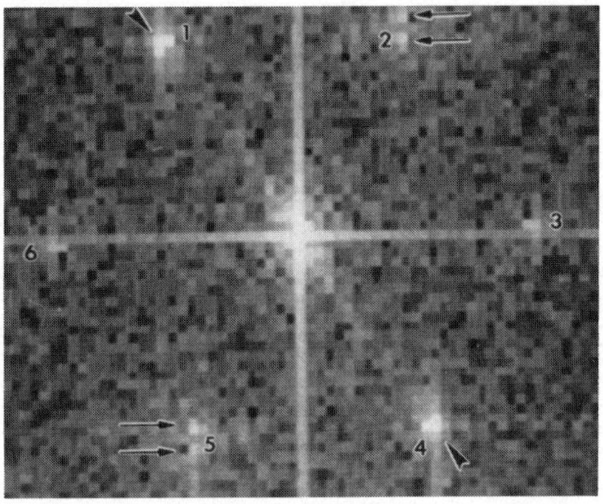

Figure 8. Fourier transform from the image shown in Fig. 9a. Observe that spots 2 and 5 are splitting and that there is a diffuse line between spots 1 and 4.

4. DISCUSSION

Several explanations for the dark line have been proposed. Specifically, that it is a remanent of a calcified organic matrix,[4] a screw dislocation,[10] a twin or grain boundary,[2] or a localized defect plane of carbonate ions coherent in the apatite structure.[11] However the (100) plane fringes are not shifted trough this line and that the (100) plane is not a twinned plane for hexagonal lattices. The fact that the defect plane sometimes ends within the crystal also indicates that it cannot be a boundary. Moreover, the absence of any known contrast when the defect plane is obliquely oriented debates these suggestions. The dependence of the line contrast on the focus suggests that the term "dark" is not correct. The out-of-focus contrast resemble the behavior of Fresnel fringes in the phase-contrast images.[6] That means that at underfocus conditions the fringe is black whereas the contrast of the virtual image, this is overfocus, the fringe is white. The lack of contrast at exact focus is due to the result that the thin specimen (phase-object) affect only the phase of the beam transmitted the specimen and not it amplitude. It worth noting the splitting observed in the Fourier transform of the processed image (Fig. 8). This kind of splitting have been interpreted by Van Dyck et al.[11] as produced by an antiphase boundary. Trying to interpret the dark line as a antiphase boundary, we modeled an antiphase boundary on a hexagonal array and with R= 1/2 [110] (Fig. 10). The Fourier transform of this model also shows a hexagonal array together with a diffuse line and splitting of two spots (Fig. 11). Therefore an antiphase boundary reproduces almost all the features observed in the "experimental" Fourier transform. However the high resolution images shows that there are any shifts across

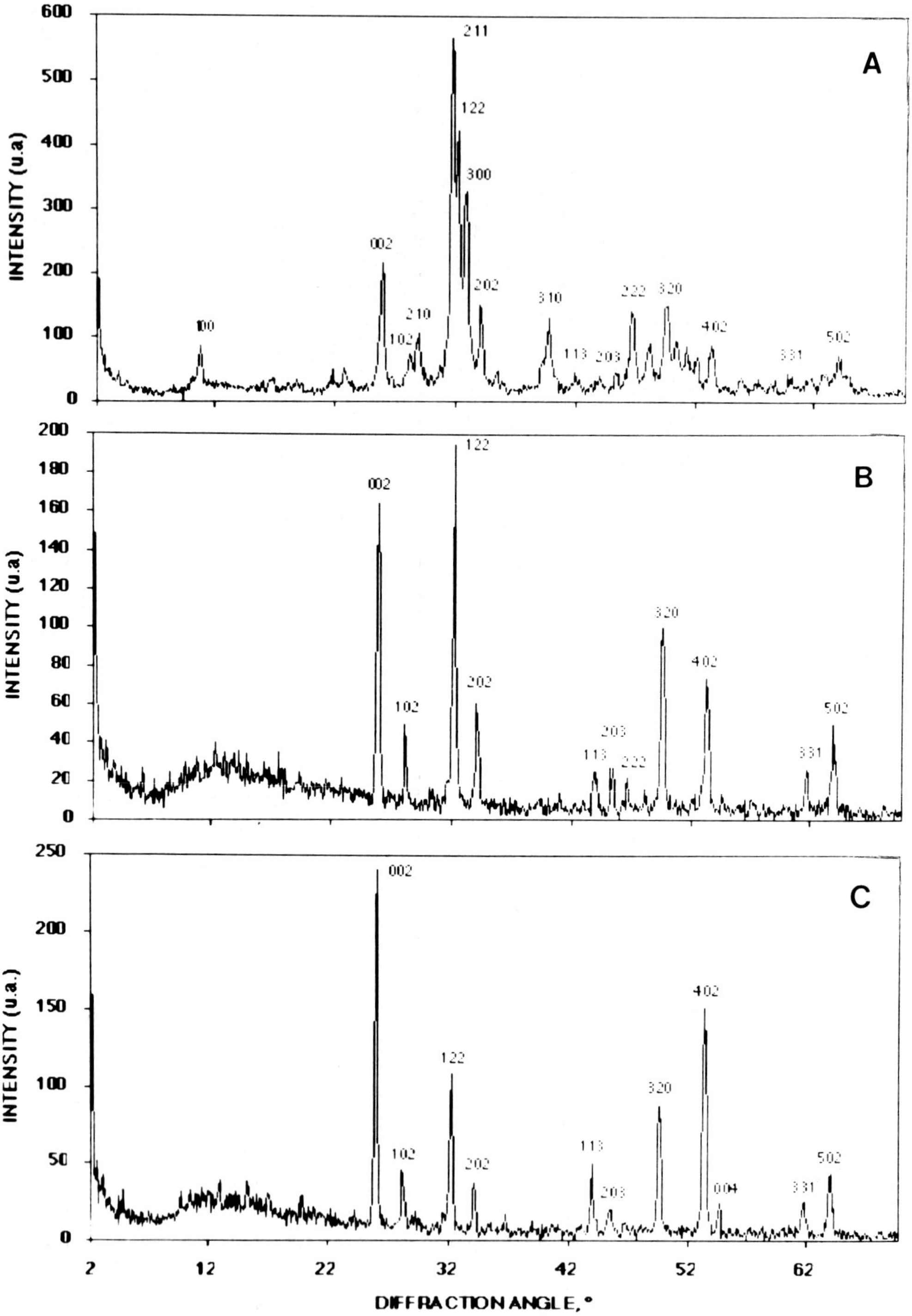

Figure 9. X-ray diffractograms from the human tooth enamel. (a) Enamel powder, (b) sagittal sample (see Fig. 11) and (c) transversal sample. Several differences are easily observed among them.

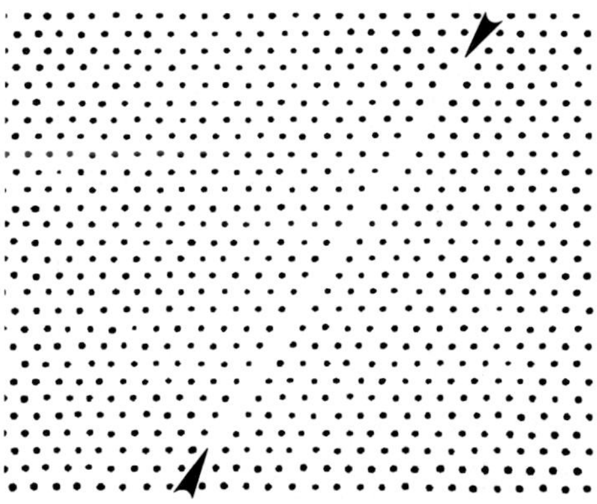

Figure 10. Optical mask consisting of a hexagonal array containing a single 1/2 $[1\bar{1}0]$ antiphase boundary in the middle.

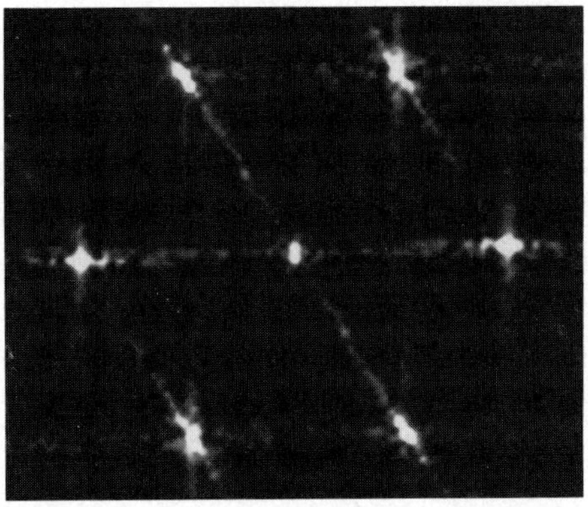

Figure 11. Fourier transform from the optical mask shown in Figure 10.

the line which our model does not predict. So, an antiphase boundary is not all the involved story. An alternative explanation is that during the process of growth of the enamel, greater amounts of impurity ions become incorporated at the center of grains.[13] Therefore the defect plane could represent a localized variation in the chemical composition of the structure. This necessarily involves constituents which commonly occur in the enamel in high amounts such as F, Cl, CO_3, Mg and H_2O ions. The defect might also represent a plane of separate phase that is coherent with hydroxyapatite. For example, octacalcium phosphate has a structure closely related to that of hydroxyapatite which might act as precursor to growth.[14] In summary, the probability that the dark line is a substitutional defect in a matrix of hydroxyapatite is high. This defect must be such that it also produces an antiphase boundary and produces a Fresnel fringe-like behavior observed in the phase-contrast images.

Acknowledgments

The authors want to thank to C. Zorrilla, E. Hernández, L. Rendón, S. Tehuacanero, A. Sanchez, J. Cañetas, L. Beltran del Rio, R. Hernández, P. Mexia, L. Quinterio, J.A. Ramirez, A. Gonzalez, A. Madrigal and V. Vazquez for technical help. This work was financially supported by CONACYT (Proyecto 1601-E9208) and DGAPA UNAM (Proyecto IN-104989).

REFERENCES

1. Ronnholm, E., J. Ultrastructur, Res. 6, 249 (1962).
2. Nylen, M. V., E. D. Eanes, and K. A. Omnell, J. Cell Biol. 18, 109 (1963).
3. Frazier, P. D., Ultras. J. Res. 22, 1 (1968).
4. Marshall, A. F., and K. R. Lawless, J. Dent. Res. 60, 1773 (1981).
5. Scott, D. B., J. W. Simmelink, and V. Nygaard, J. Dent. Res. 53, 165 (1974).

6. Hirsch, P. B., A. Howien, R. B. Nichelson, D. W. Pashley, and M. J. Whelan, "Electron Microscopy of Thin Crystals," Butterworths, London (1965).
7. Young, R. A. and J. C. Elliott, Oral. Biol. 11, 699 (1966).
8. Mackie, P. E., J. C. Elliott, and R. A. Young, Acta Cryst. B 28, 1840 (1972).
9. Kay, M. I., and R. A. Young, Nature 204, 1050 (1964).
10. Arends, J. A., B. S. H. Royce, D. O. Welch, and R. Smoluchowski, in Proc. Intern. Symp. on the Structure and Properties of Hydroxiapatite, R. A. Young (ed.) (Benjamin, New York, 1971).
11. Bress, E. F., J. C. Barry, and J. L. Hutchison, Ultramicroscopy 12, 367 (1984).
12. Dyck, D. Van., G. Van Tendeloo, and S. A. Amelinckx, Ultramicroscopy 15, 357 (1984).
13. Le Geros, R. Z., "Calcium Phosphates in Oral Biology and Medicine," San Francisco Press (1991).
14. Nelson, D. G. A., G. J. Wood, J. C. Barry, and J. D. B. Featherstone, Ultramicroscopy 19, 253 (1986).

THE IN VITRO GROWTH POTENTIAL OF HUMAN BONE DERIVED CELLS ON POLYTETRAFLUOROETHYLENE GRAFTS

M. L. Olmedo, A-P. C. Weiss, W. R. Walsh, L. Zou and M. G. Ehrlich
Orthopaedic Research Laboratories
Department of Orthopaedics
Brown University School of Medicine
Rhode Island Hospital
Providence, Rhode Island 02903

SUMMARY

This study examined the morphological changes of human derived bone cell cultures on polytetrafluoroethylene (PTFE) and polystyrene dishes (tissue culture plastic, Corning Glass Works, Corning, New York) during a three hour period using scanning electron microscopy. Since the material possesses a different configuration on each side, both sides were studied. The cells had a higher affinity for the more porous side of the material.

The morphology of the cells during the three hour period went from round attached cells at one hour to cells that projected filopodia and underwent radial spread over the three hour period. Cells plated on the polystyrene dishes attached and spread more quickly than on either of the PTFE surfaces. The cells on the outside surface of the PTFE remained mostly rounded and attached without spread during the three hour period while cells on the inner surface attached and spread within the scaffolding of the inner surface of PTFE. Clinically, these observations have implications on orthopaedic prosthesis design with regards to whether or not bone ingrowth is desired.

INTRODUCTION

Polytetrafluoroethylene was first isolated in 1938 by Plunkett.[1] Polytetrafluoroethylene is produced by the polymerization of tetrafluoroethylene at 7–70 atmospheres in the presence of water and free radical initiators (peroxy-disulphates and organic peroxidases).[2] Polytetrafluoroethylene is available in three forms: (1) granular used for molded parts and for extruding thick-walled tubing and rods; (2) coagulated dispersions (fine powder) used for extruding thin sections; (3) aqueous dispersions used for coating , impregnation, and making fibers and films.[2]
Over 5,000 kg of PTFE are used each year for medical applications in the US and Europe. PTFE is used as vascular grafts and patches, cardiac valves and aorta implants, shunts in hemodialysis equipment, bone and ligament replacements, and in injectable forms to treat dysphonia and urinary incontinence.[3]

This study was undertaken to evaluate the morphological changes of human derived bone cells in vitro and their response to differing PTFE graft

0-8493-4750-5/94/$0.00 + $.50

surfaces over a three hour period with the hope of eventually using the material for carpal replacement in an in vivo model. PTFE would be a good candidate for these carpal replacements because in its solid form it is very inert and does not cause an intense inflammatory reaction. Also the pores of the PTFE have a strong electronegative surface charge, which is thought to play a role in inhibiting cell ingrowth into the material.[4,5]

MATERIALS AND METHODS

MATERIAL

The PTFE (W.L. Gore and Assoc., Flagstaff, Arizona) used was "medical grade" with an average internodal distance on the inside of the material of 150 μm and pore sizes ranging from 2.9 μm to 18.0 μm. The outside surface of the material was composed of a less organized architecture containing areas of flattened patches of material interdigitated with fibrils. The PTFE was autoclaved and regular polystyrene tissue culture plates were prepared in a sterile manner.

CELL CULTURES

Under sterile conditions human bone was obtained from orthopaedic operations. The human osteoblast enriched cells were isolated through a standard collagenase digestion procedure. Only the 3rd and 4th digestions were used for this experiment. The cells were then grown to confluence in 75 cm flasks. The cells were harvested and plated on both sides of the PTFE and polystyrene at a cell density of 10,000 cells per cm^2. The cells were then incubated at 37 degrees Celsius and 5% CO_2 for one and three hours in F-12 with 10% fetal calf serum to allow the cells to respond to the polystyrene and PTFE samples.

SCANNING ELECTRON MICROSCOPY

Scanning electron microscopy was used to observe the morphology of the cells as they attached and spread on the polystyrene and PTFE. After one and three hours respectively the cells growing on the PTFE samples were fixed with Karnovsky's Fixative (2% PF, 2.5% GA, 0.1 M NaCaCod, pH 7.3). They were rinsed with NaCaCod buffer and post fixed with 1% osmium tetroxide for 1 hour and then rinsed again with 0.1 M NaCaCod buffer. The specimens were progressively dehydrated with EtOH, and critical point dried with liquid CO_2, before being coated with gold and observed with a Hitachi S-2700 scanning electron microscope.

DENSITOMETRY

High resolution photomicrographs were obtained from the SEM's. Each randomly selected graft-cell area was measured using a Jandel digital scanner. Determinations of the total area of cell coverage and the cell area to the total area of the material samples for one and three hours were performed.

RESULTS

	% Cell Attached	% Cell Attached and Spread	Total Cell Area (μm^2)	Total Cell Area /Total Area (%)
Control:				
1 hour	93	7	8,513.18	0.7
3 hours	79	21	28,475.90	2.6
Outside PTFE:				
1 hour	66	34	11,617.81	1.0
3 hours	70	30	14,166.77	1.2
Inside PTFE:				
1 hour	63	37	18,062.00	0.97
3 hours	48	52	14,045.16	1.2

The polystyrene control dishes at one hour had the largest percentage of cells attached, while the three hour polystyrene control had the largest percentage of total area covered by the human derived bone cells. The outside PTFE did not show an appreciable increase in the percentage of cells that just attached and those that attached and spread over the three hour time period. The inside of the PTFE did show an appreciable increase in the percentage of cells that just attached and those that did attach and spread over the three hour time course.

The cells on the polystyrene at one hour appeared round and plump as time progressed the individual cells sent out filipodias and underwent radial spread with flattening. By three hours, 2.6% of the total area we measured was occupied by cells. On the outside of the PTFE, 66% of the cells remained attached without any filipodia present. At three hours, 70% of the cells remained attached and did not send out any filipodia or spread radially. Therefore, the percentage of total area covered for one and three hours on the outside of the PTFE was 1.0% and 1.2% respectively. The inside of the PTFE had an increase in the percentage of cells that attached only and those that attached and spread over the three hour period. The percentage of cells attached and spread on the inside of the PTFE increased from 37% at one hour to 52% at three hours, and the cell area coverage increased from 0.97% to 1.2% over the three hour period.

The morphology of the cells on the polystyrene dishes at one hour demonstrated cells that were mostly round and plump with local attachment. At three hours filipodia were present surrounding a central plump nucleus, and the cells appeared to spread radially and flatten. The morphologic appearance of the cells on the outside surface of the PTFE did not change during the three hour period. The cells on the inside surface of the PTFE settled either in a internodal pore and sent filipodia out and spread between the nodes of the material, or settled on a node with filipodia projecting into the internodal fibrils.

DISCUSSION

Attachment of human derived bone cells to biomaterials entails a definite sequence of events. First, there must be adsorption of the serum proteins on to the biomaterial. Secondly, the human derived bone cells must make contact and attach. A short term tissue culture assay was used to assess cell-material interactions in this study. The process by which cells become established upon a surface in cultures involve attachment leading to cellular spread which generally occurs within three hours.[6] Finally, filipodia are sent out and radial spread occurs.[7,8] Reports indicate that porosity and pore size play an important role in bony ingrowth.[9,10] In addition, a carbon coated PTFE graft (Proplast) suggests that bony ingrowth is inhibited due to smaller interconnecting pore sizes. However, fibroblasts can grow on biomaterials with small interconnecting pores (<50 μm). [11]

The design of biomaterials must consider the form, function, and biocompatibility of the material it is replacing. PTFE can be made in different configurations and does not illicit a significant foreign body tissue response. The use of PTFE for interpositional arthroplasties or small vessel replacement may favor smaller interconnecting pore sizes (<30 μm) to prevent tissue ingrowth. However, if bone ingrowth is desired larger interconnecting pore sizes (>30 μm) would be advantageous.

A morphologic evaluation determined that the inside of the PTFE graft possessed an appropriate internodal distance and pore size to permit osteoblast ingrowth, and that if an in vivo study wanted bony ingrowth. PTFE is a promising biomaterial for a number of orthopaedic applications which requires further study.

Acknowledgement

The authors wish to thank Mr. Andrew Berman of W.L. Gore & Associates, Inc., for providing the experimental material.

REFERENCES

1. McCane, D.I., Tetrafluoroethylene polymers, in *Encyclopedia of Polymer Science and Technology, Plastics, Resins, Rubbers, Fibers*, Vol. 13, Bikales, N.M., Ed., Interscience, New York, 1970, p. 623.
2. *IARC Monographs on the Evaluation of the Carcinogenic Risk of Chemicals to Humans*, Vol. 19, 1979, p. 285.
3. Halpern, B.D., Karo, W., Medical Applications, in *Encyclopedia of Polymer Science and Technology, Plastics, Resins, Rubbers, Fibers*, Suppl. Vol. 2, Interscience, New York, 1977, p. 369..
4. Soyer, T., Lempinen, M., Cooper, P., et al., A New Venous Prosthesis, *Surgery*, 72:864, 1972.
5. Kempczinski, R., Physical Characteristics of Implanted Polytetrafluorethylene Grafts, *Arch Surg*,114:917, 1979.
6. Howlett, C.R., Evans, M.D.M., Walsh, W.R., Johnson, G., Steele, J.G., The Mechanism of initial attachment of cells derived from human bone to commonly used prosthetic materials during cell culture, *Biomaterials*, in press, 1993.
7. Grinell, F., Cellular adhesiveness and extracellular substrata., *Int. Rev. Cytol.*, 53:85, 1978.
8. Malik, M.A., Puleo, D.A., Bizios, R., Doremus, R.H., Osteoblast on hydroxyapatite, alumina and bone surface in vitro: morphology during the first 2 h of attachment, *Biomaterials* 13(2):123, 1992.
9. Homsy, C.A., Comments on "Characteristics of Tissue Growth into Proplast and Porous Polyethylene Implants in Bone," *J Biomed Mat Res* , 13:987, 1979.
10. Neel, H.B., Implants of Gore-Tex, *Arch Otolaryngol*, 109:427, 1983.
11. Spector, M., Harmon, S.L., Kreutner, A., Characteristics of Tissue Growth into Proplast and Porous Polyethylene Implants in Bone, *J Biomed Mat Res*, 13:677, 1992.

ULTRASONIC PROPERTIES OF CORTICAL BONE FOLLOWING IN-VITRO FLUORIDE ION TREATMENT

W.R. Walsh,*@ D. P. Labrador,* H. D. Kim* and N. Guzelsu#
*Biomechanics Laboratory, Department of Orthopaedics, Brown University School of Medicine, Rhode Island Hospital, Providence, RI 02903.
@Division of Engineering, Brown University, Providence, RI 02912.
#University of Medicine and Dentistry of New Jersey - SOM Biomechanics & Rutgers University Biomedical Engineering, Piscataway, NJ 08854.

INTRODUCTION

The mechanical properties of cortical bone have been examined using destructive, mechanical testing as well as non-destructive, ultrasound testing to obtain the elastic coefficients. By measuring the sample density and velocities of sound waves in a number of different directions, ultrasonic testing allows characterization of the anisotropy of a single, small specimen not possible by traditional destructive mechanical testing techniques. Furthermore, the comparison of ultrasonic and mechanical testing properties for cortical bone demonstrates that ultrasound is a high strain rate test.[1] Ultrasonic techniques offer a method to examine the high strain rate elastic properties of a single cortical bone specimen in all directions.

As a material, cortical bone is a non-homogenous, anisotropic, viscoelastic, multi-phased composite composed of a stiff inorganic bone mineral embedded in a compliant organic matrix.[2] Bone mineral, a hydroxyapatite-like material, ($Ca_{10}(PO_4)_6(OH)_2$), also contains substantial amounts of CO_3^{2-} (4-6%), citrate (0.9%), Mg^{2+} (0.5%), and Na^+ (0.7%), and trace amounts of Cl^-, F^-, K^+ and Sr^{2+}, and other metal ions.[2] The dimensions of bone mineral have been reported to be in the range of 20-40 nm in length and 2-4 nm in width.[3] Type I collagen comprises more than 90% of the organic matrix of bone.[4] The remaining 10% of the organic matrix is composed of a number of noncollagenous proteins and lipids.[4,5] The majority of the noncollagenous proteins are anionic (negatively charged)[6] and bind readily to calcium on the surface of hydroxyapatite.[6,7]

A number of studies have characterized the non-homogenous and anisotropic nature of cortical bone revealing further complexity of this tissue with respect to position (proximal, midshaft and distal) and quadrants (anterior, posterior, medial and lateral).[1,8,9] Similar to other composites, the mechanical properties of cortical bone have been demonstrated to depend on a number of factors including: constituent properties, volume fraction, orientation and, more recently, interfacial bonding interactions between the mineral and organic phases.[10-12] Using a detergent and ion-treatment protocol we have demonstrated that interfacial bonding interactions between the mineral and organic phases of bone play an important role in the mechanical properties using slow strain rate mechanical testing ($2.65 \times 10^{-3}\ s^{-1}$). Partial debonding between

0-8493-4750-5/94/$0.00+$.50

the consituents of bone have been hypothesized to play a role in the properties of aged and diseased bone.[13] Furthermore, the effects of fluoride ions on the mechanical properties of bone remain extremely controversial. Literature reports of an increase as well as a decrease in properties.[15,17] The present study examines the role of interfacial bonding on the ultrasonic properties of adult bovine cortical bone and the effects of in-vitro fluoride ion treatment.

MATERIALS AND METHODS

An adult bovine femur was obtained from a local slaughterhouse. Specimens were prepared from the medial quadrant of the central diaphysis to minimize biological variability due to position and quadrant with respect to density and mineral content.[1] The specimen was wrapped in 0.145 M NaCl soaked paper towels and stored at -20°C until use. This storage procedure does not alter the mechanical properties of bone tissue. Samples remained completely wet throughout the preparation. Forty cortical bone cubes (5 mm x 5 mm x 5 mm) were prepared by cutting on a low speed saw with a diamond disc blade (Buelher Ltd, Lake Bluff, IL) under dripping distilled water. The long bone (**Z**), circumferential (T) and radial (**R**) orientations were marked with a pencil. Samples were randomly separated into two groups (20 samples per group).

The ultrasonic velocities were obtained using 5 MHz piezoelectric transducers (Ultran Laboratories, Boalsburg, PA) in pulse-echo mode. Pulse width of 110 ns and amplitude of 200 V were employed for optimal reflection detection.[1] The longitudinal velocities in the Z, R and T directions were measured on all specimens at the start of the experiment. Transducers were placed directly on the bone with a coupling agent and the reflections recorded with a personal computer using an Ultran NDC 7000 System. The dimensions of the cubes were measured in triplicate using a digital caliper. Ultrasonic velocites were calculated by taking twice the thickness of the bone and dividing by the time of flight determined from the ultrasound reflections. Density was calculated as the hydrated tissue mass divided by the bone tissue volume. Bone tissue volume was calculated as the hydrated weight less the submerged weight. The ultrasonic modulus was calculated by multiplying the square of the velocity by the specimen density.

The detergent-ion treatment protocol developed by Walsh and Guzelsu[16] was used in this study. This protocol has been previously shown to allow ions access to the mineralized bone matrix[16] and alter mineral-organic interfacial bonding.[5-8] Cubes were treated in 0.1% Nonidet P40 (Sigma Chemical Co. St Louis MO, No. N-3516), a nonionic alcohol type detergent, for 24 hours under constant shaking at room temperature. Samples were rinsed in copious amounts of distilled water and their ulrasonic velocities in all three directions measured (day 0). Samples were then placed into either 0.145 M NaCl of 2.0 M NaF adjusted to pH 7.5. Samples were treated in these equilibration solution for 20 days under constant stirring at room temperature. The pH of the treatment solutions were measured every 24 hours using a pH electrode. The ultrasound velocities were measured at 3, 6, 13 and 20 days in treatment solutions.

Following ultrasound testing the density and ash fraction (mineral content) were determined. Samples were dehydrated in acetone for three days and ashed in a muffle furnace at 650 ^{o}C for 24 hours.[13] The ash fraction was calculated by dividing the ashed weight by the dry weight. Fourier Transform Infrared

Spectroscopy (FT-IR) was carried out in order to examine the effects that the treatment solutions had on the mineral phase of bone. Bone wafers (0.5 mm thick) were cut from the medial quadrant of a bovine femur and treated with the NP40 detergent and 0.145 M NaCl or 2.0 M NaF for 20 days. IR spectra were obtained at days 0, 3, 6, 9, 12, 20 of equilibration. Samples for FT-IR spectra analysis were ground with a mortar and pestle and prepared using approximately 0.6 mg of sample per 300 mg of KBr. FT-IR spectra were recorded with a Perkin Elmer FT-IR Spectrometer Model 1725X. Spectra were recorded from 4000 cm-1 to 400 cm^{-1} with a resolution of 2 cm^{-1}.

A fluoride ion electrode (Orion Laboratories, Boston, MA) was used to obtain the concentration of fluoride ion uptake in cortical bone specimens[17]. In addition, thirty-six bone wafers (eighteen wafers 0.5 mm x 5 mm x 5 mm and eighteen 2 mm x 5 mm x 5 mm) were cut and were equilibrated (3 wafers per group) in 2 M NaF for 0, 1, 3, 6, 9, and 12 days. Following treatments, specimens were washed twice in deionized water, dried for one hour at 60 ^{o}C, weighed, ashed at 650 ^{o}C overnight, and weighed again. Each specimen was then crushed in a mortar and pestle and then dissolved in 1 ml of 6 N HCl. Fifty ul of that solution was added to 0.95 ml distilled water. One ml of total ionic strength adjustment buffer (Orion) was added (final pH = 5.2), and the fluoride content of the sample was measured in parts per million (ppm) using the fluoride ion electrode. Furthermore, mass and volume from density measurements were used to normalize the fluoride concentrations of different specimens to be expressed as ppm per bone weight per ml HCl used (ppm/g/ml) and ppm per bone volume per ml HCl used (ppm/cm^3/ml).

STATISTICAL ANALYSIS

Statistical analysis was carried out using Statistical Analysis Software (SAS, Cary, NC). Analysis of variance (ANOVA) and multiple comparison post-hoc analyses (Duncan's Multiple Range Test, Least Significant Difference (LSD) and Bonferroni t-tests, Tukey's and Scheffe's to control for type I and type II errors) were carried out to determine the differences and levels of significance between mechanical parameters (ultimate and yield stress, elastic modulus, energy at peak load/volume) between groups. Coanalyses of variance (COANOVA) were performed using density and ash weights as covariates to account for any biological variation between groups and its influence on the differences.

RESULTS

The pH of the NaCl solution remained at pH 7.5 (±0.2) throughout the twenty day experimental period. The pH of the sodium fluoride solution rose steadily from pH 7.5 to near 10.0 after three days and remained constant. This reflects a hydroxyl ion exchange with fluoride ions consistent with our previous results[10-12] and the exchange between fluoride ions and hydroxyl ions.[18,19] The densities and ash fraction of the samples before and after the twenty day treatment did not significantly differ.

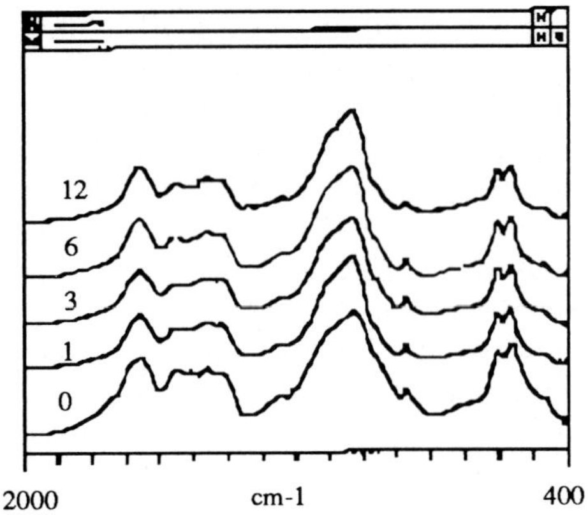

Figure 1. Infrared (IR) spectra from 2.0 mm thick bone wafers following NP40 treatment and various days of equilibration in 2.0 M NaF. The IR patterns did not demonstrate any significant variations.

Infrared (IR) spectra did not reveal any significant differences between the sodium chloride or sodium fluoride treated groups versus time (figures 1, 2). The spectra between 1200-900 cm^{-1} (v_1 and v_3 stretching mode PO_4 regions) and 700-500 cm^{-1} (v_4 bending modes PO_4 region) did not vary with respect to resolution. No change in resolution can be interpreted as no effect of treatment on the crystal size.[20] The IR spectra between 700-500 cm^{-1} did not shift to that of an amorphous calcium phosphate. Equilibration in NaF did not significantly alter the IR spectra of the mineral phase within the limitations of detection. Fluoride ion probe measurements revealed that fluoride ion concentration per dry weight of mineral (ppm/gm ashed bone) reached a steady state by three days for 0.5 mm and 2.0 mm wafers.

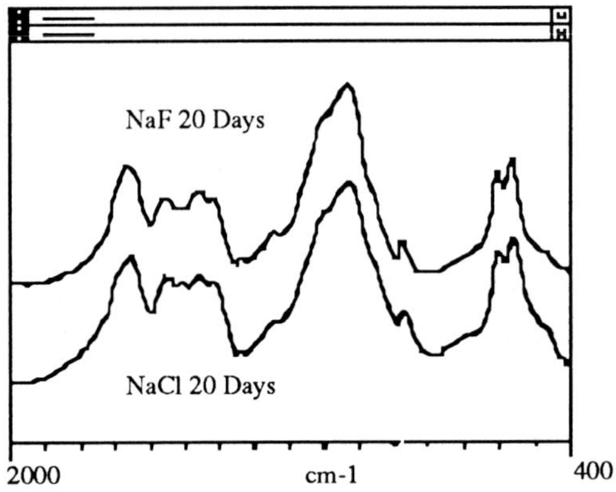

Figure 2. IR spectra for controls and NaF treated at day 20 did not demonstrate any significant variations.

The ultrasonic velocities and moduli for all time points are summarized in figures 3-5 (means and standard deviations). Moduli were highest in the Z axis followed by T and R for both groups at all time points ($p<0.0001$). ANOVA analysis at time 0 did not demonstrate any statistical differences between the NaCl and NaF samples in the Z direction. However, at time 0 the R and T NaF moduli were slightly greater than the sodium chloride controls ($p<0.05$).

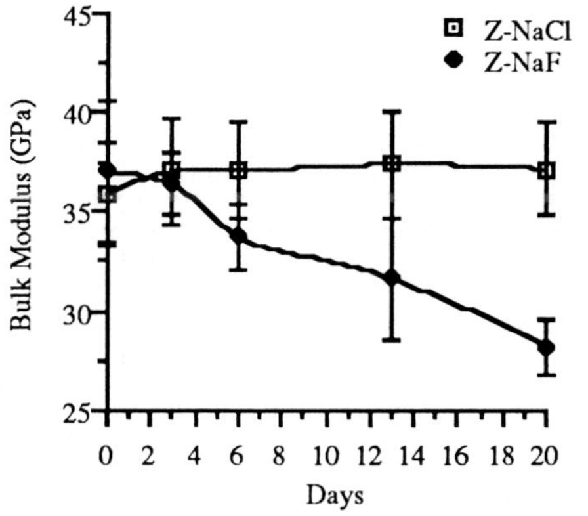

Figure 3. Ultrasonic moduli in the long bone (Z) direction is presented for 0.145 M NaCl (controls) and 2.0 M NaF treated versus time. The NaCl moduli did not differ versus time. However, NaF treatment caused a significant reduction which becomes significant after day 6 ($p < 0.001$). The modulus continued to demontrate an increase in the reduction even at day 20 ($p < 0.001$).

The Z, R and T NaCl moduli did not statistically differ during the twenty day equilibration period (figures 3-5). ANOVA analysis revealed no statistically significant differences between the NaCl versus NaF moduli in the Z, R or T directions until day 6 ($p < 0.001$) which continued at days 13 and 20. The NaF moduli in the R and T direction did not significantly change after day 6. The NaF moduli in the Z direction continued to demonstrate a reduction at days 13 and 20 ($p < 0.001$). A two-way ANOVA revealed time had a significant interactive effect on the NaF group (up to day 6 for R and T and day 20 for Z directions) but not on the NaCl samples. Coanalysis of variance (COANOVA) using ash weight and density as covariates revealed no findings not already predicted by the ANOVA.

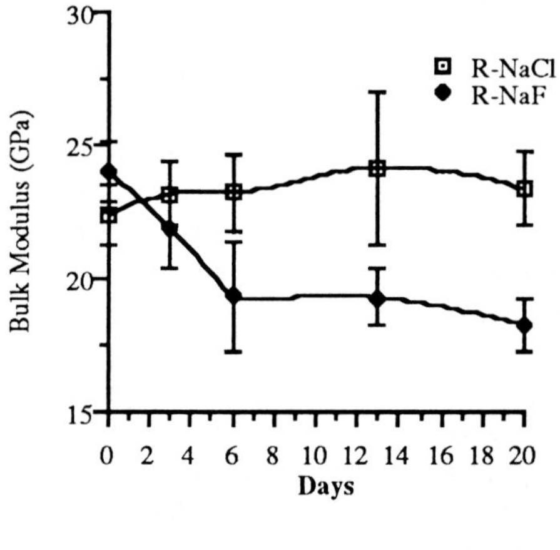

Figure 4. Ultrasonic moduli in the radial (R) direction is presented for 0.145 M NaCl (controls) and 2.0 M NaF treated versus time. The NaCl moduli did nott vary versus time. However, NaF treatment caused a reduction which became significant after day 6 ($p < 0.001$) and stabilized.

DISCUSSION

Ultrasound testing, a non-destructive technique, offers an advantage over destructive mechanical testing by enabling the properties of a single specimen to be obtained in many directions. Considering our experiment was an *in-vitro* equilibration, the biological effects of sodium fluoride on bone cells was not considered in the present study. We have previously demonstrated using slow-strain rate destructive mechanical testing that in-vitro sodium fluoride equilibration results in a reduction in the tensile[13] and compressive properties[14,15] of adult bovine cortical bone oriented in the long bone (Z) axis.

The results obtained in the present study indicate that *in-vitro* equilibration of bovine cortical bone in sodium fluoride lowers the ultrasonic properties in Z, R and T axis.

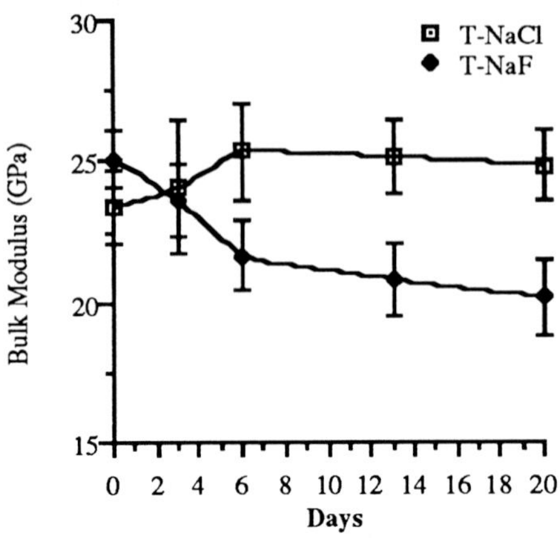

Figure 5. Ultrasonic moduli in the circumferential (T) direction is presented for 0.145 M NaCl (controls) and 2.0 M NaF treated versus time. The NaCl Moduli did not vary versus time. However, NaF treatment caused a significant reduction which became significant after day 6 ($p < 0.001$) and stabilized.

The reduction in the ultrasonic properties following fluoride ion treatment *did not* arise as a result of a reduction in density or partial demineralization or deorganification, or modification in the IR spectra in the specimens.[13-15] Rather, the reduction in the ultrasonic moduli and ultrasonic velocity may be attributed to an alteration in the interfacial bonding between the mineral and organic constituents of bone. The detergent and ion-treatment protocol allows ions access to the mineral-organic interface and alter the interfacial bonding between the mineral and organic consituents of bone.[10-12,16] Partial debonding of the matrix and fibers of a composite will significantly modify the strength and stiffness.[13]

This work presents the first data indicating that interfacial bonding between the mineral and organic constituents of bone play an important role in determining the anisotropic nature of bone. The greatest reduction in the fluoride treated sample compared to controls was observed in the Z axis. The radial and circumferential orientations revealed similar alterations compared to the Z axis, but did not continue to decrease. This may reflect the orientation of the mineral phase and the available organic bonding sites.

Interfacial bonding between the mineral and organic constituents occurs primarily through electrostatic interactions and can be altered by ions which selectively adsorb to the mineral surface. Fluoride ions are able to exchange with the hydroxyl ions of HA.[18,19] This leads to a local pH increase at the interface and an electrostatically unfavorable condition between the constituents.[11,12] These factors along with possible conformational protein charges may account for the reduction observed in the ultrasonic properties of bone following fluoride ion treatment.

REFERENCES

1. Kim, H.D. and Walsh, W.R., Mechanical and Ultrasonic Characterization of Cortical Bone, *Biomimetics,* in press, 1993.
2. Posner, A.S., Betts, F., and Blumenthal, N.C., Bone mineral composition and structure, in *Skeletal Research: An Experimentral Approach,* Simmons, D.J. and Kunin, A.S., Eds., Academic Press, New York, 1979.
3. Cowin, S.C., The mechanical properties of cortical bone, in *Bone Mechanics,* Cowin, S.C., Ed., CRC Press, Boca Raton, FL, 1989.
4. Veis, A., Bones and teeth, in *Extracellular matrix biochemistry,* Piez, K.A. and Reddi, A.H., Eds., Elsevier, New york, 1984.
5. Boskey, A.L., Mineral-matrix interactions in bone and cartilage, *Clin. Orthop. Rel. Res.,* 281:244, 1992.
6. Li, S.T. and Katz, E., On the state of anionic groups of demineralized bone and dentin, *Calcif. Tiss. Res.,* 22:275, 1977.
7. Pinto, M.R., Gorshi, J.P., Penniston, J.T., and Kelly, P.J., Age-related changes in composition and Ca^{2+} binding capacity of canine cortical bone extracts, *Am. J. Physiol.,* 255:101, 1988.
8. Ashman, R.B., Cowin, S.C., Van Buskirk, W.C. and Rice, J.C., A continuous wave technique for the measurement of the elastic properties of cortical bone, *J. Biomechanics,* 17:349, 1984.
9. Katz, J.L., and Yoon, H.S., The structure and anisotropic mechanical properties of bone, *IEEE Transactions on Biomedical Engineering,* 31:878, 1984.
10. Walsh, W.R., Ohno, M., and Guzelsu, N., Bone composite behavior: effects of mineral organic bonding, *J. Material Science - Materials in Medicine,* in press, 1993.
11. Walsh, W.R. and Guzelsu, N., Mineral organic interfacial bonding and the mechanical properties of cortical bone tissue, *Biomimetics,* in press, 1993
12. Walsh, W.R. and Guzelsu, N., Compressive properties of cortical bone: mineral-organic interfacial bonding, *Biomaterials,* in press, 1993.
13. Bundy, K.J., Determination of mineral-organic bonding effectiveness in bone - Theoretical considerations, *Ann. Biomed. Eng.,* 13:119, 1985.
14. Franke, J., Runge, H., Grau, P., Fengler, F., Wanka, C. and Rempel, H., Physical properties of fluorosis bone, *Acta orthop. scand.,* 47:20, 1976.
15. Lees, S. and Hanson, D.B., Effect of fluoride dosage on bone density, sonic velocity and longitudinal modulus of rabbit femurs, *Cal. Tiss. Int.,* 50:88, 1992.
16. Walsh, W.R. and Guzelsu, N., Electrokinetic Behavior of Intact Wet Bone: Compartmental Model, *J. Orthop. Res.,* 9:683, 1991.
17. Lundy, M.W., Wergedal, J.E., Teubner, E., Burnell, J., Sherrard, D. and Baylink, D.J., The Effect of Prolonged Fluoride Therapy for Osteoporosis: Bone Composition and Histology, *Bone,* 10:321, 1989.
18. Young, R.A., Implications of atomic substitutions and other structural details in apatites, *J. Dent. Res.,* 2:(Suppl.) 193, 1974.
19. Chander, S. and Fuerstenau, D.W., An XPS study of the fluoride uptake by hydroxyapatite, *Colloids and Surfaces,* 13:137, 1985.
20. Legeros, R.Z., Calcium phosphates in Oral Biology and Medicine, *Monographs in Oral Science,* vol. 15, Myers, H.M., Ed., Krager, Basel, 1991.

XPS STUDY OF APATITES AND RELATED CALCIUM PHOSPHATES

A. Lebugle, B. Sallek
Laboratoire des Materiaux
Institut National Polytechnique
118, route de Narbonne
F-31077 Toulouse Cedex, France

Apatites and calcium phosphates of either natural (bone, teeth) and synthetic origin, show compositions which are often complex due to the number and the nature of the elements included (with a low or high molecular weight).[1] The complexity is also due to the chemical form in which the elements are present (PO_4^{3-}, HPO_4^{2-}, CO_3^{2-}). The determination of each element, in different possible chemical forms is not easy, particularly when they are together. Thus, HPO_4 ion determination as pyrophosphate[2] is disturbed when CO_3 ions are present in apatite.[3] In the same way, HPO_4 ions interfere with the determination of CO_3 ions by IR using the band near 873 cm^{-1}.[4] Also, natural apatites often need a pretreatment in order to remove the organics which are invariably present. This treatment can affect the chemical composition of the calcium phosphate. Apatites and calcium phosphates exhibit surface reactivities which has important implications in their biological behavior.[5] The study of such properties (dissolution, adsorption of organic molecules) can not be achieved by bulk analysis.

In this paper we will firstly present, through examples concerning calcium phosphates, the main characteristics of XPS. Then, we will show how this technique allows some of the analytical problems previously been mentionned to be solved.

A. MAIN CHARACTERISTICS OF XPS

1. Principle

Briefly, x-ray photoelectron spectroscopy or XPS consists of exposing a sample to a monochromatic x-ray beam. The electrons from each atomic level (1s; 2s; 2p3/2, etc.) are ejected with a kinetic energy equal to the difference between the beam energy, and the electron binding energy. The measurement of the kinetic energies of the electrons produced allow their binding energies to be determined.[6] So the XPS spectrum of a given element is constituted of several peaks at given energies, like a finger print. In such conditions, identification of the elements present is easy.

0-8493-4750-5/94/$0.00 + $.50

2. Qualitative Analysis

The XPS spectrum of dentine is represented in Figure 1. Various atomic levels of the elements of the mineral and organic parts (Ca, P, O, C, N, etc) can be seen.[7] Furthermore, elements present in small quantities, like Mg or F for example, can also be detected. XPS can be applied to almost all elements of the periodic table. It has been applied to the study of natural concretions, such as urinary stones.[8]

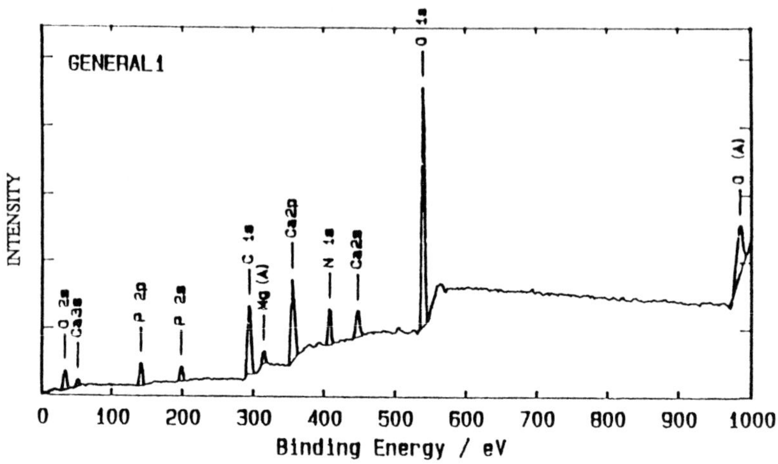

Figure 1. XPS spectrum of dentine.

3. Quantitative Analysis

The C/N and Ca/N atomic ratios of dentine were determined at two locations (near the enamel and near the pulp), by measuring the peak areas and using the Scofield sensitivity factors (Table 1). The first ratio corresponds to the composition of apatite. The second one reveals the degree of mineralization of the dentine. It is more calcified near the pulp. The difference in composition with the dentine level can be determined, because the depth of analysis is limited to about 30-40 Å, due to the electron mean free path.

Table 1.
Quantitative analysis of dentine (near enamel).

Dentine	Ca/P	Ca/N
near the enamel	1.34	1.08

4. Chemical Shift

Chemical shift is the variation of the core level electron binding energy due to the environnement in which the atom is sited, and due to its ionic charge. Although the principle is completly different, XPS can de compared to some extent to NMR due to its sensitivity to chemical environnement. Chemical shift can be exemplified in the case of monetite $CaHPO_4$, on the oxygen 1s spectrum (Figure 2). The peak is disymetric and can be decomposed into two components which are in a ratio close to 75/25. They correspond to the two types of oxygen atoms which can be distinguished in the HPO_4 groups. Three equivalent oxygen atoms are only linked to P, whereas one is linked to both P and H. The P-O-H oxygen is less charged than the P-O one, and appears at higher binding energy.

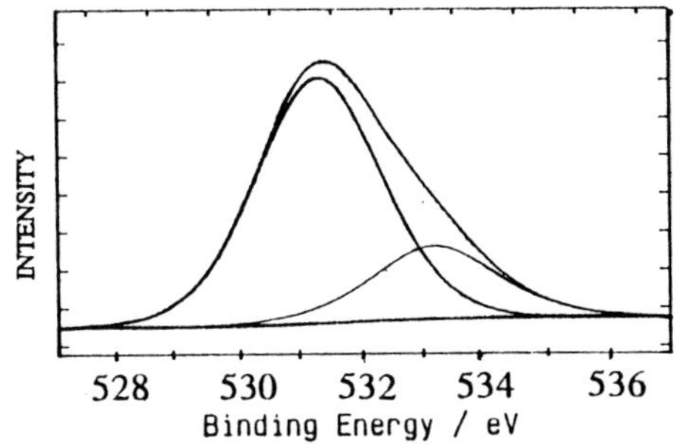

Figure 2. O 1s spectrum of monetite ($CaHPO_4$).

B. APPLICATIONS TO THE STUDY OF CALCIUM PHOSPHATES

1. Determination of the HPO_4 Content

We have seen that the oxygen 1s spectrum is disymetric, due to the two types of oxygen in HPO_4 groups. On the contrary, the O 1s spectrum of β-TCP which contains only PO_4 groups, is absolutely symetrical since the four oxygen atoms are equivalent. In the case of a deficient apatite containing both PO_4 and HPO_4 groups, such as apatitic TCP of formula $Ca_9(PO_4)_5HPO_4OH$. The oxygen 1s spectrum is disymetric and reveals more than one component (Figure 3). From the ratio of the two oxygen types (P-O-H ant P-O), it is possible to determine the HPO_4 content of this apatite (after taking in account the water contribution to the signal).

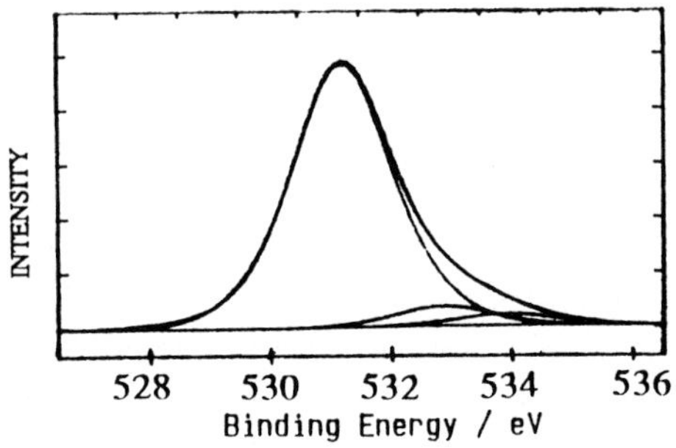

Figure 3. O 1s spectrum of apatitic TCP.

2. Determination of CO_3 Content in a Carbonated Apatite

The case of dentine will be considered. It is composed of a protein, collagen and a carbonated apatite. The C 1s spectrum of decalcified dentine presents 3 components which correspond to the main carbon atoms of a given environment in the protein:aliphatic carbon, a carbon and peptidic carbon (Figure 4). These three types of carbon atoms have differents partial ionic charges due to the electronegativity of the atoms which they are linked to.

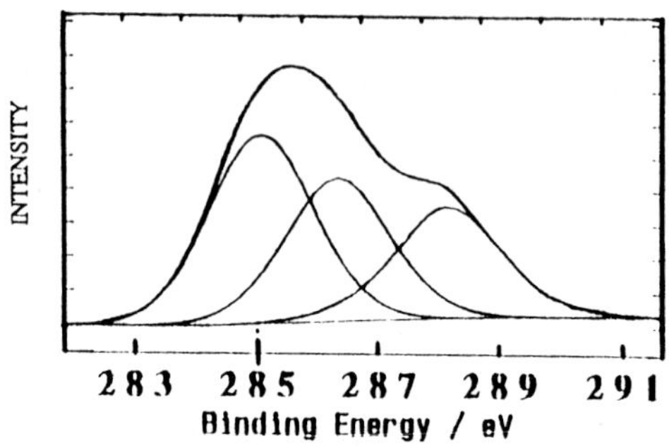

Figure 4. C 1s spectrum of decalcified dentine.

The C 1s spectrum of the initial, non-decalcified dentine, presents one component more at 289.5eV due to the carbonate ions (Figure 5). Its proportion allows the determination of the CO_3 content in apatite, without pretreatement of dentine. At the same time, the mineral/organic ratio can be evaluated.

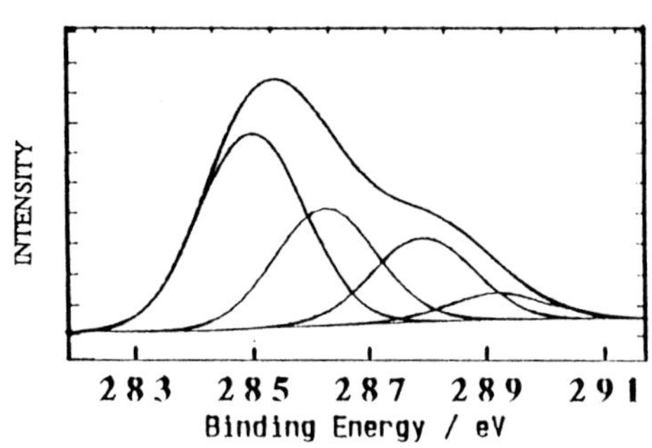

Figure 5. C 1s spectrum of initial dentine.

3. Study of Superficial Reactivity

The superficial reactivity of low specific surface area calcium phosphate can be difficult to observe. For example, after dissolution of $CaHPO_4$ at 37°C in water for 7 days, no information is obtained by bulk analysis of the solid (XRD, FTIR, chemical analysis). On the other hand, changes are observed in the solution composition. Quantitative analysis of the surface by XPS, reveals an increase in the Ca/P ratio by a factor 1.4. Furthermore, decomposition of the O 1s peak shows a decrease of the HPO_4 content. These observations indicate an evolution toward a calcium phosphate containing less HPO_4 groups, and probably apatitic.

4. Adsorption Mechanisms of Organic Molecules

The adsorption of an organic molecule containing primary and secondary amines and OH groups onto apatite was studied. The N 1s spectrum of the amine salt before adsorption, is represented in Figure 6(a). Its decomposition shows that the main peak is about 402 eV. Nearly all amines, primary and secondary, are protonated. The peak at 400 eV is due to small amounts of unprotonated amines.

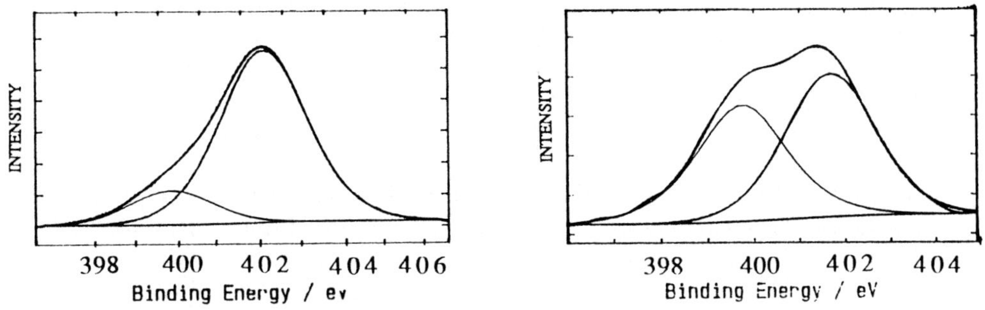

Figure 6. N 1s spectrum (a) before adsorption; (b) after adsorption.

After adsorption, there is an important increase in the peak at 400 eV as seen in Figure 6(b) and Table 2. This variation means that the amines are deprotonated to some extent. Furthermore, the deprotonated/protonated N atom ratio suggests that only the secondary amines are deprotonated during adsorption. This assumption is in agreement with their well-known reactivity.

Table 2
N 1s peak fitting.

Peak	E_b	% before adsorption	% after adsorption
1	400 eV	16	45
2	402 eV	84	55

C. CONCLUSIONS

XPS allows the qualitative and quantitative chemical analysis of either synthetic or natural calcium phosphates, (such as teeth and bone), to a depth of 30-40 Å. This technique enables the HPO_4 and CO_3 ion contents to be determined very easily, without pretreatment as in the case of dentine. The use of XPS is especially adapted to the study of reactions occurring on the surfaces of compounds with a low specific surface area. Also, organic molecules adsorbed onto mineral phases can be analysed with XPS and the groups involved in the adsorption mechanisms can be determined.

REFERENCES

1. Legeros, R., Calcium Phosphates in Oral Biology and Medicine, Editor Howard M. Myers (ed.), Karger, 1991, Chap. 6, 110.
2. Gee, A. andDeitz, V. R., J. Am. Chem. Soc., 77, 2961, 1955.
3. Greenfield, D. J., Termine, J.D., Eanes, E.D., Calcif. Tiss. Res., 14, 131–138, 1974.
4. Legeros R. Z. and Legeros, J. P., Carbonate analysis of synthetic mineral and biological apatites, J. Dent. Res., 62, 259, 1983.
5. Montel G., La cristallochimie des apatites et ses relations avec le comportement biochimique des tissus calcifiés. Information dentaire, 28, 15, 1976.
6. Siegbahn, K., Nordling, C., Falkman, A., Norberg, R., Hamrin, K., Hedman, G., Johansson, G., Bergmark, T., Karlson, S., Lindgren, I., Lindberg, B., ESCA Atomic Molecular and Solid State Structure studied by Means of Electrons Spectroscopy. Almquist and Wiksells A. B., Stockholm, 1967.
7. Elfersi, S., Lebugle, A., and Gregoire, G., Apports de la technique ESCA dans la caractérisation des surfaces dentine-adhésif-matériaux de reconstitutions coronaires esthétiques. Journal de Biomatériaux Dentaires, 7, 141, 1992.
8. Campbell, A., Gardella, J., Richardson, C., Nancollas, G. and Siorda, R., Urinary Stone Analysis by Small-Spot Electron Spectroscopy for Chemical Analysis (ESCA), Applied Spectroscopy, 44, 1015, 1990.

CALCIUM PHOSPHATE DEPOSITION IN RAT KIDNEYS

Saeed R. Khan,[a] James H. Adair,[b]
Augusto A. Morrone[b] and Guy P. Latorre[c]
Departments of [a]Pathology,
[b]Material Sciences and [c]Advanced Materials
University of Florida,
Gainesville, Florida

INTRODUCTION

Calcium phosphate (CaP) is a common constituent of human urinary stones.[1,2] It is suggested to be involved in crystallization of the predominant crystalline component of most urinary stones namely the calcium oxalate (CaOx). In most stones, CaP is present as apatite which occurs in two forms, hydroxylapatite and carbonate apatite. Hydroxylapatite is generally found in stones associated with sterile urine while carbonate apatite is found in stones associated with infection. To better understand the mechanisms involved in CaP deposition in mammalian kidneys and the role of CaP in crystallization of CaOx we are involved in a study of renal deposition of CaP and CaOx in Sprague-Dawley rats.

MATERIALS AND METHODS

Renal deposition of CaP was induced in female Sprague-Dawley rats by feeding them a calculogenic diet called AIN-76.[3] After 2 to 4 weeks on the diet rats were sacrificed. Their kidneys were fixed by perfusion with a paraformaldehyde/glutaraldehyde mixture and processed for light microscopy (LM) and scanning (SEM) and transmission electron microscopy (TEM). Kidney sections were examined by LM after histochemical staining with Periodic acid-Schiff, alcian blue or colloidal iron in addition to hematoxylin and eosin. The deposits were isolated from the kidneys by sodium hypochlorite treatment[4] and analyzed by Energy Dispersive X-ray Microanalysis, and Fourier Transform Infrared Microscopy.

RESULTS

After two weeks on the AIN diet all rats had renal calcification. CaP deposits were located exclusively in the proximal renal tubules at the corticomedullary junction of the kidney. After 4 weeks on the diet, deposits were large enough to not only obstruct the tubules they were in but also the neighboring ones (Fig. 1). They had nodular surfaces which appeared amorphous when examined by SEM. Cross sections of the deposits had a scalloped and laminated appearance (Fig. 2). TEM examination illustrated a

0-8493-4750-5/94/$0.00 + $.50

central amorphous area with cellular degradation products. Distinct needle-shaped crystals could be identified at the periphery (Fig. 2). High resolution TEM revealed well defined crystals (Fig. 3) embedded in an amorphous matrix. Energy dispersive x-ray microanalysis of the deposits demonstrated the presence of calcium and phosphorus. Analysis by fourier transform infrared spectroscopy of the isolated calcium phosphate deposits (Fig. 4) showed them to contain carbonate apatite with a high content of organic material (Fig. 3).

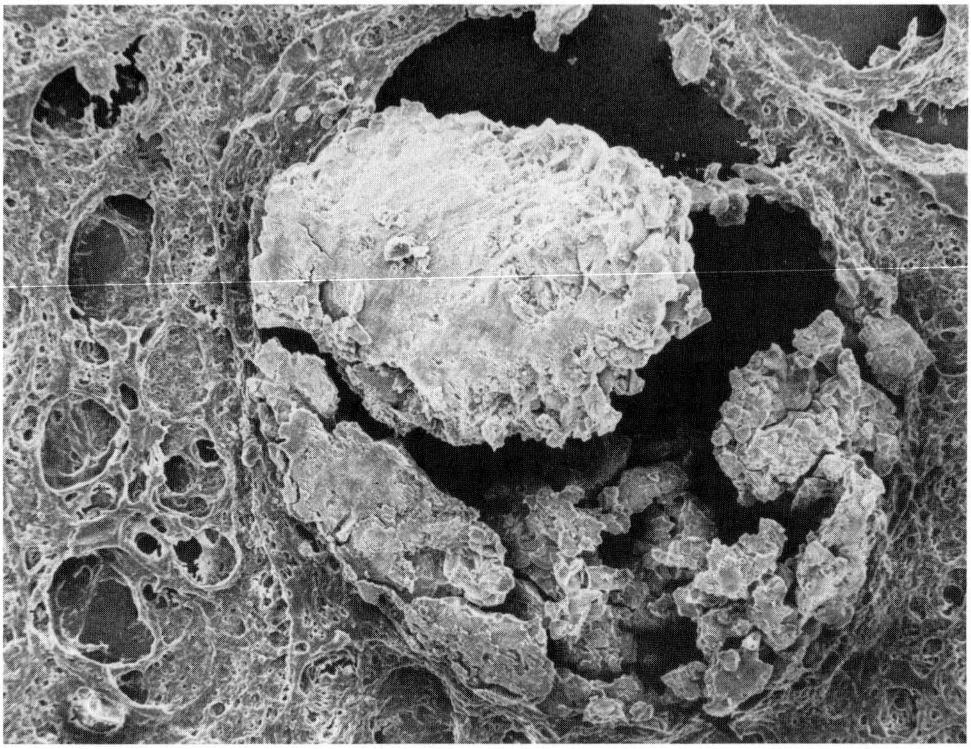

Figure 1. SEM of CaP deposit in a renal tubule. It is clear that the deposit has not only obstructed the tubule that it was in but the neighboring ones as well. Stone surface appears amorphous. X450.

Histochemical staining showed the deposits to be PAS, colloidal iron, and alcian blue positive, the later at pH 1 as well as at 2.5 indicating that the organic matrix of these deposits consisted of mucopolysaccharides and mucoproteins including the highly acidic sulfated mucoproteins.

DISCUSSION

Renal deposition of CaP is quite common in humans.[5] Deposition can start in the tubular lumen, within tubular epithelial cells, or the interstitium. It is suggested that such deposits when strategically located can provoke kidney stone formation.[6] Luminal CaP travelling down the nephron may, under suitable supersaturation and other favorable conditions, aggregate with additional

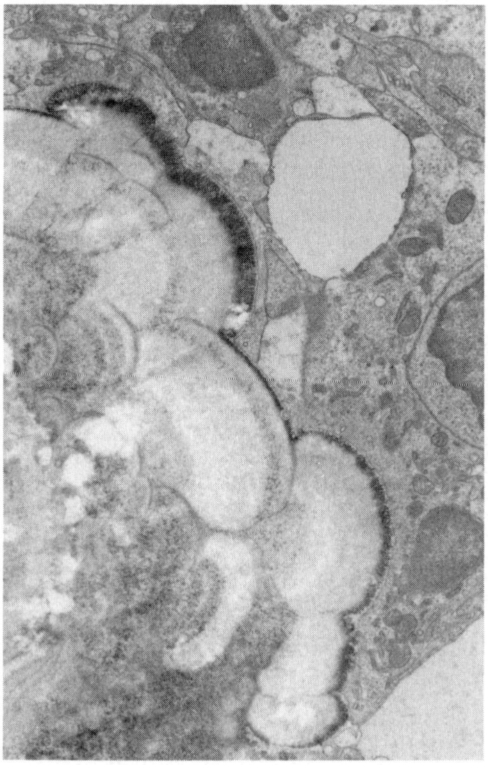

Figure 2. TEM of a cross-section through the deposit. The scalloped and laminated appearance is evident. Central area appears amorphous while the periphery is covered with dark staining needle shaped crystals. X2,000.

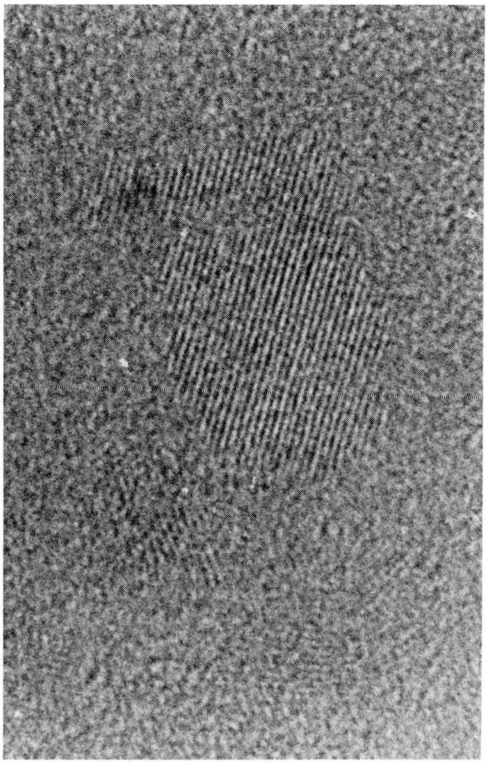

Figure 3. High resolution TEM showing crystals embedded in an amorphous matrix. X3,750,000.

crystalline and non-crystalline substances and be retained in the renal papilla where it becomes the nidus for the development of a stone. Similarly renal papillary interstitial deposits may erode through to the papillary surface exposing themselves to a supersaturated urine and initiate the development of a urinary stone. Stones formed on such nidi were shown to account for 28.4% of 500 spontaneously passed small stones examined by Cifuentes-Delatte.[7] Since CaP is the most common crystal in human urine,[8] is ubiquitous in human urinary stones,[1,2] is often seen at the center of mixed CaP-CaOx stones, and is a good nucleator of CaOx *in vitro*,[9] various forms of CaP have been proposed to act as heterogeneous nucleators of CaOx. Calcium phosphate deposits retained in the renal papilla may act as heterogeneous nucleator of CaOx and subsequently appear as the stone nucleus.

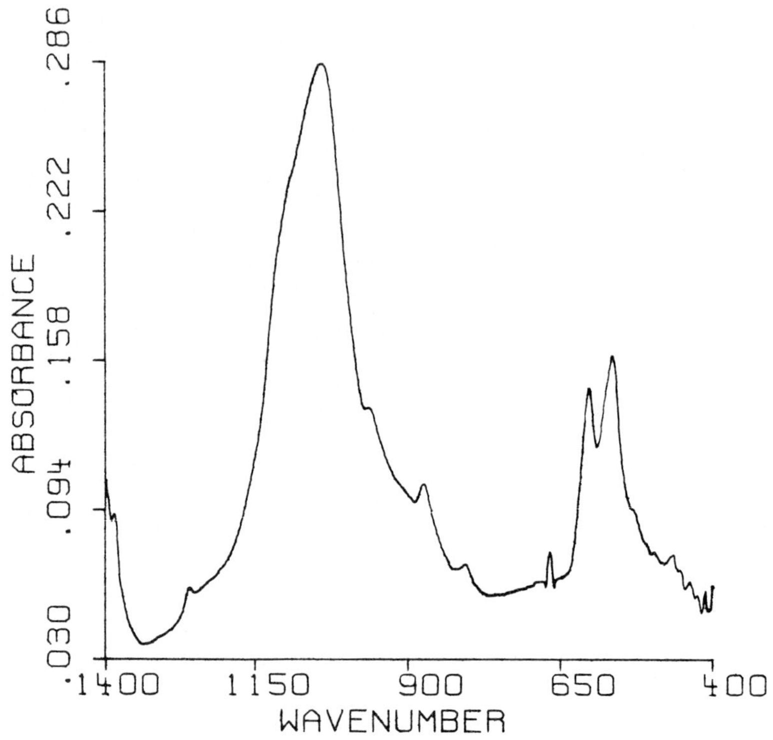

Figure 4. FTIR spectrum of CaP deposits isolated from the kidneys.

Cellular membranes and their lipids are intimately involved in both physiological and pathological calcification.[10] In a number of experimental studies of renal calcification, non-mitochondrial calcific deposits are formed in proximal tubular basement membrane in association with membrane outpouchings or in the apical vacuoles of the epithelial cells. Intraluminal CaP deposits resulting from magnesium deficiency start in association with the membranes of the apical vacuoles of the proximal tubular epithelial cells. CaP deposition in the kidneys of rats fed AIN-76 diet is also shown to be membrane mediated. Membrane-bound vesicles derived from the brush border microvilli provide the nidus for the formation of intraluminal deposits. Deposits start in the lumens of the early part of proximal tubules and travel down the nephron while at the same time accrete mass by laminar growth in which both membranous vesicles and mineral are involved. Mineral content of the deposit increases with the result that they become much more compact. Finally these deposits become too large to pass through the narrower loop of Henle and thus are retained at the junction of the proximal tubules and the loop.

FTIR analysis of the deposits indicates that carbonate apatite is probably the major mineral phase present. Earlier studies of nephrocalcinosis in female rats also identified the mineral as apatite.[3,11] Crystalline material appeared embedded in an amorphous matrix suggesting that perhaps calcification started as deposition of amorphous mineral which later matured into a more crystalline form.

ACKNOWLEDGEMENTS

Supported in part by NIH grants #RO1 DK414345 and PO1 DK20586.

REFERENCES

1. Khan, S.R., Structure and development of Calcific Urinary Stones, in *Calcification in Biological Systems,* Bonnuci, E, Ed., CRC Press, Boca Raton, Florida, 1992, 345.
2. Otnes, B., Urinary stone analysis, methods, materials and value, *Scand. J. Urol. Nephrol., Suppl. 71, 1, 1983.*
3. Nguyen, H.T. and Woodard, J.C., Intranephronic calculosis in rats, *Am. J. Pathol.,* 100, 39, 1980.
4. Moradian-Oldak, J., Weiner, S., Addadi, L., Landis, W.J. and Traub, W., Electron imaging and diffraction study of individual crystals of bone, mineralized tendon and synthetic carbonate apatite, *Conn. Tissue Res.,* 25, 219, 1991.
5. Laberke, H.G., Pathological anatomy, etiology, and pathogenesis of nephrocalcinosis, in *Nephrocalcinosis, Calcium Antagonists, and Kidney,* Bichler, K.H. and Strohmaier, W.L., Eds., Springer-Verlag, Berlin, Heidelberg, New York, 1988, 67.
6. Randall, A., The origin and growth of renal calculi, *Ann. Surg.,* 105, 1009, 1937.
7. Cifuentes-Delatte, L., Minon-Cifuentes, J. and Medina, J.A., New studies on papillary calculi, *J. Urol.,* 137, 1024, 1987.
8. Werness, P.G., Bergert, J.H. and Smith, L.H., Crystalluria, *J. Crystal Growth,* 53, 166, 1981.
9. Meyer, J.L., Bergert, J.H. and Smith, L.H., Epitaxial relationships in urolithiasis, calcium oxalate monohydrate- hydroxyapatite system, *Clin. Sci. Mol. Med.,* 49, 369, 1977.
10. Boskey, A.L., Phospholipids and calcification, in *Calcified Tissue,* Hukins, D.W.L., Ed, CRC Press, Boca Raton, Florida, 1989, 215.
11. Geary, C.P. and Cousins, F.B., An oestrogen-linked nephrocalcinosis in rats, *Br. J. exp. Path.,* 50, 507, 1969.

ISOLATION OF CALCIUM-PHOSPHATE CRYSTALS OF MATURE BOVINE BONE BY REACTION WITH HYDRAZINE AT LOW TEMPERATURE

Hyun-Man Kim, Christian Rey,* and Melvin J. Glimcher
Laboratory for the Study of Skeletal Disorders and Rehabilitation
Department of Orthopaedic Surgery
Harvard Medical School
The Children's Hospital
Boston, MA 02115

I. INTRODUCTION

Despite recent advances in our knowledge of the chemistry, structure and short range order of the calcium-phosphate crystals of apatite in the mineralized tissues of vertebrates, there still remain a number of critical important characteristics which need to be explored, not only for the sake of a clearer understanding of the intimate nature of the inorganic crystals *per se*, but also to help elucidate the biological functions of the crystals. These commonly accepted functions have now been extended to include mineral-cell interactions, either directly or via the binding of specific protein components through the mineral crystallites and the interaction of such mineral-bound proteins with the surrounding cells; for example, the role of mineral-bound osteocalcin in recruiting and facilitating differentiation of mononuclear cells to osteoclasts and their participation in bone resorption.[1] Further progress especially in the elucidation of the fine structure and short range order of the bone crystals has been seriously limited, however, by the fact that the inorganic crystals are anatomically intimately related at the ultrastructural level to the major organic constituents of the extracellular matrix, viz., their location *within* the collagen fibrils of bone, dentin, cementum, and within the protein rich "tubules" of enamel.[2] Moreover, it is very likely that there are strong chemical bonds formed between the mineral crystallites, collagen and other protein components of the organic matrix, as well. The organization at the ultrastructural level of the major organic matrix components and the inorganic crystals, not only prevents a direct visualization of individual crystals necessary to determine the size and shape of the crystals and any changes in these parameters with maturation and aging, for example, but seriously interferes with techniques such as Fourier transform infrared spectroscopy (FTIR) and nuclear magnetic resonance (NMR) used to explore the fine, short range order of the crystals. The purpose of this research progress was to develop methods to isolate the crystals of bone and other mineralized tissues essentially free of organic constituents without altering the

---

* Laboratoire des Materiaux–Physicochimie des Solides, Toulouse, France.

0-8493-4750-5/94/$0.00 + $.50

chemical composition or structure of the crystals, and to disperse the crystals so that they can be examined visually by high resolution transmission electron microscopy and by electron diffraction and microprobe analyses.

There have been a number of studies conducted in the past in attempts to accomplish this task but both criteria, i.e. isolation of the crystals essentially free of organic matrix constituents, and their dispersion as well as the maintenance of crystal structure and order have not been met previously. A major obstacle has been the limitation imposed by the necessity to employ chemical techniques which are completely non-aqueous. Otherwise, the use of highly polar organic solvents rapidly results in complete or partial crystal dissolution, re-crystallization, formation of additional non-apatitic calcium phosphates in addition to apatite, etc. Secondly, it is also necessary to carry out such experiments at low temperature in order to prevent significant changes in both the composition and structure of the crystals. These limitations are especially important when dealing with the extremely small crystals of bone and other collagenous, calcified tissues. For example, ethylenediamine was used to isolate the crystals from such tissues.[3-5] This procedure produced significant structural and chemical changes in the crystals. Other investigators have utilized NaClO in aqueous solutions.[6] However, in addition to the extensive exposure of the crystals to water, the ionic and sharply alkaline and oxidant solution of NaClO inevitably causes both chemical dissolution and chemical transformation of the mineral phase.[7] Plasma ashing has also been utilized,[8] but even at what was considered low temperature, local temperatures produced by the plasma ashing were quite high, sufficient to alter crystal structure. Attempts to utilize the water-free solvent hydrazine have been reported,[9] but at the temperatures and time of reaction used significant alterations of the crystals are induced. More recently, Rey et al.[10] reacted bone and cartilage at approximately 25°C without producing any measurable changes in the crystals measured by FT-IR analysis or by x-ray diffraction, but the crystals were not dispersed and the tissues still contained a significant amount of organic matrix constituents.

In the present study, we have been able to disaggregate, isolate and disperse the Ca-P crystals of adult bovine bone, essentially free of the organic matrix component without introducing significant chemical or structural or short range order changes in the crystals. This has been accomplished using non-aqueous hydrazine at ~4°C to degrade the proteins[11] for a relatively long period of time. The use of water is completely avoided both in the initial preparation of the bone samples from the animals, in the subsequent washing of the bone powder, and in the removal of the hydrazine, by using only absolute ethanol at 4°C. The crystals were further disaggregated and dissociated and dispersed from the partially proteinized bone particles by low power sonication for short periods of time in absolute ethanol at ~4°C.

II. MATERIALS AND METHODS

Sources of Bone and Isolation of Bone Crystals

Bovine cortical bone from freshly slaughtered two to four year old animals was used. Defatted bone powder was produced by milling small pieces of the bone in liquid nitrogen. The bone powder was reacted with anhydrous hydrazine at 4°C for 24–72 hours, and the hydrazine was removed by repeated washing with absolute ethanol. The partially de-proteinized bone was then sonicated at low energy in absolute ethanol at 4°C, and for short periods of time. The partially deproteinized and loosely disaggregated bone particles were again extracted with anhydrous hydrazine at 4°C, washed again with absolute ethanol and dried under vacuum. Bovine bone crystals were also obtained (but with a very much lower yield) from samples of bovine bone particles by sonication alone in absolute ethanol at ~4°C without reaction with hydrazine and used as native crystals. Their characteristics were compared with crystals obtained by treatment with hydrazine and sonication in absolute ethanol. In addition, synthetically prepared, extremely small crystals of apatite were subjected to the same procedures as the bovine bone samples. The untreated milled bone powder and the untreated synthetic apatite crystals were also used for chemical and structural analyses as additional controls and after being subjected to the same procedures on the bone powder.

Analytical and Morphogenic Analyses

Residual protein associated with the isolated apatite crystals was determined by amino acid analysis carried out on a Beckman 121-M amino acid analyzer after hydrolysis of the crystals at 110°C in 6N HCl. Ash weight was determined after heating the samples at 600°C for 24 hours. The habit and dimensions of the crystals were analyzed morphometrically by transmission electron microscopy: the crystals were dispersed in absolute ethanol, loaded onto a carbon coated formvar grid, and examined in a JEOL 100C electron microscope equipped with a liquid nitrogen cooling device. The maximum length and maximum width of the crystals were measured on photographs at 102,000X magnification. Ca was analyzed by atomic absorption spectroscopy and P by a colorimetric method using ammonium molybdate.[12] Long range order of the crystals and short range order of crystals were analyzed by x-ray diffraction, electron diffraction, and computer resolution enhanced Fourier transform infrared spectroscopy (FT-IR) on a Perkin Elmer 1700 spectrometer. Deconvolution of FT-IR spectra, intensity ratios and resolution factors were calculated as previously reported.[13,14]

C. RESULTS

Treatment with low temperature hydrazine removed the vast majority of the proteins associated with the crystals when compared with crystals isolated solely by sonication (Table 1). The procedure was even more effective when compared to the protein content of the original native bone powders.[15,16] The additional 7.9% of the weight of the crystals which was removed from the isolated crystals after muffle furnace ashing at 600°C was due to the release of carbonate ions present in the apatite crystals.[17] The habit of the isolated crystals was that of somewhat irregular, very thin plates whose average length and width were unchanged by treatment with hydrazine (Figure 1, Table 2). X-ray diffraction studies of the isolated crystals were, unchanged after treatment with hydrazine. FT-IR studies of the isolated bovine crystals also showed no significant change in the spectra or in the short range order or crystallinity of the mineral phase (Figures 2a and 2b, Table 3) except for a small decrease in the labile P.

Table 1
Chemical effects on mineral crystals before and after treatment of bovine bone mineral crystals with low temperature hydrazine.

	Ca[a]	P[b]	Ca/P	proteins (%)	ashing (%)
sonicated only	262.3	108.1	1.82	28.0	33.4
hydrazine plus sonicated	312.2	153.9	1.52	0.2	7.9

a. atomic absorption spectroscopy (μg/mg)
b. colorimetric spectroscopy (μg/mg)

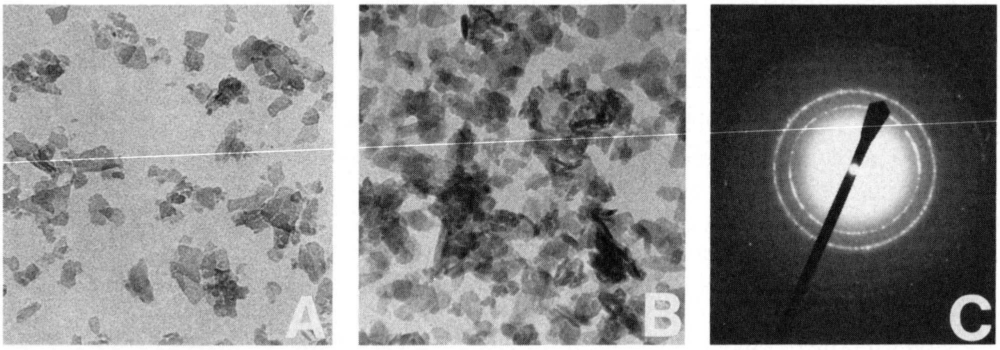

Figure 1. Electron micrograms and electron diffraction of the mineral crystals well dispersed before (A) and after (B) the treatment of bovine mineral crystals with hydrazine at low temperature, x 102,000. The crystals isolated by the treatment with hydrazine and sonication are wide plates in shape and generate diffraction pattern of apatite (C) (80kV, 45 cm).

Table 2
Dimensions of mineral crystals before and after treatment by hydrazine.

	width	length	w/l
sonicated only	20.4 ± 9.8	32.8 ± 14.4	0.65 ± 0.21
hydrazine plus sonicated	21.7 ± 9.5	32.8 ± 13.5	0.68 ± 0.18

n=111, average ± S.D. nm

D. DISCUSSION

The procedures outlined in this report have permitted us to isolate and disperse the Ca-P apatite crystals from native, mature adult bovine bone, essentially free of organic matrix constituents, and without significant alteration of the chemistry, chemical composition or structure of the crystals. The approximately 7-8% of additional loss of weight after calcination at 600°C of the crystals isolated by reaction with hydrazine and sonication in ethanol is due to the expected loss of crystal carbonate. This not only substantiates the maintenance of carbonate in the crystals[17] during the procedures carried out to isolate them from the organic matrix constituents, but is also consistent with the findings obtained by amino acid analyses of the isolated crystals, viz., that the crystals are essentially free of the organic matrix constituents initially present in the bone tissue.

Table 3.
Phosphate and carbonate environment of mineral crystals before and after hydrazine treatment measured from the data of deconvoluted FT-IR. [a]

	labile P	PO_4RF^b	labile CO_3	$v2\ CO_3$ RF
sonicated only	0.40	0.76	0.50	0.53
hydrazine plus sonicated	0.30	0.79	0.48	0.54

a. [13,14]
b. RF: resolution factor

Another important finding is that the crystal habit and particularly the crystal size was not affected by treatment with hydrazine, another indication that there was little, if any, alteration chemically or structurally of the crystals, even as concerns their surface area, an important consideration with regard to their biological and biomechanical functions.

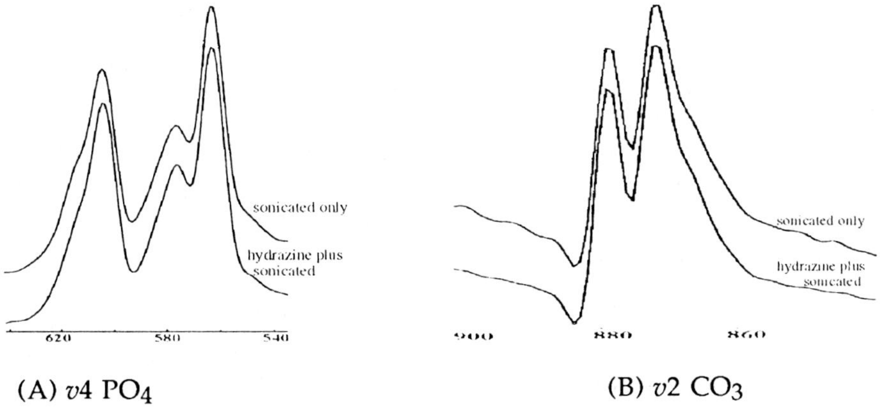

Figure 2. $v4\ PO_4$ (A) and $v2\ CO_3$ (B) of deconvoluted FT-IR before and after the treatment of hydrazine at low temperature.

With regard to the intimate chemical constituents, fine structure and short range order of the crystals, there were no significant changes noted after reaction with hydrazine, except for the small diminution of the labile phosphate groups. The exact nature of this labile phosphorus environment is presently unknown, although it may in part be contributed to by the interaction by phosphate groups with specific proteins such as glycosylated phosphoprotein and osteocalcin.[18-20] There was also no evidence for the presence of crystalline Ca-P solids other than apatite.

Current studies on crystals of bone from other species and other calcified tissues have provided similar results as are reported here for adult bovine bone. In the case of very young, newly mineralized bone, the procedures must be modified in order to obtain the isolated crystals free of organic matrix components. In addition, we have also been able to utilize low energy, short time period, very low temperature plasma ashing as an additional technique which in selected instances reduces the organic matrix components even further.

REFERENCES

1. Glowacki, J., Rey, C., Glimcher, M.J., Cox, K.A., Lian, J., A role for osteocalcin in osteoclast differentiation, *J. Cellular Biochem.* 45, 292-302, 1991.
2. Travis, D. F., Glimcher, M. J., The structure and organization of the relationship between the organic matrix and the inorganic crystals of embryonic bovine enamel, *J. Cell Biol.* 23, 447-497, 1964 .
3. Williams, J. B. and Irvine, J. W., Preparation of the inorganic matrix of bone, *Science* 11, 771-772, 1954.
4. Peckham, S., Losee, F. L., Ettleman, I., Ethylenediamine versus potassium hydroxide glycol in the removal of organic matter from dentin, *J. Dent. Res.* 35, 947-949, 1956.
5. Amstrong, W. D. and Singer, L., Composition and constitution of the mineral phase of bone, *Clin. Orthop.* 38, 179-190, 1967.
6. Weiner, S. and Price, P. A., Disaggregation of bone into crystals, *Calcif. Tiss. Int.* 39, 365-375, 1986.
7. Sakae, T., Mishima, H., and Kozawa, Y., Changes in bovine dentin mineral with sodium hypochlorite treatment, *J. Dent. Res.* 69, 1229-1234, 1988.
8. Frazier, P. D., Brown, F. J. , Rose, L. R., and Fowler, B. O., Radio frequency oxygen excitation apparatus for low-temperature ashing, *J. Dent. Res.* 46, 1098-1101, 1967
9. Termine, J. D., Eanes, E. D., Greenfield, D. J., Nylen, M. U., and Harper, R. A., Hydrazine-deproteininzed bone mineral: Physical and chemical properties, *Calcif. Tiss. Int.* 12, 73-90, 1973
10. Rey, C., Boshah, K., Griffin, R., and Glimcher, M. J., Structural studies of the mineral phase of calcifying cartilage, *J. Min. Bone Res.* 6, 515-525, 1991
11. Akabori, S., Ohno, K., and Narita, K., On the hydrazinolysis of proteins and peptides: A Method for the characterization of carboxyl -terminal amino acids in proteins, *Bull. Chem. Soc. Jap.* 25, 214-218,1952.
12. Bartlett, G. D., Phosphorus assay in column chromatography, *J. Biol. Chem.* 234, 466-468, 1959.
13. Rey, C., Shimizu, M., Collins, B., and Glimcher, M. J., Resolution-enhanced Fourier transform infrared spectroscopy study of the environment of phosphate ions in the early deposits of a solid phase of calcium-phosphate in bone and enamel, and their evolution with age. I: Investigations in $v4$ PO_4 domains, *Calcif. Tiss. Int.* 46, 384-394, 1990

14. Rey, C., Renugopalakrishnan, B., Collins, B., and Glimcher, M. J., Fourier transform infrared spectroscopic study of the carbonate ions in bone mineral during aging, *Calcif. Tiss. Int.* 49, 251-258, 1991
15. Cohen-Solal, L., Lian, J. B., Kossiva, D., Glimcher, M. J. , Identification of organic phosphorus covalently bound to collagen and non-collagenous proteins of chicken-bone matrix: the presence of O-phosphoserine and O-phosphothreonine in non-collagenous proteins, and their absence from phosphorylated collagen, *Biochem. J.* 177,81-98,1979
16. Glimcher, M. J., Lefteriou B, Kossiva D. On the problem of covalent linkages between phosphoproteins and collagen in bovine dentin and bone, *J. Bone Min. Res.* 1, 509-522, 1986
17. LeGeros, R. Z., Balmain, N., and Bonel, G., Structure and composition of the mineral phase of periosteal bone, *J. Chem. Res. Synop.* 1, 8-9, 1986
18. Lee, S.L., Glonek, T., Glimcher, M. J., ^{31}P nuclear magnetic resonance spectroscopic evidence for ternary complex formation of fetal phosphoprotein with calcium and inorganic orthophosphate ions, *Calcif. Tissue Int.* 35, 815-818,1983
19. Lee, S.L., Kossiva, D., Glimcher, M.J., Phosphoproteins of bovine dentin: evidence for polydispersity during tooth maturation. *Biochemistry* 22, 2596-2601, 1983
20. Glimcher, M. J., Recent studies of the mineral phase in bone and its possible linkage to the organic matrix by protein-bound phosphate bonds, *Phil. Trans. Roy. Soc. London B* 304, 479-508,1984

AUTHOR INDEX

SUBJECT INDEX